Pediatric Ophthalmology

A Clinical Guide

Pediatric Ophthalmology

A Clinical Guide

Pamela F. Gallin, M.D.
Director, Pediatric Ophthalmology
Associate Clinical Professor of Ophthalmology
Edward S. Harkness Eye Institute
Associate Clinical Professor of Pediatrics
Babies and Childrens Hospital of New York
Columbia Presbyterian Medical Center
New York-Presbyterian Hospital
Columbia University, College of Physicians
    and Surgeons
New York, New York

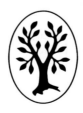

2000
Thieme
New York • Stuttgart

Thieme New York
333 Seventh Avenue
New York, NY 10001

Editor: Andrea Seils
Editorial Assistant: Michelle Carini
Developmental Manager: Kathleen P. Lyons
Director, Production and Manufacturing:
  Anne Vinnicombe
Marketing Director: Phyllis Gold
Sales Manager: Ross Lumpkin

Chief Financial Officer: Seth S. Fishman
President: Brian D. Scanlan
Cover Designer: Michael Mendelsohn at MM
  Design 2000, Inc.
Compositor: Prepare
Printer: Götz, Ludwigsburg

0027436

Library of Congress Cataloging-in-Publication Data

Pediatric ophthalmology : a clinical guide / [edited by] Pamela F. Gallin.
    p. ; cm.
  Includes bibliographical references and index.
  ISBN 0-86577-768-3 (TNY : alk. paper)
   1. Pediatric ophthalmology--Outlines, syllabi, etc. I. Gallin, Pamela.
  [DNLM: 1. Eye Diseases--Child. 2. Eye Diseases--Infant. WW 600 P37135 2000]
  RE48.2.C5 P433 2000
  618.92'0977--dc21

                                                            00-056810

Important note: Medical knowledge is ever-changing. As new research and clinical experience broaden our knowledge, changes in treatment and drug therapy may be required. The authors and editors of the material herein have consulted sources believed to be reliable in their efforts to provide information that is complete and in accord with the standards accepted at the time of publication. However, in view of the possibility of human error by the authors, editors, or publisher of the work herein, or changes in medical knowledge, neither the authors, editors, publisher, nor any other party who has been involved in the preparation of this work, warrants that the information contained herein is in every respect accurate or complete, and they are not responsible for any errors or omissions or for the results obtained from use of such information. Readers are encouraged to confirm the information contained herein with other sources. For example, readers are advised to check the product information sheet included in the package of each drug they plan to administer to be certain that the information contained in this publication is accurate and that changes have not been made in the recommended dose or in the contraindications for administration. This recommendation is of particular importance in connection with new or infrequently used drugs.

Some of the product names, patents, and registered designs referred to in this book are in fact registered trademarks or proprietary names even though specific reference to this fact is not always made in the text. Therefore, the appearance of a name without designation as proprietary is not to be construed as a representation by the publisher that it is in the public domain.

Printed in Germany

5 4 3 2 1

TNY ISBN 0-86577-768-3
GTV ISBN 3-13-111391-X

Dedication

To my best teachers, Laura, Abigail, Hilary, and Peter, and my beloved husband, Leonard H. Yablon. And to my parents, Saara and Martin Gallin, who instilled a love of learning in their children.

Contents

Contributors

Deborah Alcorn, M.D.
Director of Pediatric Ophthalmology
Department of Ophthalmology and Pediatrics
Stanford University Medical Center
Stanford, California

J. Bronwyn Bateman, M.D.
Professor and Chair of Ophthalmology
Department of Ophthalmology
University of Colorado School of Medicine
Denver, Colorado

Darel M. Benaim, Ph.D.
Developmental Clinical
   Psychologist and Psychoanalyst
New York, New York

Richard E. Braunstein, M.D.
Assistant Clinical Professor of Ophthalmology
Department of Ophthalmology
Edward S. Harkness Eye Institute
Columbia Presbyterian Medical Center
New York-Presbyterian Hospital
Columbia University, College of Physicians
   and Surgeons
New York, New York

Christina Butera, M.D.
ONSLOW Ophthalmology
Jacksonville, North Carolina

Emily J. Ceisler, M.D.
Assistant Clinical Professor of Ophthalmology
Assistant Director of Pediatric
   Ophthalmology and Strabismus Service
Department of Ophthalmology
New York University School of Medicine
New York, New York

Stanley Chang, M.D.
Professor and Chair of Ophthalmology
Department of Ophthalmology
Edward S. Harkness Eye Institute
Columbia Presbyterian Medical Center

New York-Presbyterian Hospital
Columbia University, College of Physicians
   and Surgeons
New York, New York

Kim L. Cooper, M.D.
Department of Opthalmology
Stanford University
Stanford, California

Arthur M. Cotliar, M.D.
Associate Clinical Professor
Department of Ophthalmology
Edward S. Harkness Eye Institute
Columbia Presbyterian Medical Center
New York-Presbyterian Hospital
Columbia University, College of Physicians
   and Surgeons
New York, New York

Stella Douros, M.D., P.C., F.A.C.S.
Clinical Instructor
Department of Ophthalmology
Mount Sinai Medical Center
Department of Ophthalmology
Lenox Hill Hospital
New York, New York

Rehlie Eis-Figueroa, B.S., M.S.N., C.P.N.P.
Lecturer
Departments of Nursing and Pediatrics
Edward S. Harkness Eye Institute
Columbia Presbyterian Medical Center
New York-Presbyterian Hospital
New York, New York

George S. Ellis Jr., M.D.
Associate Clinical Professor of Ophthalmology
   and Pediatrics
Tulane University School of Medicine and
   Louisiana State University School of
   Medicine
Children's Hospital
New Orleans, Louisiana

**John Figueroa, B.A., M.S.W., A.C.S.W.,
  L.C.S.W.**
Lecturer
Departments of Pediatrics and Social Work
Edward S. Harkness Eye Institute
Columbia Presbyterian Medical Center
New York-Presbyterian Hospital
New York, New York

John T. Flynn, M.D., C.O.
Anne Gohen Professor of Pediatric
  Ophthalmology and Strabismus
Department of Ophthalmology
Executive Director, Pediatric Ophthalmology
Edward S. Harkness Eye Institute
Columbia Presbyterian Medical Center
New York-Presbyterian Hospital
Columbia University, College of Physicians
  and Surgeons
New York, New York

Thomas E. Flynn, M.D.
Assistant Clinical Professor of Ophthalmology
Department of Ophthalmology
Edward S. Harkness Eye Institute
Columbia Presbyterian Medical Center
New York-Presbyterian Hospital
Columbia University, College of Physicians
  and Surgeons
New York, New York

C. Stephen Foster, M.D., F.A.C.S.
Professor of Ophthalmology
Director of the Ocular Immunology and
  Uveitis Service
Department of Ophthalmology
Harvard Medical School/Massachusetts Eye
  and Ear Infirmary
Boston, Massachusetts

Douglas R. Fredrick, M.D.
Assistant Clinical Professor of Ophthalmology
Department of Ophthalmology
University of California, San Francisco,
  School of Medicine
San Jose, California

Pamela F. Gallin, M.D.
Associate Clinical Professor of Ophthalmology
Department of Ophthalmology
Edward S. Harkness Eye Institute
Associate Clinical Professor of Pediatrics
Department of Pediatrics
Babies and Childrens Hospital of New York

Columbia Presbyterian Medical Center
New York-Presbyterian Hospital
Columbia University, College of Physicians
  and Surgeons
New York, New York

B. David Gorman, M.D.
Assistant Clinical Professor of Ophthalmology
Department of Ophthalmology
Edward S. Harkness Eye Institute
Columbia Presbyterian Medical Center
New York-Presbyterian Hospital
Columbia University, College of Physicians
  and Surgeons
New York, New York

Albert J. Hofeldt, M.D.
Associate Clinical Professor of Ophthalmology
Department of Ophthalmology
Edward S. Harkness Eye Institute
Columbia Presbyterian Medical Center
New York-Presbyterian Hospital
Columbia University, College of Physicians
  and Surgeons
New York, New York

Creig S. Hoyt, M.D.
Professor of Ophthalmology
Department of Ophthalmology
University of California, San Francisco
  Medical Center
San Francisco, California

San Deep Jain, M.D.
Cornea Fellow
Cornea Service Department
Massachusetts Eye and Ear Infirmary
Boston, Massachusetts

Michael Kazim, M.D.
Associate Clinical Professor of Ophthalmology
Associate Clinical Professor of Surgery
Edward S. Harkness Eye Institute
Columbia Presbyterian Medical Center
New York-Presbyterian Hospital
Columbia University, College of Physicians
  and Surgeons
New York, New York

Erik F. Kruger, M.D.
Fellow, Retina Research
Department of Ophthalmology
The New York Eye and Ear Infirmary
New York, New York

Martin L. Leib, M.D.
Associate Clinical Professor of Ophthalmology
Director, The Orbit and Ophthalmic Plastic
 Surgery Service
Edward S. Harkness Eye Institute
Columbia Presbyterian Medical Center
New York-Presbyterian Hospital
Columbia University, College of Physicians
 and Surgeons
New York, New York

Irene H. Maumenee, M.D.
Ort Professor of Ophthalmology
Professor of Genetics
Professor of Pediatrics
Professor of Medicine
Department of Ophthalmology
The Johns Hopkins Center for Hereditary
 Eye Diseases
Baltimore, Maryland

Sally A. Moore, B.S., C.O.
Clinical Professor of Ophthalmology
Department of Ophthalmology
Edward S. Harkness Eye Institute
Columbia Presbyterian Medical Center
New York-Presbyterian Hospital
Columbia University, College of Physicians
 and Surgeons
New York, New York

Quan Dong Nguyen, M.S., M.D.
Chief, Fellow in Immunology and Uveitis,
 Fellow in Ophthalmology
Department of Ophthalmology
Harvard Medical School/Massachusetts Eye
 and Ear Infirmary
Boston, Massachusetts

Marc G. Odrich, M.D.
Assistant Professor of Ophthalmology
Department of Ophthalmology
Edward S. Harkness Eye Institute
Columbia Presbyterian Medical Center
New York-Presbyterian Hospital
Columbia University, College of Physicians
 and Surgeons
New York, New York

Steven A. Odrich, M.D.
Assistant Professor of Ophthalmology
Department of Ophthalmology
Edward S. Harkness Eye Institute

Columbia Presbyterian Medical Center
New York-Presbyterian Hospital
Columbia University, College of Physicians
 and Surgeons
New York, New York

Ilene Pardon, M.D.
Practice
New Jersey

Marshall M. Parks, M.D.
Clinical Professor of Ophthalmology
George Washington University Medical Center
Washington, District of Columbia

Louis D. Pizzarello, M.D., M.P.H
Associate Clinical Professor
Department of Ophthalmology and
 Public Health
Edward S. Harkness Eye Institute
Columbia Presbyterian Medical Center
New York-Presbyterian Hospital
Columbia University, College of Physicians
 and Surgeons
New York, New York

James L. Plotnick, M.D.
Arizona Pediatric Eye Specialists
Scottsdale, Arizona

Cindy Prichard, C.O., C.O.T.
Clinical Instructor of Ophthalmology
Tulane University
Children's Hospital of New Orleans
New Orleans, Louisiana

Renee Richards, M.D.
Surgeon Director
Director of Strabismus Department
Manhattan Eye, Ear, and Throat Hospital
New York, New York

Richard M. Robb, M.D.
Associate Professor of Ophthalmology
Harvard Medical School
Ophthalmologist-in-Chief
Children's Hospital
Boston, Massachusetts

William Schiff, MD
Assistant Professor of Ophthalmology
Department of Ophthalmology
Edward S. Harkness Eye Institute
Columbia Presbyterian Medical Center
New York-Presbyterian Hospital

Columbia University, College of Physicians
and Surgeons
New York, New York

Caroline J. Shea, M.D.
Assistant Professor of Ophthalmology
Department of Ophthalomology
University of Colorado School of Medicine
Denver, Colorado

Carol L. Shields, M.D.
Associate Surgeon
Department of Oncology Service
Willis Eye Hospital
Associate Professor
Jefferson Medical College
Thomas Jefferson University
Philadelphia, Pennsylvania

Jerry A. Shields, M.D.
Director
Department of Oncology Service
Willis Eye Hospital
Professor of Ophthalmology
Jefferson Medical College
Thomas Jefferson University
Philadelphia, Pennsylvania

Hermann D. Schubert, M.D.
Professor of Ophthalmology
Department of Ophthalmology
Edward S. Harkness Eye Institute
Columbia Presbyterian Medical Center
New York-Presbyterian Hospital
Columbia University, College of Physicians
and Surgeons
New York, New York

Kuldev Singh, M.D., M.P.H.
Associate Professor of Opthalmology
Director, Glaucoma Service

Department of Ophthalmology
Stanford University
Stanford, California

Stephen L. Trokel, M.D.
Clinical Professor of Ophthalmology
Department of Ophthalmology
Edward S. Harkness Eye Institute
Columbia Presbyterian Medical Center
New York-Presbyterian Hospital
Columbia University, College of Physicians
and Surgeons
New York, New York

David S. Walton, M.D.
Associate Clinical Professor
of Ophthalmology
Department of Ophthalmology
Harvard University/Massachusetts Eye
and Ear Infirmary
Boston, Massachusetts

Michael J. Weiss, M.D.
Associate Professor of Clinical
Ophthalmology
Director of Uveitis Service
Department of Ophthalmology
Edward S. Harkness Eye Institute
Columbia Presbyterian Medical Center
New York-Presbyterian Hospital
Columbia University, College of Physicians
and Surgeons
New York, New York

Thom J. Zimmerman, M.D., Ph.D.
Professor and Chair
Department of Ophthalmology
and Visual Sciences
University of Louisville
Louisville, Kentucky

Foreword

This book was conceived by Dr. Gallin. She recognized that a text was needed to teach ophthalmology residents beginning pediatric ophthalmology and pediatricians and family practitioners to diagnosis and treat ophthalmic diseases in children. She called upon her teachers, friends, peers, mentors, and students—some of the best minds in pediatric ophthalmology—to help her address this need. What she came up with is a text that is factual, accurate, comprehensible, and good reading.

"Pam" has been like a member of our family since she moved to St. Louis (Washington University) from New York with the intent of becoming a biomedical engineer. While on an elective period, she spent a few months on the neuro-ophthalmology consultation service at Washington University Medical Center. She became intrigued and, before anyone could develop a rational set of arguments to the contrary, she decided to take a second major in biology. During this elective period, she also wrote an honors thesis with me on optic nerve function in patients with retrobulbar neuritis that is considered a classic and is still quoted.

Pam has always learned from others—among them her Harkness colleagues in general and Phil Knapp in particular—and so honed her clinical skills.

She has also always been aware of the importance of excellence in science as a precursor to excellence in medicine and of the need for humanism as a backbone of life.

Ronald M. Burde, M.D.
Montefiore Medical Center

A Parent's Perspective on Patching

Having to have an eye patched for the first time is one of the most frightening experiences a young child can undergo. It is especially difficult when the parent and the child are not really able to communicate. It is therefore very important that a parent understand that the child will pick up on any ambivalence the parent may be feeling. The parent needs to approach patching with confidence and determination in order to make the experience as comfortable as possible. After patching my daughter for 4 years (since she was 3 months old), I have learned a few things that have helped make the experience less stressful.

One of the first things I did was to try a patch on my own eye when my daughter could not observe me. I made sure that I used the same brand that she would be using and tried to proceed with a normal routine. It was extremely irritating and I was very relieved when it was time to take the patch off. After a half hour, I had a much better understanding of the ordeal my daughter would be facing. I also realized that her experience would be even worse because her unpatched eye did not have perfect sight. I was more sympathetic and patient with her while her eye was patched because I knew how it felt. I did not allow my other children to experiment with the patch in front of my daughter because they had the option to remove the patch while my daughter did not.

The first few times I patched my daughter were very difficult for my entire family. While she was an infant, I needed another person to hold her head still while I attached the patch. I found that once the patch was properly placed I had to hug my daughter immediately. Not only did it help calm her down, it helped stop her from trying to rip the patch off her eye. We

stopped patching my daughter for almost a year, and so when we resumed patching her (as a toddler), I found I had to pin her down on the ground in order to place the patch on her. Her screams while we were putting the patch on greatly upset my other children. It took me awhile to be able to look at my baby with the patch on her eye without becoming upset myelf. Getting the patch on was very stressful for everyone.

Patching a child is very time consuming in the beginning. My daughter needed to be held the entire time for the first week which I had not factored into my week's schedule. My other children began to resent the time I had to spend with my daughter, and I found I had to adjust my normal routine. I had to build up to the amount of required time gradually because my daughter often became exhausted long before it was time to take the patch off. It was easier to patch her in the morning when she was not as tired and I tried to time the other activities during the day when she was not patched. Car trips posed a special dilemma because my daughter would fall asleep and when she awakened she would scream because the patch was still on. As she grew older, I found that she preferred not to wear the patch to morning preschool so as not to attract attention. We patched her immediately after lunch. It was also difficult for her to become involved in small motor activities when patched because her vision was less than perfect. Going to the playground, baking, or even going shopping was much less frustrating.

The quality of the eye patch is also important. While there are a number of choices, I chose the one that stayed in place most securely—especially since there were many tears. In addition, the non-adhesive section of the patch needs to cover the eye and the eyebrow so that removing the patch is not painful.

The best way a parent can help a child through the patching experience is to be firm and loving—many hugs and a lot of patience are the most reassuring way to alleviate a child's fear and annoyance while patched.

Rosemary Roberto

Introduction for Residents

The children that physicians see in clinics are no different than we were. They have the same fears, curiosity, and shyness that we did. Their responses, attention span, and communication skills are quite different than those of an adult. Therefore, it is no wonder that a subspecialty in ophthalmology was created particularly for children. Much information has been written on examination techniques and ocular disorders involving children. As a beginning ophthalmology resident, I found the wealth of information and techniques overwhelming. One approach was to learn pediatric ophthalmology from the many textbooks. Another more hands-on method was to learn by doing examinations in the clinic.

With the basic knowledge of ophthalmology, keen perception, and patience, a doctor can learn and diagnose many findings in a child during a first visit. Creating a good first impression and establishing rapport with the child patient is an important step before doing any sort of evaluation. Whether the child is playful, shy, or scared, it is important that both the child and doctor are comfortable from the start. Once this occurs, the doctor should watch and observe the child before doing anything else. This allows the child to act naturally in the situation as well as giving the child more time to become comfortable. The doctor can observe how a child sees objects or whether he or she is cooperative or not. This gives clues to whether or not a more playful approach as opposed to a direct approach is needed in the exam.

Having a child that is cooperative and comfortable is vital in any pediatric ophthalmic exam. The resident physician may need to tailor his or her image to a level that is appropriate to the age of the child. Playng with the patient using bright, interesting toys might get the attention needed. In addition, since children love games, this can be used to advantage in performing basic routine tests on children such as visual acuity, slit lamp examination, indirect ophthalmoscopy, stereo acuity, evaluation of ocular motility, and so forth. Sometimes having the child patient touch and play with the examining instruments will reduce anxiety he or she may have while being examined with the equipment.

One important aspect of pediatric ophthalmology involves the parents or guardians. Parents can help facilitate the history and exam as they are often keen observers. Many times parents also know how to obtain cooperation and increase comfort in the child during the exam. Active participation from parents can help speed many exams. This may also help make parents feel more responsible for the care of their children, especially when follow-up is needed. Since parents act both as an observer and enforcer for the follow-up care, a thorough explanation of the diagnosis and treatment plan should be given to parents to ensure compliance is maintained.

One of the fascinating aspects about pediatric ophthalmology is the interdisciplinary topics that are involved. The use of prisms for measurement of strabismus and glasses for refractive errors all require an understanding of optics. Many of the optical illusions involving stereoacuity are utilized to evaluate the degree of visual fusion and amblyopia. The surgical aspects of strabismus correction require a fundamental understanding of orthoptics for measurement and a basic knowledge of ocular anatomy. A genetic understanding of certain inherited ocular diseases is needed to aid in the diagnosis of diseases. The retina, uveitis, glaucoma, and neuro-ophthalmology must have special attention because of unique characteristics and presentation in the young population. Pediatric ophthalmology also plays an important role in promoting eye safety in sports as well as in diagnosing cases of subtle child abuse.

Overall, pediatric ophthalmology is diverse and challenging. Children are unique individuals who can present with a vast variety of ocular diseases and disorders. Patience, creativity, and flexibility are key ingredients for obtaining a successful history and physical exam. Relax and enjoy what can be a worthwhile lifetime experience.

Pamela S. Gallin

Preface

This text is intended as a guide for residents and practitioners in ophthalmology and for pediatricians. Its purpose is to provide an outline of pediatric ophthalmology with detailed descriptions of its major topics. Although many excellent definitive texts delve into and describe this fascinating subject, a need exists for an intermediate transitional text to decode and reorganize the extensive subject matter of pediatric ophthalmology. The goal of *Pediatric Ophthalmology: A Clinical Guide* is to fill that void. Collectively the senior authors of the chapters have at least 400 years of wisdom and judgment. Their expertise has been applied to sorting the most important topics and fine points within ophthalmology.

The book can be used as a first pass at understanding pediatric ophthalmology and a refresher for general ophthalmologists now seeing children. Pediatricians should find this useful as a reference book as well. The authors organize the information decision tree as if the physician were examining a patient, instead of the physician needing to reorganize the facts in the book to apply to the patient before them.

Key chapters include how to conduct a child's eye exam, how to perform retinoscopy, and how to treat amblyopia. Child abuse, a heinous crime, is described by the former Section Chief at the Babies and Children's Hospital of the Columbia Presbyterian Medical Center in great detail as it applies to ophthalmology. Learning disabilities are a topic often confronted by general and pediatric ophthalmologists. A special detailed chapter is included to give historical background and an understanding of current concepts in that burgeoning field.

The chapter on lasers by Dr. Marc Odrich and Dr. Stephen Trokel, who holds the patent on the excimer laser, describes current applications. Future uses of lasers in ophthalmology are described as well; these applications will become commonplace over the next few years.

Writing this book has been thrilling for me. Many of the professors with whom I had the honor to study as a medical student, resident, and during my fellowship honored me by writing chapters. Other authors were residents and fellows when I was an undergraduate and later a medical student at Washington University in St. Louis. Some were fellows with Dr. Marshall Parks and Dr. Philip Knapp, the two champions of pediatric ophthalmology and strabismus, who have had the most profound influence on this field and me personally. Colleagues at the Edward S. Harkness Eye Institute have made this text a collective effort.

Pamela S. Gallin

Acknowledgments

My editor Andrea Seils had the unique ability to cajole, coax, encourage, support, and criticize (gently) simultaneously. Miss Jennifer Charton, organizer and friend par excellence, made this book become a final text—without any more changes.

Arthur Cotliar, M.D., was instrumental in organizing the concepts to be included in this text. Dr. Cotliar also was key in determining the tenor of the text and the approach taken toward the patient—that of a superb general ophthalmologist who has made many babies see. Dr. Steven Obstbaum, former President of the American Academy of Ophthalmology and present Director of Ophthalmology at Lenox Hill Hospital, was the spark for this text. To all of them, I wish to say a special thanks.

Pamela S. Gallin

Pediatric Ophthalmology
Edited by P. F. Gallin
Thieme Medical Publishers, Inc.
New York © 2000

1
■ ■ ■

Pediatric Eye Examination

PAMELA F. GALLIN AND ILENE PARDON

The examination of the pediatric patient brings a host of challenges not incurred during the adult examination. Children are able, even from infancy, to give us a large amount of information. All children, independent of age, can have a complete ophthalmological examination. It is our job as ophthalmologists to learn how to glean this information effectively. There are significant differences between the design and function of the adult and pediatric exam. It is the goal of this chapter to arm the general ophthalmologist and ophthalmologist-in-training with the techniques needed to perform a standard eye exam on children of all ages. This chapter is a guide to the eye exam and must be adapted to specific problems and situations.

To begin, it is important to be equipped with some essential tools. It is highly recommended that you assemble the following "shopping list" before embarking on your first exam. You can create many items on this list inexpensively on your own.

Two or three medium-sized colorful toys—
   plush stuffed animals work well
Three or four tongue depressors decorated
   with a variety of cartoons
Pictures (near targets)
Tongue depressor with number chart or letters

Occluder with and without pinhole
Wall eye charts, including Snellen, Illiterate
   E, and Allen figures
Hand-held Allen cards
Prism bars or individual prism box
Pediatric trial frames
Titmus test
+3.50 spectacles (single vision)

■ Rapport

Once you have obtained the necessary materials for a pediatric exam, it is important to establish the appropriate rapport with a child. Good rapport can allow you to gain the most information. A child who is made to feel comfortable will assist the examiner during the exam. The following are several guidelines, which we have found as effective techniques to decrease a child's anxiety level and increase his or her interactions with the examiner.

1. Make the child feel comfortable as soon as he enters the room. A cheerful and friendly hello immediately places the child and parent at ease.
2. Ask the child a question to which he knows the answer. Once a child begins to

speak, his anxiety level decreases dramatically. In addition, a question that he knows the answer to will build confidence. School-aged students usually respond to questions about grade, teacher, and favorite subject. Younger children enjoy telling you about their favorite television program or their age. Ask them if they are older than you know they are.

3. Allow the child to be comfortable in the examination chair. Offer young children the opportunity to sit on a parent's lap.
4. Do not talk "down" to older children. Try to speak to them in an age appropriate manner and avoid a sing-song voice.

■ History

It is vital when examining children not to miss a window of opportunity. Most children have a limited attention span, and, once they have lost interest in the examination, obtaining information becomes very difficult. Therefore, it is not recommended to start your examination with a long history-taking session between yourself and the parent.

History can be obtained by a questionnaire distributed to a parent in the waiting area. The sample included here can be adapted for your particular practice situation (Fig. 1–1). It is important to include pregnancy and delivery information (including medications). A family history of strabismus and amblyopia as well as developmental and family histories are important. The past medical and ocular histories are also necessary. A parent's statement of the chief complaint is helpful and ensures that you will address the parent's primary concern.

It is important to understand that the indirect nature of the history (mainly from parents) presents unique problems in the pediatric exam. Children will rarely complain of unilateral visual loss and surprisingly do not usually complain of severe bilateral visual loss. Therefore, the pediatric exam may yield surprises that are not presented during history taking.

■ Examination

Visual Acuity

The pediatric ophthalmic exam should begin as soon as the patient enters the room. Observing the patient's approach to the examination chair allows the examiner to note head position, eye position, gait, and other clues to the diagnosis of ocular disease. Watching a child inspect your office can also yield important clues.

Visual acuity in a child should always be assessed by the ophthalmologist. The examiner's subjective assessment is extraordinarily important. This is used as a standard against which the results are measured. Children are eager to please; therefore, poor vision in one eye may be missed by the child's peeking around the occluder (Fig. 1–2). Always watch a child while checking visual acuity. In addition, decreased visual acuity due to occlusion nystagmus may be missed by a technician. Also, it is important to be aware that some children must be constantly coaxed throughout checking visual acuity. A few words of encouragement can sometimes move a child ahead several lines. A suspicion of malingering can also be noted at the time visual acuity is checked. Inconsistent acuities may clue the examiner to this situation. The acuity can be repeated again later in the examination beginning with the "worse" eye.

Visual acuity testing must be tailored to the child's age and ability. Infant visual acuity is the most challenging for an examiner, but important information may be gleaned from observing the infant. The ability to fix and follow an object should be present by 2 to 3 months of age (Fig. 1–3). Yet it can be present at birth in a very healthy, alert infant. Unfortunately, infants from birth to several months of age often show no response to inanimate objects such as toys or a flashlight. The human face is generally the strongest visual stimulus for the young infant. It is important to be aware that young infants may not be capable of producing the normal slow, smooth pursuit movements seen in older children and adults.

Pediatric Ophthalmology Exam

Patient's name _____

Age _____   Date of birth _____

Reason for today's visit

_____

_____

_____

Birth history (if complications, give details below)

Child's weight at birth _____

Was the child premature?   ❏ Yes   ❏ No

If premature, how many weeks premature?

Any complications with the delivery?   ❏ Yes   ❏ No

Any difficulty with feeding or eating initially?   ❏ Yes   ❏ No

Any early developmental delays with sitting, walking, or talking?   ❏ Yes   ❏ No

Any difficulties in school?   ❏ Yes   ❏ No

_____

_____

_____

Hereditary disease   ❏ Yes   ❏ No

Other disease   ❏ Yes   ❏ No

Disease   Relationship to patient

_____

_____

_____

Eye history (if yes, give details below)

Any previous eye examinations?   ❏ Yes   ❏ No

Are glasses worn?   ❏ Yes   ❏ No

Any previous amblyopia treatment such as patching or drops? ❏ Yes   ❏ No

Any eye surgery in the past?   ❏ Yes   ❏ No

Any eye injury in the past?   ❏ Yes   ❏ No

Details: _____

_____

_____

_____

FIGURE 1–1. Sample parent questionnaire used to obtain patient history.

Ask the parent if the child "sees" his or her face. In the case of a "blind" baby the parents will answer "no" or be uncertain. Young infants may display jerky, hypometric saccades in the same direction as the target. By 6 months of age, the average child should be able to fixate on moving toys and small targets within 6 feet.

Fixation of each eye should be evaluated separately. One technique to evaluate fixation is central steady maintained (CSM).

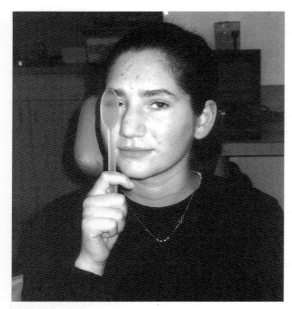

FIGURE 1–2. Peeking around occluder.

1. Central—as opposed to eccentric fixation
2. Steady—as opposed to nystagmus
3. Maintained—if fixation is held by the eye even when the other is uncovered

Cover the left eye first and note if the child follows a light or an object. It is also helpful to gauge how disturbed the infant is when the eye is covered. An infant with a severely amblyopic eye may become very anxious when his pre-ferred eye is covered. An infant will push away the patch when the seeing eye is covered, yet remain passive when the same is done to a poorly seeing eye. Check for occlusion nystagmus at this time. In a strabismic patient, you must watch both the covered and the uncovered eyes closely, especially as the occluded eye is uncovered. The assessment of vision in an infant is very subjective and exceedingly difficult, requiring much judgment.

Optokinetic nystagmus (OKN) can be used as evidence of very gross visual acuity. The examiner may use an OKN drum or tape to elicit OKNs in an infant. A simple method of eliciting OKNs is to carefully turn the infant while the examiner holds the infant approximately 10 to 15 inches from the face. Also, visual evoked responses (VERs) may be used to assess vision. These techniques use checkerboard or striped gratings of various spatial frequencies combined with electrode monitoring of the brain. (See Chapter 21 on visual acuity testing.)

Preferential looking is based on observations that infants are more interested in looking at a pattern than at homogeneous fields. The infant is exposed to a particular black and white striped pattern and an identically sized gray field of equal luminance. The observer under specific lighting conditions and at a fixed distance quantifies the amount of time that the infant focuses on each field. Preferential looking is useful in the evaluation and follow-up

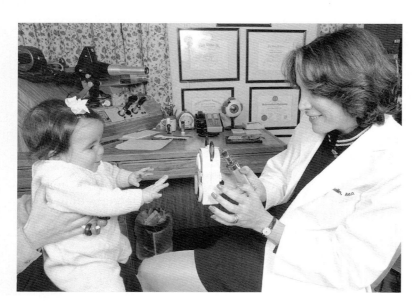

FIGURE 1–3. Baby looking at near target.

of preverbal patients with disorders affecting visual acuity. It is especially useful to compare relative acuity between the two eyes. Unlike VER, preferential looking is dependent upon eye movements.

Snellen Visual Acuity

The American Academies of Ophthalmology and Pediatrics recommend a vision screen at the age of 3. The age at which a child can participate in acuity testing varies widely. Some 2-year-olds can read the Snellen letter or number chart, whereas some 6-year-olds cannot. A hierarchy of increasing difficulty and accuracy in testing begins with the Allen cards (Fig. 1–4). The illiterate E game is extraordinarily accurate, although some 3-year-olds cannot cooperate. Often a normal child with a perfectly normal exam will only read up to the 20/30 line. **Symmetry in acuity on vision screens is of more importance than the actual acuity.** In young children this is a soft test result unless the final acuity is 20/30 or better. As well, note that the left eye acuity is often worse than the right because the kids have become inattentive. Combined with a normal exam and retinoscopy,

these kids should return for acuity testing of the "worse eye" first on a subsequent exam or later during the same exam. Often "the problem" evaporates, or not, in which case more sophisticated tests can be undertaken.

Snellen letter charts can be difficult for international patients and kids with learning disabilities. Often the 4- to 6-year-olds prefer the Snellen numbers, as there are only 9 digits to choose from instead of 26 letters. Other optotype tests include the Landolt C, HOTV, and Sheridan STYCAR. Be aware that amblyopes may demonstrate a "crowding phenomenon" in which the acuity is one to three lines worse than when single individual letters are presented. (i.e., with individual letters they "see" one to three lines more).

All tests and methods of tests should be noted. When an asymmetrical acuity is suspected and these very charming cheaters try to peek and memorize the chart promptly, an occlusive patch in conjunction with a hand (so they don't peel if off) may be useful.

Testing should be done at distance and near but is often done at distance only in a screening situation. Do not try to have them read every letter, as you will lose their attention.

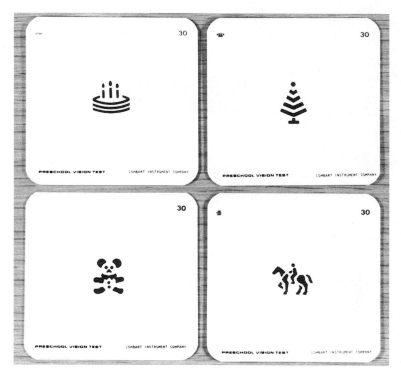

FIGURE 1–4. Allen cards.

Rapidly skip downward toward the 20/60 lines and then 20/50 to accurately assess their acuity. Do not forget head posture. Children with nystagmus and null points may need to be tested in their null points. Occlusion nystagmus may require both eyes open with a dark filter or blur over the eye not being tested. In severe nystagmus, one must often "infer" the range of their vision with both eyes open.

Strabismus Testing

The type of testing used to elicit strabismus must also be tailored toward the child's age. With infants and uncooperative children, corneal light reflection tests are the methods of choice. **The simplest and least accurate is the Hirschberg test** (Figs. 1–5 and 1–6). The patient fixates on a light source, and the amount of corneal decentration of the light reflex is noted. One should note the amount of decentration

in millimeters and multiply each millimeter of decentration by 15 prism diopters to obtain a rough approximation of the deviation. **A second, more accurate method of measuring deviations utilizing corneal reflexes is the Krimsky test** (Fig. 1–7). In this test, a prism is used to center the corneal light reflection. The prism is changed until the corneal reflexes are symmetrically centered. Most infants can cooperate sufficiently for this test.

For older children, the cover test and alternate cover test are routinely used to detect strabismus. **The cover test** (Fig. 1–8) **is used to detect manifest deviations.** It is performed first by having the child look at a distant target. The examiner places an occluder before one eye and watches the other uncovered eye for any shift in fixation. A shift in fixation implies that the patient has a tropia (a manifest deviation). The test is then completed by covering the other eye. The patient should be returned to a

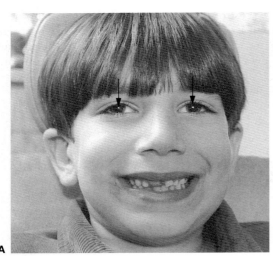

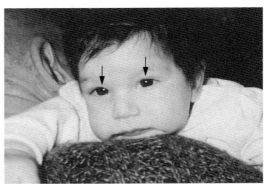

FIGURE 1–5. (A) Hirschberg reflex—eyes straight. **(B)** Hirschberg reflex—eyes straight.

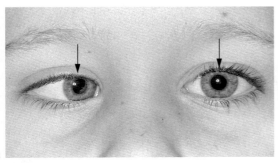

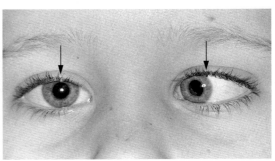

FIGURE 1–6. Hirschberg reflex—eyes esotropic. **(A)** Fixing with left eye. **(B)** Fixing with right eye.

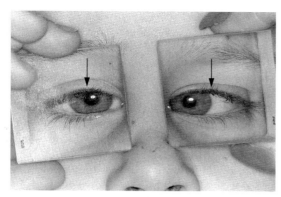

FIGURE 1–7. Krimsky test.

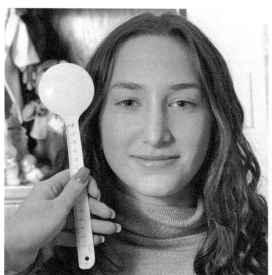

A

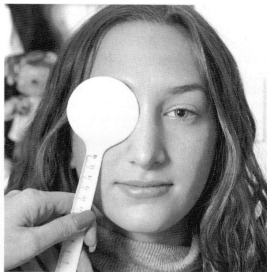

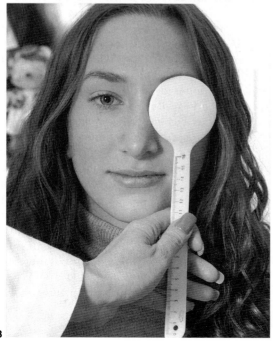

B

FIGURE 1–8. (A) Uncover/cover using occluder.
(B) Alternate cover.

binocular condition prior to testing the other eye. The cover test should be repeated to be sure that a subtle rapid switch in fixation did not take place unnoticed during the binocular interval. This is especially important in children who readily alternate fixation.

The next test in the series is the alternate cover test. **The alternate cover test is a method of detecting a latent deviation (a heterophoria).** The alternate cover test is performed by moving the occluder from one eye to the other without allowing an interval of binocular viewing. This technique is able to detect phorias because it interrupts fusion. If no shift occurs as the occluder is passed from eye to eye, then the eyes are considered aligned and termed orthophoric. If a shift does occur, then a heterophoria is detected. It is important to consider these results in relation to the cover test. Alternate cover test does not diagnose a phoria alone without the use of the cover test to rule out a tropia.

After the diagnosis of a deviation, the alternate cover test combined with prisms may be used to measure the deviations. A prism is held before either eye with the apex of the prism pointing toward the deviation while the alternate cover test is performed. The correct prism has been chosen when no movement is detected. The correctly chosen prism will deflect light from the target onto the fovea of the deviating eye, making a shift unnecessary. The measurements should be made with the patient fixating on a near and distant target. Different patterns of tropias should also be noted at this time. A- or V-pattern tropias should be noted, and measurements in different fields of gaze should be recorded.

The simultaneous prism/cover test may be used to quantify the tropic component of a deviation. The test is performed by simultaneously introducing the occluder before the fixating eye and a correctly chosen prism before the deviating eye. If the prism neutralizes the refixation movement, then the prism accurately reflects the tropic component of the deviation.

It is important when choosing a treatment plan to differentiate among an accommodative tropia, a partially accommodative tropia, and a nonaccommodative tropia. Placing +3.50 lenses on a child while measuring the near deviation

will help to clarify the diagnosis. The single-use +3.50 lenses in a single-use spectacle is a trick taught to us by Sally Moore, professor of ophthalmology at the Harkness Eye Institute. These can be used easily if the child does or does not wear spectacles. It is easier than holding up two +3.50 lenses. The lenses will relax a child's accommodation, effectively neutralizing its participation in a tropia. The deviation will be decreased in cases of partially accommodative esotropias, but nonaccommodative deviations will not be affected by +3.50 lenses.

■ Versions and Ductions

Versions are the range of motion of the eyes used together. This examination may be easily conducted by having the patient follow a colorful object in the nine cardinal fields of gaze: primary, up, down, right, left, supertemporal, supernasal, inferotemporal, and inferonasal (Fig. 1–9).

■ Color Vision

In children capable of color vision testing, it is important to incorporate this testing into the examination. Nearly 10% of normal males have color vision abnormalities, which should be recognized at an early age as they may affect school performance in certain activities. Commonly used clinical color vision tests include the full and concise editions of Ishihara's Tests for Color Blindness. (There are four editions, with 10, 14, 24, and 38 plates.) For screening purposes, the concise edition is ideal. Children, especially those younger than 6, will most commonly confuse the numbers four and seven. The number four is stylized and not used by this generation of children. Finger tracing of numbers and patterns can be used for nonverbal children, although oil spots remain on the pages. The American Optical Color Plates will detect red and green color vision defects, which are the most common hereditary defects found in children. Hardy-Rand Ritter pseudoisochromatic plates will detect both red–green and blue–yellow defects, but these are no longer commercially available. Detailed color tests use the Farnsworth Munsell 15 and 100 hue tests in research conditions.

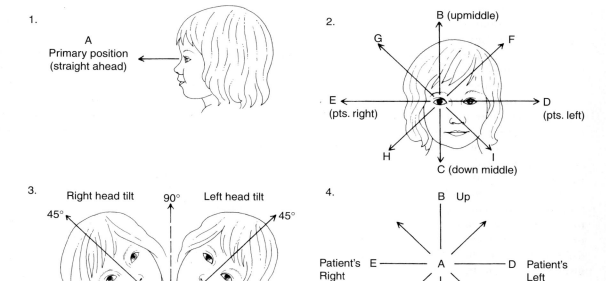

1.

A
Primary position
(straight ahead)

2.

B (upmiddle)

G   F

E
(pts. right)   D
(pts. left)

H   I

C (down middle)

3.

Right head tilt   90°   Left head tilt
45°   45°

4.

B   Up

Patient's   E —————— A —————— D   Patient's
Right   Left

C   Down

FIGURE 1–9. Cardinal field drawing.

■ Stereoacuity

Stereoacuity is one of the most fundamental sensory tests. A child must have excellent acuity to participate in this test. The test should be done with the best correction in place. These tests measure peripheral retinal fusion (gross) and a more refined central (macular) fusion measured in degrees (seconds of arc). A stereoacuity of 60 seconds or better shows bifoveal fusion. **The Titmus test is the most commonly used near test today and is designed for children** (Fig. 1–10). To be accurate, the test must be conducted with adequate illumination, and the distance from the eyes to the test must be held constant. Polaroid glasses are placed on the child's nose, over existing spectacles, if present. The Titmus test has a large housefly with wings that present a test of gross stereopsis representing 300 seconds of arc. Asking the child to grab the fly's wings is the best way to determine if a child has stereoacuity. Children below the age of 6 usually do not understand the ques-

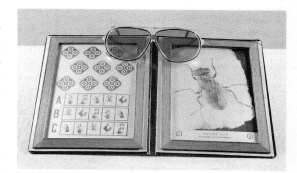

FIGURE 1–10. Titmus test.

tion, "Are the wings standing up or coming out at you?" A frightened or excited response may be further evidence that the child does indeed have stereoacuity. As a check of accuracy, the examiner may turn the fly picture sideways. The fly cannot be seen stereoscopically sideways because the disparity is now vertical as opposed to the usual horizontal disparity.

A positive response to the fly and the larger figures on the Titmus test proves at least peripheral fusion. The patient needs to show recognition of circles 7, 8, and 9 to definitely have bifoveal fixation (circle 9 is equal to 40 seconds of arc). Only older children can understand the circle section of the Titmus test, therefore, only peripheral fusion can be absolutely proven in younger children. It is possible for patients with bifoveal fixation to fail the stereoacuity test simply because they did not understand the test or were bored with the examination by this time. The patient's best acuity is required, e.g., an uncorrected myope is not being accurately tested.

The A-O Vectographic Project-O-Charter Slide is the most commonly used distance stereopsis test in the United States. Distance stereopsis may be very useful when there is a difference in fusional status at distance and near. Stereopsis testing may occasionally be possible in children as young as 3 years but becomes much more reliable around the age of 5 or 6. Several other sensory tests are available to assess stereoacuity and central suppression, but they are beyond the scope of the routine pediatric examination.

■ Slit Lamp Examination

As with all other aspects of a pediatric examination, a slit lamp examination can be adequately performed with patience and usually with speed. If a slit lamp examination needs to be performed, it is conducted much in the same way for older children as it is for adults. Younger children may want to sit on a parent's lap and often need to be coaxed to the slit lamp by a promise of seeing something exciting in the slit lamp such as a pretty light or target. Having the parent show "how much fun" it is by putting his chin in the slit lamp is also quite helpful to convince a child to investigate the slit lamp. Infants can usually be supported by the parent with one hand under the buttocks and the other hand on the back of the head. A second adult can hold the head fixed with both hands on the ears. An examiner can hold the eyelids open. Ignore screams—you are not hurting the baby.

Slit lamp examinations do not need to be performed on all children, but certain circumstances require closed inspection. For example, all patients with juvenile rheumatoid arthritis require a slit lamp exam to rule out anterior uveitis. Children with leukocoria and a poor red reflex should also be examined with biomicroscopy. Children with systemic diseases that may lead to lenticular abnormalities (e.g., Marfan syndrome) are another group that should routinely undergo slit lamp exam. Also, trauma to the eye is another reason to perform a slit lamp exam on a child. It is important not to defer a needed examination because the patient is an uncooperative young child or an infant. If available, a portable slit lamp can be used while a child is papoosed to remain still.

Applanation tonometry can also be accomplished at the time of the slit lamp examination. Obviously, not all patients will be cooperative enough for applanation tonometry. Again, as in the slit lamp examination, intraocular pressure (IOP) only needs to be checked in a patient with a specific cause for concern. For example, pressure should be checked in patients with a family history of congenital or pediatric glaucoma. In an otherwise normal infant or child, some pediatric ophthalmologists record that each eye is soft to palpation. Infant IOP can be checked with a Perkins hand-held applanation tonometer, or Tono-Pen X-L (Mentor). It is important that the child not be squeezing the eyelids during the pressure check or the IOP may be falsely elevated. It is helpful if the infant is sleeping when the IOP is checked, which often occurs just after feeding.

■ Dilation

The choice of dilating drops is very important in children. It must be tailored to a child's age and reason for dilation. **All infants and children should undergo cycloplegia to be accurately refracted owing to their tremendous accommodative abilities.** The relationship between refractive state and horizontal strabismus makes it essential to accurately assess a child's refraction. It is mandatory that all children entering an ophthalmologist's office for any reason have a complete cycloplegic examination. It is imperative to assess cornea, lens, and vitreous clarity and the presence or absence of potentially life-threatening tumors, such as retinoblastoma.

Mydriacyl 1% (tropicamide)alone does not provide adequate cycloplegia in children. It is often used in conjunction with cyclopentolate (cyclogel). Cyclopentolate 1 to 2% in conjunction with Mydriacyl 1% is the preferable route for routine cycloplegia in the office. Cyclopentolate has a rapid onset of action and is less toxic than some of the other agents. Cyclopentolate provides a cycloplegic effect that is similar to atropine. Atropine ointment is another good method of cycloplegia, but the onset of cycloplegia takes several hours, and recovery of accommodation can take several days after the last instillation. The duration of action makes atropine especially troubling to school-aged children.

Cyclopentolate is used as 0.5% solution in infants and a 1% solution after the age of 6 months. The cycloplegic effect achieves its maximal level within 30 minutes. The dilation effect is enhanced by the instillation of 2.5% phenylephrine, which will stimulate the pupillary dilator muscles. If atropine is to be used, the drops are the preferred route of administration over ointment. The dosage of the drops can be more accurately given. Atropine is usually given one or two times a day for 3 days before the examination, often in children who are difficult to examine.

Side effects of the cycloplegic agents include topical sensitivity and parasympatholytic effects following systemic absorption. Systemic side effects include facial flushing, tachycardia, dry mouth, and mild central nervous system disturbances. Transient psychosis has been described. Children with Down syndrome are exceedingly sensitive to atropine, and therefore it is not recommended for them.

■ Retinoscopy

Retinoscopy can be performed on the vast majority of infants and children (Fig. 1–11). If all the lights are turned off except that of the retinoscope, most infants and children will look at the retinoscope. Making creative noises, such as buzzing or clicking, will also enhance the child's participation in the exam. Some young children will be frightened by the hand-held lenses; therefore, estimation techniques may be used initially. Trial frames can be used in slightly older and more cooperative children.

Of note, **retinoscopy is the most accurate when performed on an unrestrained cooperative patient.** The use of eyelid speculums or eyelid squeezing often results in distortion of corneal curvature. Off-axis retinoscopy is a problem with restrained patients. Therefore, this part of the exam is one in which patient cooperation is most crucial. It is generally better to perform retinoscopy prior to fundus examination because a child's cooperation is often lost after indirect ophthalmoscopy. The

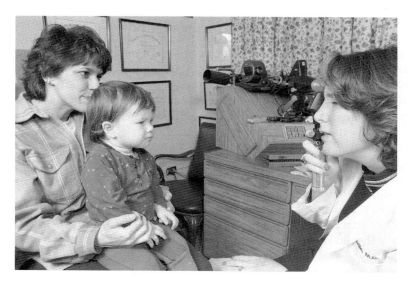

FIGURE 1–11. Retinoscopy.

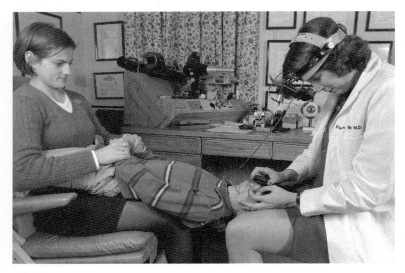

FIGURE 1–12. Indirect ophthalmoscopy. (Position can also be used for retinoscopy.)

retinoscope is extremely useful in assessing the visual significance and size of corneal or lenticular opacities. If a child is cooperative and because it is mandatory to obtain at least an estimated retinoscopy, we employ the following positions. (1) Start with the child in a bear hug with parent (chest to chest). Have child lie down face up in examiner's lap with legs around parent. Hold child's head between examiner's knees. Parent holds hands. Examiner opens eyelids (Fig. 1–12). (2) Papoose is often helpful. (3) Wrap child on flat surface with sheet below neck encircling arms.

■ Fundus Examination

A good fundus examination with the indirect ophthalmoscope is an essential component of the initial pediatric ophthalmology exam. Obviously, children will not allow the examiner the liberty of time for close inspection. Therefore, it is important to gain a general overview quickly and efficiently. Before beginning the exam, turn the light on the ophthalmoscope lower than usually used with a compliant adult. Positive encouragement before the examination will help to gain a child's confidence. With older children, it is helpful if you explain that this is only a bright light and the exam should only

last for a minute. Younger children can be coaxed to look at the light by telling them to find their favorite characters in the light (Barney, Mickey Mouse, etc.). A very uncooperative child can be placed in his parent's lap with his back to the examiner and his legs straddled around the parent's waist. The child is then gently laid back until his head rests on the examiner's lap (Fig. 1–12). This technique works very well with cooperative parents and a quick examiner.

Newborn infants at risk for retinopathy of prematurity require a topical anesthesic, lid speculum, and scleral depression for an adequate assessment. New parents are often very upset by the lid speculum; therefore, it is sometimes advisable to ask for an assistant to hold the baby. Always give parents the option to stay or leave the room during the exam.

An initial screening with a 28-D lens works very well. This lens gives a broad view well beyond the vascular arcades. If any retinal pathology is noted, the examiner should change to a 20-D lens or even a 14-D lens for greater enlargement, particularly of the foveal area or optic nerve. In older children, the examiner can usually get beyond the posterior pole by using a 20-D lens while the child voluntarily moves the eye to the appropriate positions. Younger children will not move their eyes as directed, and the examiner must change position often to get an adequate fundus view.

■ Conclusion

A pediatric ophthalmic exam, similar to a physical exam given by an internist, has a few basic components: a check of visual acuity and alignment, retinoscopy, assessment of the visual axis, and indirect retinoscopy. The exam is then expanded in certain areas, depending on the chief complaint and findings. In particular, we recognize that the exam is quite complex and difficult to administer.

SUGGESTED READINGS

Catalano R, Nelson LB, eds. *Pediatric Opthalmology: A Text Atlas.* Stanford, CT: Appleton & Lange; 1994.

Crawford J, Morin J, eds. *The Eye in Childhood.* New York: Grune & Stratton; 1983.

Tasman W, Jaeger EA, eds. *Duane's Clinical Ophthalmology.* Philadelphia: Lippincott-Raven; 1995.

Nelson LB, Harley RD, eds. *Harley's Pediatric Ophthalmology,* 4th ed. Philadelphia: WB Saunders; 1998.

Parks MM. *Atlas of Strabismus Surgery.* New York: Harper & Row; 1983.

Von Noorden G, Maumenee AE, eds. *Atlas of Strabismus,* 3rd ed. St. Louis: Mosby; 1997.

Wright K, ed. *Color Atlas of Strabismus Surgery.* St. Louis: Wright Publishing; 2000.

Wright K, Stone E, Ellis F, et al, eds. *Pediatric Ophthalmology and Strabismus.* St. Louis: Mosby; 1995.

Pediatric Ophthalmology
Edited by P. F. Gallin
Thieme Medical Publishers, Inc.
New York © 2000

2

Visual Assessment

GEORGE S. ELLIS JR. AND CINDY PRITCHARD

Vision testing in children is often the most challenging part of a comprehensive eye examination. Assessing the visual acuity of infants and young children is an art. The detection of physical abnormalities is only a clue to visual function. Obtaining a quantitative or qualitative assessment of visual function requires a skill that is developed utilizing a repertoire of techniques.[1,2] Until the age of 5 or 6 years, the assessment of vision is frequently dependent on the examiner's clinical judgment and expertise.

In this chapter, we address the art of vision testing and describe approaches to assessing the visual function of infants, preliterate children, and developmentally delayed older children.

■ General Principles

The examination should begin as a child he enters the exam room. This may be your best opportunity to evaluate vision. Be alert to visual attentiveness of a child. Specifically, be aware of head position, nystagmus, photophobia, or strabismus. Establishing a good rapport with a child is key to obtaining cooperation for subsequent testing. Incorporate the establishment of rapport with the actual examination; make the exam fun. For example, while showing the child a small toy, the examiner can be evaluating fixation patterns (Fig. 2–1). Leading the child into a conversation about the toy establishes the dia-

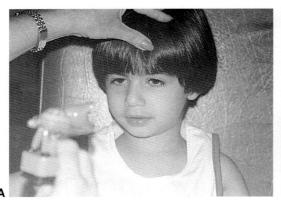 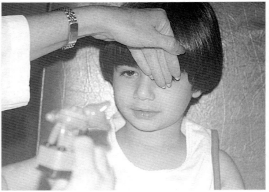

A **B**

FIGURE 2–1. Child fixates on a small toy while the examiner evaluates fixation preferences. A cover, uncover test is being performed.

logue needed for a later objective vision test. Conversation centered around a toy not only helps to relax the child but also provides an opportunity to evaluate the cooperativeness and developmental level of the child. This knowledge will help direct you toward the appropriate method of visual assessment.

Choose the appropriate method of testing based on the level of cooperation and on the developmental rather than chronological age. It is common to encounter bright 3- and 4-year-olds who are prepared to read Snellen letters. However, one also must be alert to developmentally delayed 6- and 7-year-olds who require preliterate testing methods. **It is important to emphasize that the child's developmental age will determine which tests will be most appropriate.**

■ Neonates

Assessing the visual function of the neonate or very young infant is often limited by the lack of attention by the patient or by lack of patience by the examiner. In the first few weeks of life, an infant sleeps frequently, and it can be difficult to sufficiently arouse her for vision testing. **In the most unarousable infant, pupillary responses may be the only measure of visual function available.** Multiple visits may be necessary. It can be helpful to see the child when he or she is hungry and is more likely to be alert. Do not confuse a somnolent recently fed baby with one who is neurologically delayed.

The alert neonate with normal visual functions should respond to lights and to faces. The infant's gaze should fixate on and follow the face of the examiner as the examiner moves in various directions, positioned rather closely to the face of the infant (recorded as Fix and Follow Face). Some infants will also look at the direction of a light source but will not follow the movement of the light source (recorded as Fix, No Follow Light). When no fixation or following movements can be elicited, room lights can be turned on and off. A consistent reaction to the change in room illumination is a gross measure of visual response (recorded as Responds to Room Lights). Avoidance reactions to light of the indirect ophthalmoscope are also useful (recorded as Avoids Bright Light). Observations

from home by parents can be an adjunct to the clinician's observations. Question the parents regarding the infant's responses to faces and lights. Be careful to eliminate voice recognition. In this age group do not assume that a lack of response is due to inability to cooperate. Most children choose to participate in the examination—even neonates.

Electrophysiological testing or preferential looking testing can be utilized when a quantitative value is necessary. These tests are generally more useful when the infant reaches an age when he or she is more alert. Visual evoked potentials (VEPs) and electroretinograms (ERGs) will be discussed in more detail in Chapter 21. Theoretically, these tests can be performed at any age. However, in neonates these tests can often suggest misleadingly poor visual function. The results, particularly of VEP testing, should, in such cases, be interpreted with caution. An examiner's judgment often is the most useful test.

There are a number of available tests utilizing a preferential looking technique. These are based on the principle that an infant will "preferentially" look toward a pattern. The patterns are most often gratings or checks. A card is presented to the infant with a pattern on one side of the center and a gray field on the other. The Teller acuity cards, for example, are a series of cards with variously sized gratings. By determining the finest grating to which the infant will consistently direct his or her gaze, acuity can be extrapolated relatively accurately (Fig. 2–2).

Such tests can be administered in any clinical setting by an ophthalmic assistant with minimal training. They serve as a quantitative vision test for patients of all developmental ages and have, in fact, been utilized for vision testing of premature infants shortly after birth in studies of retinopathy of prematurity. These tests, however, have limitations with respect to interpretation and decreased sensitivity to amblyopia.

The recording of neonatal acuity is often descriptive in nature, although preferential looking and VEP results are recorded in cycles/degree, which allows for translation to Snellen acuity. Acuity might otherwise be recorded as "follows faces," "responds to light," "avoids bright light," or "no fixation or following." Normal neonatal acuity is gross and difficult to quantitate.

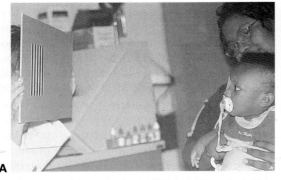

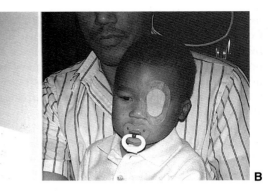

A

B

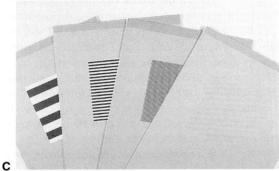

C

FIGURE 2–2. (A) A child with one eye patched views a Teller Acuity Card while the examiner evaluates the infant's visual preference for the right or left side of the card. If the child prefers viewing the side of the card with the stripes, the infant is judged to have resolution acuity based on the stripe width. **(B)** A child with horizontal nystagmus can be tested with the cards held vertically. **(C)** A display of some of the Teller Acuity Cards showing the range of stripe width.

The visual acuity of a neonate is most often inferred by the physical exam and gross response to light and faces. For instance, if a baby is not responding to your face, your conclusion will vary depending upon whether a lens opacity or significant pathology is present. With a large central opacity, for example, the lack of response would be corroborative. In the absence of an opacity, the lack of response would be perplexing, and an explanation would be necessary.

Assessment of acuity is dependent more upon physical findings and upon evidence of potential abnormalities that could be caused by central nervous system defects or other medical problems. A careful birth and family history should be obtained, and an appropriate follow-up plan to assure optimal visual development is recommended. Fortunately, infants develop at a rapid rate, allowing more detailed assessment to be obtained as described in the following section of this chapter.

■ Infants

At a few months of age an infant is more consistently responsive on a visual and sensory basis. A few classes of convention are used in the assessment. One convention is fixation behavior, as described above. Another, central-steady-maintained, which incorporates fixation preference, is often recorded as CSM.

CSM Classification

C = Central	Is the visual axis central in each eye, in contrast with eccentric (recorded as nC) fixation? If so, the macula is fixating.
S = Steady	Is the monocular fixation without movement, or does the eye wander? Is the globe bobbing up and down or back and forth as in nystagmus? If not steady (recorded as nS), the type of movement must be described. In nystagmus the fixation can often be steady at the null point but not elsewhere.
M = Maintained	Can the fixation be maintained with each eye individually under binocular viewing? In strabismus, the amblyopic eye may not maintain fixation under binocular conditions, and the patient will preferentially fixate with the dominant or sound eye. In a neurologically impaired child maintenance of fixation due to a lack of vision versus central neurological suppression (seizures) must be sorted out.

Determining whether fixation is central and steady tests each eye individually (monocular testing), whereas determining whether fixation is maintained compares the vision of each eye (a binocular test). The evaluation of fixation maintenance (M) allows for better assessment of relative visual acuity and therefore more sensitive detection of amblyopia.

The second classification uses one eye essentially as a control. The "M" of CSM is the most important segment of the fixation description when amblyopia is suspected. The "M" refers to "maintained" and specifically addresses the relative acuity between the eyes. An infant who has a manifest strabismus is forced to choose to fixate with one eye or the other because both eyes cannot be simultaneously directed at the object of regard. If the child alternates fixation between the eyes freely, equal vision is assumed. If, however, the infant has a strong preference for fixation with one particular eye, the other eye is presumed to be amblyopic or to have organic loss of vision.

The parents may offer their observations regarding which eye the infant "crosses." The examiner might observe that the infant spontaneously shifts fixation from one eye to the other, suggesting that acuity is probably equal in the two eyes, and the acuity could be recorded as in each eye.

To test for amblyopia, the preferred eye is covered, usually with the examiner's hand, forcing the infant to take up fixation with the nonpreferred eye. With the preferred eye covered, the object of regard, usually a small toy, is moved horizontally or vertically. The fixating eye should make appropriate following movements to insure that the child is, indeed, fixating and allow the examiner to evaluate whether the fixation in the nonpreferred eye is central and steady.

When the cover is removed, the infant can only do one of two things: (1) continue to fix with the nonpreferred eye or (2) shift back to the preferred eye. If the infant immediately shifts back to the preferred eye, fixation with the nonpreferred eye is described as not maintained (recorded as nM) or fixation with the preferred eye is described as "strongly preferred," implying that the infant sees more clearly with the preferred eye and has significant amblyopia in the nonpreferred eye.

When the infant does not immediately switch back to the preferred eye upon removal of the cover, fixation is described as maintained in the nonpreferred eye. Maintained fixation in the nonpreferred eye may be graded or subdivided. To further qualify how well the child will maintain fixation with the nonpreferred eye, the examiner should continue to observe the infant after removing the cover to see how long he or she will continue to fixate with the nonpreferred eye. The blink reflex should be incorporated into the description of fixation preference. The infant might continue to hold fixation with the nonpreferred eye after a blink (recorded as "M through a blink"), also described as mild preference for the preferred eye. The infant may switch fixation back to the preferred eye immediately following a blink (recorded as "M to a blink"), or the preferred eye may be described as "moderately preferred." The infant might hold fixation with the nonpreferred eye for a very short time after the cover is removed, which is before the blink occurs (recorded as "M few seconds") in which case the preferred eye would be described as "strongly prefers."

By describing the strength of fixation preference in terms of relationship to a blink, density of amblyopia can be estimated and responses to therapy evaluated. Using these notations amblyopia treatment is modified as fixation preference changes. The ability to make this distinction is of paramount importance. This test is very useful for large deviations but is less useful for deviations that are small, less than about 10 prism diopters, and those in the monofixation range.

Base-Down Prism

When the infant does not have a large, obvious manifest strabismus, relative acuity (fixation preference) can be determined by inducing a strabismus by placing a large, usually 20 prism diopter base-down prism in front of one eye. The infant can then be tested for alternating fixation as described previously. One will often observe vertical saccades equal in amplitude to the size of the prism suggesting equal vision. A preference for fixation would suggest a possibility of poor vision in one eye. Visual preference should be evaluated

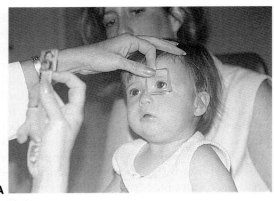 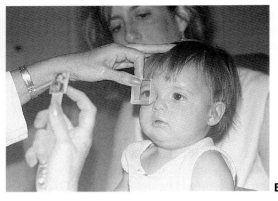

A   **B**

FIGURE 2–3. 20° base-down prism test. A preverbal child fixates on a small toy through a 20° base-down prism held in front of one eye. If both eyes shift up to view the displaced image through the prism, the child is using the eye behind the prism. **(A, B)** Each eye is tested individually.

twice, once with the prism over each eye to control for artifactual responses from prism blur (Fig. 2–3).

Four Diopter Base-Out Prism Test

Another test that can be used to help detect asymmetric acuity (fixation preference) in the infant with straight eyes is the 4 diopter base-out prism test. This test is less frequently performed because it is more difficult to assess the infant's response. In addition to detecting the presence of a fixation preference, it also tests for motor fusion. A 4 or 6 diopter base-out prism is placed in front of one eye. The normal response is to see a fusional convergence eye movement. If, however, there is consistently a version movement (both eyes move in the same direction, right or left) in the direction of the apex of the prism when it is placed in front of one eye and there is no movement when placed in front of the other eye, poor vision in the eye with no response should be suspected.

Tests for a fixation preference are more easily performed on a near target. In the older and more alert infant, testing can also be performed on a distant target by having a parent or older sibling hold an object of interest at the end of the room while verbally trying to keep the infant's attention.

Testing for a fixation preference is extremely important because amblyopia cannot be diag-

nosed by physical examination of the eye alone, yet amblyopia requires early detection and treatment for recovery of vision. Fixation preference testing is especially important for those infants with amblyogenic conditions such as strabismus or anisometropia. Other clinical findings that should be considered amblyogenic include unilateral or asymmetric cases of ptosis, glaucoma, media opacities, or fundus pathology.

How one approaches an infant is relevant to maximizing cooperation and attention. With the infant on the parent's lap, adjust the height of the chair to place the infant's eyes at the examiner's eye level or higher. An infant tends to look down. As you greet the parent and child make eye contact with the infant, smile and coo like a loving doting grandparent or relative. Touch the child's head early in the interaction as a love pat. These techniques will give the child the security to let you touch the head/face to occlude a place of prism. Occlusion of the visual axis of one eye can be accomplished with your hand 6 to 12 in from the child's face without touching.

Testing for a fixation preference can in some cases be very difficult or impossible because the infant violently resists occlusion. Resistance to occlusion can, in itself, be a useful observation tool in assessing infant acuity. If the infant consistently objects more to occlusion of one eye than the other, suspicion should arise regarding the possibility that vision is poor in the eye with which the infant offers the least resistance to occlusion.

Bruckner Simultaneous Red Reflex Test

This test works well in infants over 2 months of age and can detect potential amblyogenic conditions (anisometropia, strabismus, and media opacities). This test is performed in a darkened room. The examiner observes both of the child's red reflexes simultaneously at a distance of arm's length, while the infant fixates on the light of the ophthalmoscope. Notice the pupillary constriction. If with that constriction you observe any differences in size, shape, color, or brightness of the reflex, the child *may* have an amblyogenic condition, and a more careful visual assessment is indicated.

Optokinetic Drum (OKN)

Special testing may be required for the uncooperative, inattentive, or very young infant. By 4 to 6 months of age infants should have a brisk response to optokinetic stimulation. A pediatric OKN drum (Fig. 2–4) rotated slowly induces optokinetic nystagmus. The OKN drum is particularly useful in the low vision infant who does not display central and steady fixation or the infant with nystagmus. In patients with nystagmus, the ability to superimpose vertical OKN on a horizontal nystagmus suggests that the infant is developing useful vision. Although the ability for the infant to respond to the OKN stimulus is a gross measure of acuity, response to the OKN drum is sometimes the only clinical method of determining with certainty that the infant does, indeed, see.

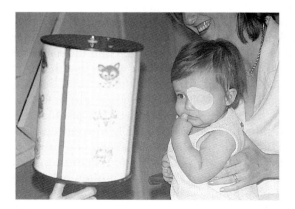

FIGURE 2–4. A preverbal child monocularly viewing the pediatric OKN drum.

Doll's Head Maneuver

Eliciting vestibular nystagmus while spinning a child indicates a gross level of visual function. The examiner performs the test by holding the infant head up, feet down at eye level and at arm's length. With the examiner as the hub, the child is rotated around an arc in a circle. A vestibular nystagmus is created. When the examiner stops rotating, a child with a higher level of central visual development will have rapid dampening of the vestibular nystagmus. The ocular motor system must be intact for this test to be of value.

Other Tests

When there is no evidence of visual response to optokinetic or vestibular stimulation, it may be necessary to rely on pupillary responses or responses to bright lights, room illumination changes, or threat (a hand rapidly approaching the eyes) for observation of behavioral responses (i.e., blink or grimace).

■ Preverbal Child

Language skills usually begin to develop prior to the age of 2 years. Between the ages of 2 and 3 years, however, spoken vocabulary may be too limited for many preliterate acuity charts. The child does often have adequate understanding of language to respond in other ways to simple quantitative acuity tests.

Finger mimicking is a test that can be applied to very young children, sometimes prior to the age of 2 years. The examiner holds up one finger, two fingers, four fingers and a thumb, or a fist and prompts the child by asking in a playful tone, "Can you do this?" or "Show me this" or other similar instruction that encourages the child to show that she can see how many fingers are being presented. Have the parent use a hand or a tissue as an occluder. By gradually increasing the distance between the examiner and the child by repeating the "game," a measure of acuity can be obtained for each eye. Obviously, finger mimicking at 20 ft is a gross measure, but it allows for a comparison of performance between eyes and a comparison of acuity from one visit to the next to help evaluate response to therapy.

Other preliterate acuity tests are available that require the child's development to be at a level of understanding the concept of "same" as with finger mimicking. One of the more commonly used tests of this type is the HOTV test. With this test, the child holds a card on which are printed four large letters: H, O, T, and V. The examiner holds an acuity chart that appears similar to the Snellen letter chart but has only the letters H, O, T, and V as optotypes. The chart is designed for testing at 10 ft; however, testing can begin at shorter distances while the child is learning the "game" of matching the letter to which the examiner is pointing with the same letter on his card. With this test, the child needs only to point to the correct letter on his card so that it is not necessary for him to know the letter, and he in fact does not need to speak at all. For this reason, the HOTV test and other similar tests are not only useful for preverbal children but such tests are useful for older children who are too shy or frightened to speak or for speech- and hearing-impaired children.

The goal of vision testing in this age group is not necessarily to demonstrate that the child can see 20/20 but rather to determine equality of vision. There should be more concern for the child who has 20/20 vision in one eye and 20/40 in the other eye than for the child who has 20/40 vision in both eyes.

When cooperation is poor, objective tests described earlier in this chapter can be applied to this age group. Once again, it is most important to determine whether the vision appears to be equal in both eyes.

■ Verbal Preliterate Children

There are a number of preliterate vision charts available for the pediatric population. Some, like the HOTV test described in the previous section, do not require a verbal response. Others require the child to name pictures. A number of studies have compared the reliability of various tests: however, it is beyond the scope of this chapter to review the literature on that subject. Instead, the focus will be on testing tech-

niques and techniques for maximizing cooperation and reliability when measuring acuity with the various tests commonly used in clinical practice.

To enhance attentiveness, it may be necessary to shorten the distance between the child and the test figures. This can easily be accomplished by using printed charts instead of projected charts. It might also be necessary to present the test target in an isolated format, such as with the Allen cards. Unfortunately, when amblyopia is present, visual acuity with isolated optotypes can be much better than linear acuity, sometimes to the degree that the diagnosis of amblyopia is missed when acuity measurement is obtained using isolated figures. Therefore, visual acuity assessment should progress to a linear format as soon as possible.

Probably the most widely used tests involve the identification of a picture. Allow a child to misname pictures. For example, if the child calls a duck a "dinosaur," it is not necessary to correct her as long as she is consistent throughout testing. With a sample of each picture photocopied together on a sheet of paper, the examiner can alternatively measure acuity by having a child match the test picture to a picture on the sheet the child is holding, similar to testing with the HOTV test described earlier in this chapter. This works well with the child who will not or cannot verbally interact with the examiner. The paper with the samples of pictures can also be given to parents to take home to teach the child the names of the pictures for subsequent visits.

When a child is first introduced to a picture chart, it is useful to allow the child to binocularly name the pictures on the largest three lines of the chart. This will give the examiner an opportunity to teach the child the names of the pictures or to learn the words that the child chooses to use to identify the pictures. Encourage the child with each answer, right or wrong. As the child becomes more comfortable with testing binocularly, gradually introduce occlusion. There are a number of methods for maintaining cooperation while occluding, but making it part of the "game" is often helpful, as is identifying occlusion as a form of assistance by saying "let me help you" as you occlude one eye. Encourage the child to guess when he says he cannot see it or it is too small. Testing of one or both eyes may need to be repeated later during the examination if cooperation and attention are lost.

Other common tests that do not require verbal interaction but are designed for the verbal preliterate age group are the E game and the Landolt rings. Testing requires that the child identify the direction of the open part of the E or ring. These tests are more difficult for children to perform and may only be applicable to older children. The child also tends to get bored more quickly with the E game format.

Although some children learn to identify numbers before the alphabet, they seem to have difficulty distinguishing numbers that appear similar and will often resort to guessing to alleviate frustration. Unless the child is very confident with identifying numbers, a picture chart may be preferable. The number and alphabet Snellen charts are more accurate than the picture chart.

It is important to always record which test was used to obtain acuity (Allen, numbers, letters, Es, Cs, or pictures) and how the test was performed (isolated, linear, or matching). It can also be useful to comment on level of cooperation and reliability as this can fluctuate from visit to visit and affect recorded acuity and interpretation of comparison of acuity.

As the child gets older, assessment of acuity will progress from isolated to linear figures and later from illiterate test figures to Snellen letters. Whenever a test or technique is changed, the acuity should also be measured with the previous technique or test to allow for a more accurate comparison of acuity from one visit to the next. For example, if a child was tested with linear Allen figures at the last visit and now has learned the alphabet, acuity should be measured with Snellen letters and with pictures. In deciding if there has been a change in the child's acuity, the picture acuities should be compared. At the next visit, only Snellen letter acuity need be tested as there will now be a previous Snellen letter acuity for comparison. Similarly, the examiner must take into consideration the level of cooperation of the child. With this information recorded at each visit, incorrect impressions regarding improvement or loss of vision can be minimized.

■ Occlusion Techniques

Occluding one eye is very often the most difficult maneuver in testing acuity in children. The occluder itself is often viewed as either threatening or more interesting than the fixation target or vision chart. In short, the occluder becomes a serious distraction.

The importance of adequate occlusion cannot be overstated. If the child is inadvertently allowed to peek, poor vision in one eye can go undetected, delaying treatment, potentially allowing a dense amblyopia to develop.

In place of the occluder the palm of the hand of the examiner, parent, or child may be used. If the fingers are used, there may be a small gap either between the fingers or between the fingers and bridge of the nose. If the eye being occluded is the stronger eye, the child will very easily find the gap and peek. It is advisable to place a tissue between the hand and the eye for added prevention of peeking.

The best method of occlusion, when tolerated, is an adhesive eye patch. This will allow the child to have more freedom of movement. The examiner can then observe the child for any abnormal head posturing that might be associated with dampening of nystagmus or compensation for ptosis.

When no form of occlusion is tolerated, test acuity binocularly. Certainly, obtaining a binocular acuity is better than obtaining none at all, and it will give the child practice with the testing procedure.

■ Visual Field Testing

Confrontation visual field testing is quite easy to perform with the pediatric patient. With the infant's or child's attention drawn to an object of interest in center gaze, a second object is slowly brought in toward the center from each of the peripheral four quadrants. Detection of the peripheral object is determined by watching the patient's direction of gaze. If the child consistently ignores the peripheral object in one or more quadrants, but consistently directs his/her gaze to the object in the other quadrants, a field defect may be present. The older child can be tested in the four quadrants with the finger counting or finger mimicking method. Some children can be tested on the Goldmann perimeter with the examiner constantly monitoring fixation, using a switch of fixation from the central target to the test target as a method of determining isopter thresholds. This, however, requires a great deal of patience and a fair amount of experience on the part of the examiner.

■ Answering Parents' Questions

Often, parents will have good questions regarding their child's vision. They may want to know why the vision is not 20/20. Because children develop 20/20 Snellen letter acuity in the 4- to 6-year age range, it is appropriate to say that 20/30 Allen vision is normal for 3-year-old children and that children do not develop 20/20 vision until they are older. When an acuity is not available, it helps to explain that, although we do not have a number to describe the child's acuity, all of the structures look normal and the behavior is normal, so the child's vision seems to be on track for his or her age. Similarly, one might explain to the parent of a child with a unilateral vision deficit that the child appears to have normal visual behavior with one eye but does not see well with the other. Although the terminology is simple, it is most often sufficient to satisfy the parents. If the child is globally developmentally delayed, one can explain that the vision may improve as the developmental delay improves. In answering questions, the ophthalmologist may be limited to placing the child's visual status into one of four categories: normal, abnormal, improving, and getting worse. By applying the techniques described in this chapter, categorizing the patient in such a way should be possible.

REFERENCES

1. Wagner RS. Pediatric eye examination. In: Nelson LB, ed. *Harley's Pediatric Ophthalmology*, 4th ed. Philadelphia: WB Saunders; 1998:82–96.
2. Day S. History, examination, and further investigation. In: Taylor D, ed. *Paediatric Ophthalmology*, 2nd ed. London: Blackwell Science; 1997:77–93.

Pediatric Ophthalmology
Edited by P. F. Gallin
Thieme Medical Publishers, Inc.
New York © 2000

3

∎∎∎

Practical Pediatric Refraction

RICHARD M. ROBB

Determining refractive errors in children nearly always requires an objective method of measurement. Subjective refractions prior to 10 years of age are unreliable. Although autorefractors are widely available and are commonly used for adult refractions, children have difficulty maintaining consistent central fixation in these instruments, and the measurements are therefore variable. Retinoscopy has been and remains the standard technique for pediatric refractions. It not only provides the desired information about the focus of the eyes but at the same time it allows the examiner to assess the clarity of the cornea and the lens and the quality of the fundus light reflex.

∎ Central Role of Retinoscopy

An important advantage of the retinoscope is that the light of the retinoscope can be directed toward the child's eye and can follow it when the child moves. Fortunately, most children, especially young infants, will look at the retinoscopic light without much prompting. Central fixation is critical for accurate retinoscopy.[1] This fact can quickly be appreciated by noting the change in the character of the retinoscopic reflex when the child looks away from the light. With central fixation the corneal reflex is centered in the pupil, except for small displacement due to variations

in the anatomic and visual axis, and the fovea is aligned with the retinoscopic beam. In cases of unsteady or eccentric retinal fixation in one eye, this eye can be more accurately refracted by allowing the preferred fellow eye to fix on a distant animated target (e.g., toy or video screen) while the examiner moves to a position from which the corneal reflex of the eccentrically fixing eye is centered in the pupil. In other cases of strabismus, with central and steady fixation in each eye, the eye not being refracted can be occluded by the examiner's hand or by an occluder in the trial frame while the fellow eye looks directly at the retinoscope (Fig. 3–1). Not only is it critical that retinoscopy be performed in the visual axis but it is also important to read the central portion of the retinoscopic reflex rather than the peripheral reflex, especially when the pupil has been dilated for refraction. The periphery of the reflex may be less hyperopic than the center, exhibiting an "against" movement while the central reflex is still a "with" movement. **The central reflex is the more accurate indicator of the true refractive error.**[2]

∎ Cycloplegia

Because the accommodative state of the eye can vary with any change of fixation or attention, cycloplegia is required for pediatric refractions.

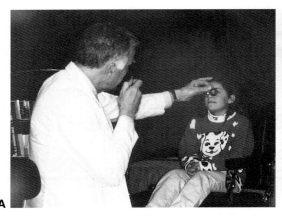 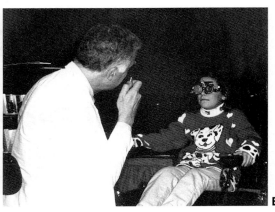

A   B

FIGURE 3–1. (A) Retinoscopy being performed on the left eye of a patient while the crossing right eye is occluded by the examiner's hand. **(B)** A trial frame with an occluder over one eye can also be used to assure central fixation of the fellow eye on the retinoscope.

Cycloplegia is also required for any refraction under anesthesia because anesthetic agents induce changes in the state of contraction of the pupil and ciliary body at various planes of anesthesia.[3] Cyclopentolate is an effective cycloplegic agent for most refractions.[4] Two drops of 1% solution in each eye is the usual dose. Stronger concentrations or more frequent applications have been associated with psychic effects, including convulsions. The drug requires approximately 30 minutes to achieve maximum cycloplegia. It is more rapidly effective in blue- rather than brown-eyed patients. One percent atropine ointment is an alternative agent and the standard by which other cycloplegics are measured. It is reliably effective in eyes of any pigmentation and will uncover from one third to one half diopter more hyperopia than cyclopentolate in hyperopic patients.[5] The major disadvantage of atropine is that it has a duration of action of up to 1 week. Tropicamide is effective as a mydriatic agent, but its cycloplegic action is weaker and shorter in duration than that of cyclopentolate.[6] **All pediatric patients who have an ophthalmic examination should have a cycloplegic examination with retinoscopy and indirect ophthalmoscopy. Anisometropes with attendant amblyopia are often diagnosed in this way, especially in preverbal children in whom a formal visual acuity cannot be obtained. Furthermore, the retina must be inspected for tumors and other anomalies. Partial lens opacities can also be uncovered by this technique.**

■ Advantage of Trial Frame and Hand-Held Lenses

Retinoscopic refractions of young children are best done with hand-held lenses. The spherical and cylindrical lenses can be directly superimposed, making it easy to compare meridians and to refine the axis of astigmatism and to standardize the distance between the vertex of the cornea and the posterior surface of the trial lens. Variations in this distance can significantly alter the spherical power required for neutralization when the ametropia is greater than plus or minus 4 diopters.[7] Retinoscopy can, of course, be performed with a phoropter, but positioning the very young pediatric patient behind a phoropter and maintaining this position is difficult. It is not surprising that most pediatric ophthalmology examining lanes do not include a phoropter as standard equipment.

■ Hyperopic Corrections

Straight-Eyed Hyperopes

When hyperopia is found in a patient whose eyes are straight and binocular, the decision to prescribe glasses depends on the amount of hyperopia and the age of the child. Infants under 1 year of age with 3 or 4 diopters of hyperopia are not generally enthusiastic about wearing glasses, whereas at 4 years they may find correction with glasses quite helpful. Hyperopia of 5 diopters or more is usually corrected whenever it is found, even if the patient is apparently asymptomatic.

Symptoms of reduced visual acuity or blurring in the near range are found only in older children, but when present they should prompt the prescription of a hyperopic correction. It is often theorized that an early glass correction for hyperopia will prevent the development of accommodative strabismus and amblyopia, but controlled trials have failed to show a clear difference in groups of patients managed without spectacles.[8] Rather large hyperopic errors found in the early months may diminish or disappear by 1 year of age, so watchful waiting and repeat refraction are appropriate management in this situation.[9]

On the other hand, hyperopia present after age 1 year may increase with age until approximately the end of the 7th year.[10] Beyond age 7 years, hyperopia usually stabilizes or begins to diminish. In the latter case, glass prescriptions must be reduced to avoid blurring at a distance. Straight-eyed hyperopes are usually corrected with something less than their full cycloplegic measurement. This is certainly true if atropine has been used for cycloplegia, but, even if cyclopentolate has been used, one half to one diopter of plus power can be cut when writing a prescription. **The same reduction should be made for both eyes**.

Hyperopia Associated with Partly or Fully Accommodative Esotropia

When hyperopia is associated with overt esotropia or even large esophoria, a full cycloplegic correction should be prescribed. There is no need to subtract power from a refraction done with cyclopentolate. This is a common error. Because, as mentioned previously, atropine cycloplegia uncovers on average one half diopter more hyperopia than cyclopentolate, one may choose to subtract this amount from the atropine refraction, but in many cases even the full atropine refraction can be given without a postcycloplegic overcorrection.

Esotropia may be caused by a wide range of hyperopic refractive errors.[11] When the amount of hyperopia is modest, there is usually a high

accommodative convergence to accommodation (AC/A) ratio, so even small corrections in the range of +1.50 to +2.00 diopters may afford a significant straightening effect. Larger amounts of hyperopia are usually associated with a normal AC/A ratio, and the straightening effect of glasses rests on the large amount of accommodation that is relieved.

It is advisable to repeat the cycloplegic refraction every 6 months because the hyperopia is often found to have changed in that interval, and the glasses may be accordingly changed in strength. If a patient is not compliant, refusing to wear the prescribed glasses, there are two choices. The first choice is to prescribe 1% atropine drops or ointment (bid × 1 day, then q hs × 1 week) to paralyze the accommodation. The glasses then become mandatory for the child to see clearly. As the atropine-induced cycloplegia wears off, the child will be accustomed to wearing the glasses and will be comfortable with them.

The second choice is to reduce the strength of the prescription slightly to ease the way to full-time wear. A second, more complete correction of the hyperopia is then given to eliminate fully the accommodative element of the deviation. This approach requires two sets of lenses.

In any event, it is wrong to discount the effect of glasses completely in a noncompliant patient and to proceed with strabismus surgery on the basis of the uncorrected angle of deviation. This often results in a variable postoperative deviation, and, when such patients finally tolerate glasses, the original surgery may have produced an overcorrection that requires reoperation. It is mandatory to delay surgery until glasses are worn full time to eliminate any accommodative element preoperatively and to have correct and reliable measurements.

Bifocals may be used to control a residual esotropia in the near range if the distant deviation is fully straightened by glasses. If there is a residual esotropia at a distance and a lack of binocularity, adding bifocals for the near deviation is an empty exercise. Some ophthalmologists prefer the executive type of bifocal extending the full width of the spectacle. The margin is usually placed high, at the lower edge of the undilated pupil (Fig. 3–2). The

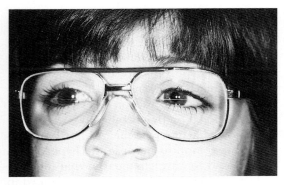

FIGURE 3–2. Flat top bifocal placed so that the upper margin of the bifocal is at the lower edge of the undilated pupil.

placement and type of bifocal must be stated on the prescription. An executive bifocal is often difficult to obtain in high powers in polycarbonate lenses. Other ophthalmologists prefer the option of a large flat top (29 mm) bifocal bisecting the pupil can be an acceptable substitute. Progressive bifocals are not very satisfactory for accommodative esotropia because of their weak correction in the upper region of the bifocal. The maximum bifocal strength is +3.50 diopters, but, for older children, whose working distance is beyond 33 cm, less strength is preferable. Bifocals of less than +2.00 diopters are ineffective and not worthwhile.

The choice of the exact bifocal add may be made by having the patient hold a fixation target at $\frac{1}{3}$ m on the examiner's nose. Successively +2.50, +3.00, +3.50 adds are placed in the trial from over the full cycloplegic retinoscopy. The associated esotropia measurement is noted. The add prescribed is the least amount of plus needed to give the smallest angle of esotropia.

It may be possible to reduce the strength of the hyperopic correction toward the end of the first decade while maintaining straight alignment, and, of course, this will have to be done if the hyperopia itself decreases. Bifocals are often eliminated in the teenage years, even if this results in occasional crossing in the near range. Spectacle corrections can be replaced with contact lenses in properly motivated patients with no loss of straightening effect. **It is not advisable or possible to substitute strabismus surgery for the effect of glasses or contact lenses at any age**.

Attempts to do so have ended with the finding that glasses continue to be required for satisfactory stable alignment.[12]

Hyperopic Anisometropia

Inequality of hyperopia in the two eyes of a patient presents some management difficulties. The less hyperopic eye is generally preferred for fixation. The more hyperopic eye may develop refractive amblyopia or may deviate, usually inward, adding strabismic amblyopia to the visual deficit. However, there can be some variation in this course. The anisometropia may disappear or even reverse in the early years, and it is not clear that early glass correction improves clinical outcome.[13] When amblyopia does develop in the more hyperopic eye, it is usually difficult to eliminate. Glasses should be prescribed, including the full cycloplegic correction if esotropia is present. A small and equal amount of plus power can be subtracted from each eye if the eyes are straight and binocular, thus reducing the risk of noncompliance with glass wear due to overcorrection. Occlusion or other amblyopic treatments of the less hyperopic eye are required for treatment of any amblyopia. The visual acuity is rarely equalized in this kind of anisometropia, but it can often be improved and stabilized in the more ametropic eye with persistent effort. Adult patients find the peripheral vision from the amblyopic eye very helpful.

■ Myopic Corrections

Symmetrical Myopia

When myopia is discovered in childhood, the first question is whether to prescribe glasses. The amount of myopia, the age, and whether the child is having difficulty seeing in everyday life are the factors to consider. More than 1.50 diopters of myopia in a school-aged child generally affects performance, but this would not be so in a child under 3 years of age. Myopia discovered on a routine preschool vision test or on a pediatrician's annual well-child examination may not be symptomatic in the child's usual daily activities. On the other hand, 0.50 diopters of myopia in a high school or college student may impede board work and warrant at least part time correction. **Uncorrected myopes may be unaware that it is possible to see clearly at a distance, and only when they have looked through corrective lenses do they realize the extent of their myopic blur.** Because myopia acquired toward the end of the first decade tends to increase with time, if the indications for glass wear are equivocal on initial examination, a repeat examination in 6 months or 1 year may reveal enough additional myopia to make prescription of glasses clearly useful. On the other hand, myopic errors found in the early years may actually decrease with time, **so repeat refractions are useful in virtually all patients.**

Performing the refraction of myopes under cycloplegia is usually advisable to guard against overaccommodation. The full cycloplegic correction can almost always be given in the initial prescription for a child, but overcorrections should be avoided. Bifocals are not generally necessary in myopic prescriptions. (If a child is already wearing a myopic prescription with bifocals to reduce the accommodative demand at near, it may be well to leave the bifocal in place until you are sure the patient will be comfortable without it.) Children accept myopic corrections with varying degrees of enthusiasm, and there is usually no reason to push glass wear beyond what they will accept as a means of seeing more clearly. On the other hand, wearing glasses does not need to be avoided for fear of inducing more myopia. There is no convincing evidence that wearing glasses speeds the progression of myopia beyond what would occur in time without glasses.

Myopic corrections have been used in patients with intermittent exotropia in the hope that they will allow better control of the deviation,[14] but they are not as effective in this regard as plus lenses are for patients with the combination of hyperopia and esotropia. Overcorrecting with minus lenses has occasionally been recommended to avoid an early operation, but animal studies showing the induction of refractive errors by deliberate optical defocus raise concerns about this practice.[15]

Contact lenses are an attractive option for some older children with myopia, usually beyond 11 or 12 years of age. The lenses can be fit earlier than this, but there is some advantage in waiting until the child can handle the lenses without parental involvement. Daily wear soft contact lenses are the type of lens most used in the United States at this time. Refractive surgery is not an option for children with myopia because their refractive state does not stabilize until after the childhood years (see Chapter 25 on use of lasers in pediatric ophthalmology).

Myopic Anisometropia

A difference in spherical equivalent of 1.50 to 2.00 diopters between the two eyes may be considered anisometropia. Mild myopic anisometropia in this range, however, is not usually associated with refractive amblyopia. In fact, if a patient has unilateral acquired myopia of this magnitude and the visual acuity is correctable to 20/20 in both eyes, glasses can be deferred. The more troublesome circumstance, and one not infrequently encountered, is a difference in the range of 6.00 or more diopters between the two eyes. If the eyes are straight, such anisometropia is often uncovered at 4 or 5 years of age on a routine vision screening exam, but it was presumably early in onset. The more myopic eye can be expected to have refractive amblyopia. Despite a full prescription correction, the vision in the highly myopic eye remains subnormal. Doctors Hubel and Weisel won the Nobel Prize in 1981 for detailed analysis of cortical changes in amblyopia. Patching of the better eye should be undertaken, but even with occlusion therapy the acuity of the more myopic eye frequently remains less than that of the fellow eye. Amblyopia therapy must be maintained until 9 years of age. Strabismus may be present before any treatment is started, or it may become apparent in the course of occlusion therapy. The presence of strabismus in addition to the myopic anisometropia is not a favorable sign for recovery of vision in the amblyopic eye. Spectacle correction of the anisometropia should not induce a difference in retinal image size (anisoconia) if the myopia is axial in origin,[16] but, as a practical matter, with such a large difference in strength between the two lenses, contact lenses may be more acceptable for correction than spectacles.

■ Astigmatism

Astigmatism with a minus cylinder axis at 90 degrees (against the rule) has more of an impact on visual acuity than that with an axis at 180 degrees (with the rule). Likewise, correction of astigmatism at 90 degrees is more likely to improve the visual acuity. Astigmatic errors can be fully corrected in children with their first glasses, whereas older individuals may require an incremental approach. Astigmatism in childhood is not ordinarily progressive, as is myopia, but it may change with growth. The early against-the-rule astigmatism of infancy is especially likely to improve with time, so repeated measurements are helpful.[17]

The astigmatism associated with corneal limbal dermoids and with hemangiomas of the eyelids has a characteristic orientation with respect to the location of these lesions and therefore can be anticipated. In older children increasing and irregular astigmatism may be a sign of keratoconus.

Large amounts of astigmatism are not easily corrected with contact lenses, although toric soft contact lenses are available and may be tried in older children.

■ Spectacles for Children

Light and durable glasses for children are obviously desirable. The frames for young children's glasses need to be small enough that the lenses can be centered on the visual axes, thereby avoiding prismatic effects. A frame with a built-up nasal bridge is also helpful for young infants, whose noses are characteristically flat. Lenses made of polycarbonate are routinely recommended for children because of their resistance

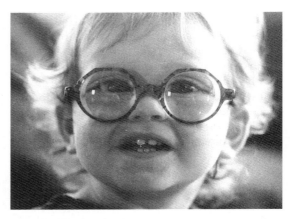

FIGURE 3–3. Lenticular lenses often fill most of a standard pediatric frame, as in this aphakic child, and they allow lens thickness to be reduced.

to breakage. These and any other lenses can be scratched with rough handling, and eventually they simply need to be replaced. Lenticular lenses will fill most of a standard pediatric frame (Fig. 3–3) and provide a convenient way to reduce the thickness of strong plus lenses, especially aphakic corrections.

Sunglasses are occasionally very helpful for children. Congenital achromatopsia is perhaps the most dramatic instance in which this is so. However, there are other children without identifiable eye disease who are bothered by bright sunlight. Some protection is afforded by wearing a cap with a visor. The use of clip-on sunglasses is another option if glasses are already worn, but they are difficult to obtain in small sizes. If either over-the-counter or prescription sunglasses are used, they should provide protection against ultraviolet light, a feature that does not affect the color or appearance of the lenses.

Finally, children who engage in activities in which the eyes might be struck with a ball or other object should use sports frames (Fig. 3–4). These frames are designed to withstand considerable force, and they hold the lenses securely so that they cannot be driven back onto the eyes (see Chapter 5). The American Academies of Ophthalmology and Pediatrics have formalized the recommendations for protective lenses in children in a position paper in *Pediatrics*[18].

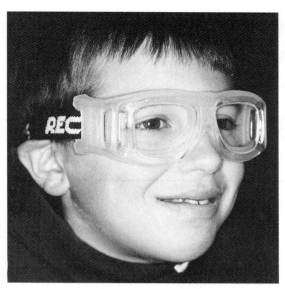

FIGURE 3–4. Sports frames with polycarbonate lenses should be used for children who engage in activities in which the eyes might be struck with a ball or other object.

REFERENCES

1. Copeland JC. The refraction of children with special reference to retinoscopy. In: Apt L, ed. *Diagnostic Procedures in Pediatric Ophthalmology.* Boston: Little,Brown; 1963:263–274.
2. Sloane AE. *Manual of Refraction.* Boston: Little, Brown; 1961;1:53.
3. Dripps RD, Eckenhoff JE, Vandam LD. *Introduction to Anesthesia: The Principles of Safe Practice.* 4th ed. Philadelphia: WB Saunders; 1972:203.
4. Gordon DM, Ehrenberg MH. Cyclopentolate HCl: a new mydriatic and cycloplegic agent, a pharmacologic and clinical evaluation. *Am J Ophthalmol.* 1954;38: 831–838.
5. Robb RM, Petersen RA. Cycloplegic refractions in children. *J Pediatr Ophthalmol.* 1968;5:110–114.
6. Beitel RJ. Cycloplegic Refraction. In: Tasman W, Jaeger EA, eds. *Duane's Clinical Ophthalmology.* Philadelphia: J.B. Lippincott; 1995;1:ch 41.
7. Ruben ML. *Optics for Clinicians.* 2nd ed. Gainesville, FL: Triad; 1974:143–145.
8. Ingram RM, Walker C, Wilson JM, et al. A first attempt to prevent amblyopia and squint by spectacle correction of abnormal refractions from age 1 year. *Br J Ophthalmol.* 1985;69:851–853.
9. Ingram RM, Barr A. Changes in refraction between the ages of 1 and 3 ½years. *Br J Ophthalmol.* 1979;63: 339–342.
10. Brown EVL. Net average yearly changes in refraction of atropinized eye from birth to beyond middle life. *Arch Ophthalmol.* 1938;19:719–734.
11. Parks MM. Abnormal accommodative convergence in squint. *Arch Ophthalmol.* 1958;59:364–380.
12. Albert DG, Lederman ME. Abnormal distance-near esotropia. *Doc Ophthalmol.* 1973;34:27–36.
13. Abrahamsson M, Fabian G, Sjostrand J. A longitudinal study of a population based sample of astigmatic children. II. The changeability of anisometropia. *Acta Ophthalmol.* 1990;68:435–440.
14. Von Noorden GK. *Binocular Vision and Ocular Motility.* 4th ed. St. Louis, MO: Mosby; 1990:331.
15. Hung L, Crawford MLJ, Smith EL. Spectacle lenses alter eye growth and the refractive status of young monkeys. *Nature Med.* 1995;1:761–765.
16. Ruben ML. *Optics for Clinicians.* 2nd ed. Gainesville, FL: Triad; 1974:212–214.
17. Dobcon V, Fulton AB, Sebris SL. Cycloplegic refractions of infants and young children: the axis of astigmatism. *Invest Ophthalmol Vis Sci.* 1984;25:83–87.
18. American Academy of Pediatrics Committee on Sports Medicine and Fitness, American Academy of Ophthalmology Committee on Eye Safety and Sports Ophthalmology. Protective eyewear for young athletes. *Pediatrics* 1996;98:311–313.

Pediatric Ophthalmology
Edited by P. F. Gallin
Thieme Medical Publishers, Inc.
New York © 2000

4

Amblyopia

PAMELA F. GALLIN

Amblyopia is defined as a two-Snellen line difference of acuity (best corrected) from one eye to another. According to Duke-Elder,[1] amblyopia is classified as

    I. Amblyopia ex anopsia (anterior segment)
    II. Congenital (organic; posterior segment)
    III. Strabismic amblyopia
    IV. Anisometropic amblyopia

Predominantly, strabismus and anisometropia (greater than a spherical equivalent of 1.5 diopters in general) are the most frequent causes of amblyopia. Structural anomalies contribute to amblyopia also.

In a nonstrabismic child it is difficult to diagnose amblyopia. In a preliterate child, amblyopia is often inferred from retinoscopy, fixation preference, and an intraocular examination. The determination of fixation preference in an infant is exceedingly difficult to assess, thus requiring judgment from an examiner schooled in assessment of vision in preliterate children.

When a child is able to read a Snellen chart of any type, one can appreciate the large or subtle differences of acuity. When the acuity differences become minimal, it is important that the second or nonseeing eye be evaluated on more than one occasion to determine that these are real lab data. Often children are less cooperative when their second eye is tested. Conversely, they are sometimes skittish when the first or initial eye is examined.

■ Etiology

The exact etiology of the amblyopia determines the treatment. In the case of structural problems, it is imperative that these anomalies such as a cataract be removed prior to the onset of the amblyopia treatment. In the case of strabismus, it is imperative that the amblyopia be resolved prior to any surgical procedures (with some exceptions). In the case of anisometropia, spectacle correction is necessary to ensure a focused image on the eye that has the greatest refractive error.

Our practical treatment of amblyopia is based on the work of Doctors Hubel and Wiesel, for which they won the Nobel Prize in 1981. Through their work with macaques and kittens they were able to determine that amblyopia is a structural change in the cerebral cortex at a microcellular level. These authors concluded that there is an initial window following birth at which time vision is formed in the occipital cortex in the absence of structural anomalies. If there is asymmetry in the presentation of a clear image to one retina, then on a cellular level the occipital cortex layers correlating with that eye become severely disorganized. If there is bilateral masking of the maculae and thus cerebral cortex, when this mask is removed, the vision in fact can turn on equally and at an excellent (but not perfect) level. When there is asymmetry in the vision beginning from birth and the occlusion is removed from one eye (lid unsutured), there can be reformatting on a microcellular basis of the occipital cells; however, this is never identical to the preferred eye but can yield excellent vision.[2–7]

There are numerous windows of time in the development of vision. The first window, which determines the onset of vision, is within days and weeks. This is the determining factor in the urgency of congenital cataract extraction. If the vision then goes unopposed for many structural, strabismus, or refractive etiologies, the poor vision will become entrenched within a few months' time. However, if there is a bilaterally symmetric obstacle such as those listed previously, then the vision in the cortical cells is "suppressed," and reorganization begins anew when the obstacle is reversed.

The amylogenic window for all children exists from birth to approximately 7.5 to 9 years of age. This end point is not crisp but is the clinically accepted end point at this time.

The basis for amblyopia treatment is to take away vision from the preferred eye and thus make the second eye (poorly seeing eye) work harder. Through the use of this added effort, the cells reorganize in the occipital cortex. This assumes a perfectly focused image on the macula of the poorly seeing eye.

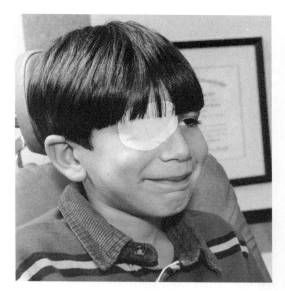

FIGURE 4–1. Occlusive patch on child.

■ Treatment

Classic (Occlusion)

The classic amblyopia therapy is that of an occlusive patch of which there are two types readily available in the United States, Elastoplast and Coverlet (Fig. 4–1). The initial treatment regimen is for full-time occlusion. This means that **the child wears the occluder on a full-time basis during waking hours except for 1 hour per day. The child is patched 1 week per year of life.** In the event that the child does not return for examination following this interval, the possibility of occlusion amblyopia occurs. Occlusion amblyopia is an amblyopia that develops in the previously preferred eye due to overpatching the preferred eye such that the poorly seeing eye then becomes the preferred eye. All patients undergoing occlusion therapy must be warned to remove the patch if they miss the follow-up visits. Full-time occlusion has numerous difficulties, most significantly including occlusion amblyopia and cooperation.

One of the many difficulties in patients who occlude full time is that functionally they cannot see the field in the patched eye. Children are forced to use a relatively nonseeing eye to fulfill their daily tasks. This is quite difficult for children and their families. In addition, at times, the adhesive from the patch can become quite irritating to the skin, thus requiring either cessation of patching or at times medical treatment to excoriated skin.

However, full-time occlusion in almost all amblyopia treatment is the initial treatment of choice. This treatment will yield the largest improvement in acuity in the smallest time interval due to the fact that the less preferred eye must be used to function on a full-time basis. **It is quite extraordinary that the occipital cortex is plastic up until the advanced age of at least $7\frac{1}{2}$ to 9 years of age.**

For example, a 6-month-old infant who has a fixation preference due to an esotropia will be patched only 3 days prior to the next visit for fear of an occlusion amblyopia. The fixation in young children is extraordinarily plastic such that fixation can change within hours, thus requiring short-term follow-up. A baby's visual demands are less significant than those of a 5-

year-old. Therefore, with the rapid increase in vision and the lower visual demands, a baby will become more comfortable with occlusion therapy in a relatively short interval than will a school-aged child who is learning to read and is subject to social comments (Fig. 4–2).

With all children, the initial phases of the amblyopia treatment are the most difficult. Parents need much support and cajoling to realize the effectiveness of this treatment. In the extreme, one can explain that, if the treatment is not followed, the child will be effectively a one-eyed patient and, in the event of an injury to the preferred eye, will not be able to function at the same level as they would with at least one eye with excellent vision.

Often, in the case of anisometropia, children are identified on 4-year-old or kindergarten vision screen examinations. Much to the horror of their parents, it is determined that the vision in one eye is in the range of 20/80 to 20/100 while the other eye is 20/20. The parents are quite concerned that this has never been brought to their attention and only on a recent vision screen. These children are difficult to treat and constitute the significant majority of amblyopes determined on incidental eye examinations. It is necessary for them to use the spectacle in the one eye, which often has either an oblique astigmatism or significant myopia or hyperopia relative to the eye for one time interval prior to the use of the occlusion therapy. At times this intermediate-level treatment can facilitate the reversal of amblyopia, thus delaying or eliminating the need for occlusion.

Often the patients have difficulty with occlusion therapy because they prefer to use their better-seeing eye. The children are quite vociferous in their protests against occlusion of their better eye. One trick is to instill atropine 1% drops into the preferred eye. Use of atropine 1% drops used twice a day for 1 or 2 days and then each night for 1 week has the effect of blurring the vision in the preferred eye such that the vision in the less preferred eye becomes relatively better. When children pull off the occluder, they cannot see well. This can be used to get the children to accept their spectacles and to accept the patch in the early and most difficult phases of treatment. Although it is a "dirty trick," it works and can be justified in comparison with a one-eyed patching failure.

Some physicians use occlusion therapy on a few-hours-per-day basis as an initial treatment regimen. This dosing is essentially ineffective. Either one provides full-time occlusion and achieves an excellent quality of vision with subsequent tapering or no patching should be undertaken. The exception to this can be seen in very young infants.

Bangerter Films

An alternative to full-time occlusion therapy, which, stated previously, is the preferred initial treatment of choice, is Bangerter films. These are plastic squares available in Switzerland where Dr. Bangerter first began using them in 1956 (Fig. 4–3).[8] These films are used essentially in anisometropes as they mount on a spectacle lens (Fig. 4–4). The Bangerter film functions to switch the fixation to the less preferred eye when the acuity hits a specific threshold (Fig. 4–5). Specifically, if a patient sees 20/20 in the right eye and 20/60 in the left eye, the right eye vision is blurred to two lines worse than 20/60 or, for example, 20/100.

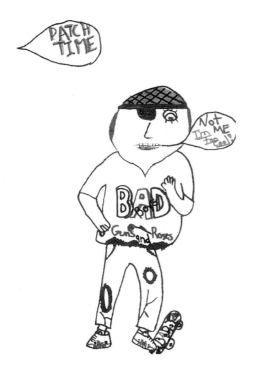

FIGURE 4–2. No patching.

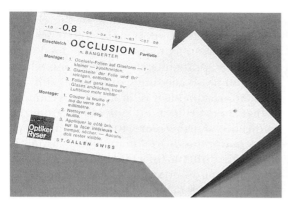

FIGURE 4–3. Bangerter film.

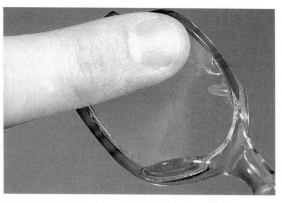

FIGURE 4–4. Bangerter film on spectacle.

A Bangerter film giving 20/100 vision is placed on the right eye. For a large target the child will see with both eyes. For smaller targets they will see with the left or less well seeing eye. Bangerter films come in nine densities, which occlude different levels of image clarity. As vision improves, the Bangerter film can be weakened such that more light gets into the eye. Ultimately, if the child is 20/20 in the preferred eye and 20/30 in the now poorly seeing eye, the preferred eye can be blurred to a level of 20/60.

Bangerter films are excellent with middle-range visions and for maintenance until 9 years of age, when an excellent acuity has been procured.

Bangerter films are available in intensities of 0.9, 0.8, 0.7, 0.6, down to less than 0.1.

Bangerter films are an excellent adjunct in the treatment of amblyopia. School-aged chil-

dren often prefer these films as their vision is improving. First, they can see from both eyes for large targets. Second, it is cosmetically acceptable. School-aged children can be quite brutal when a child wears the patch, and Bangerter films are not cosmetically objectionable. Most children do not notice that their colleague is wearing one. Third, as the vision improves, the Bangerter film can be downwardly titrated. Fourth, when the child has achieved a final vision in the amblyopic eye, a very mild Bangerter film can be used to tip the balance in favor of the preferred eye, when looking at very fine targets.

Optical Penalization

Optical penalization is a pharmacologic or optical blur to the preferred eye.

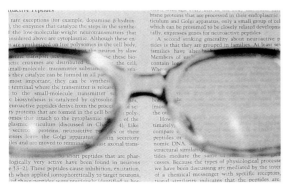

FIGURE 4–5. Blurred vision through right lens with Bangerter film and fixation switch to left "other" eye.

Pharmacologic

In Europe, a pharmacologic blur through the use of atropine 1% drops in the preferred eye is used frequently. This allows the preferred eye to see clearly only at near and the amblyopic eye to see at both distance and near with and without spectacle correction. The frequency of visits can be diminished and the intervals enlarged as the treated eye is not subject to an occlusion amblyopia to the same degree as with a full-time patch. This can be very useful in preverbal children who are resistant to occlusion therapy. It is quite wonderful as an adjunct to spectacles or occlusion.

Optical

Another type of optical penalization was described by Dr. David Guyton et al.[9] Optical penalization was created to use an optical blur in the preferred eye to switch fixation to the less preferred or second eye. Specifically, using the American Optical Vectographic Stereopsis slide, the cycloplegic refraction is placed in a trial frame over which Polaroid glasses are placed. Beginning with approximately +1.50 diopters at +0.25-diopter intervals, the lenses are added to the preferred eye until the fixation as determined by the vectographic slide is switched to the other eye (Fig. 4–6). This is then prescribed to the patient.

By using the spectacles, the patient uses the less preferred eye for distance and the preferred eye for near. Again, there is less of a chance of occlusion amblyopia, and the patient can tolerate these well. This is tolerated on a cosmetic basis by school-aged children without difficulty and is comfortable for them.

All of the penalization treatments follow a period of initial occlusion. They are most effective when the acuity is in the 20/80 or better range. All of these techniques require great understanding of the dynamics of the specific child–parent interaction. Some parents do not want a patch, and other parents do not want a pharmacologic treatment. It is quite important to discuss the need for amblyopia treatment with the parents and have the child begin adjusting the acuity early on. When the child is older, it is important to provide choices as to which modality the child would prefer as this often changes over the course of the child's development. It is important to remember that amblyopia treatment must be maintained until the child is approximately 9 years of age, which is, of course, exceedingly difficult as this is a constant treatment. It is an invisible treatment in that there are not any side effects from the medication. Furthermore, the treatment needs to be maintained over many years, which is extremely difficult for children. Giving them the option of different treatment modalities at different times makes it more acceptable to them.

The goal is vision of 20/20 in the amblyopic eye. Even when a child achieves a vision of 20/20, on direct questioning they may say that it is less preferable to the better eye. This is due to the fact that, on a microcellular basis, the cellular reorganization is not identical to the preferred eye.

■ Patching Failures

Many children are "patching failures" (Fig. 4–7). This occurs due to the difficulty of having a child of any age function with a poorly seeing eye. In Army induction studies in the United Kingdom[10] and Viet Nam,[11] approximately 2 to 7%[7] of their incoming healthy 18-year-old men had difficulty seeing. Amblyopia is a silent disease.

FIGURE 4–6. American Optical Vectographic Projection slide.

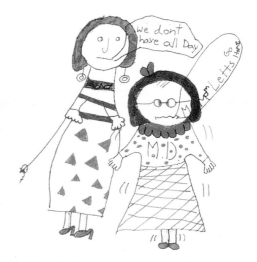

FIGURE 4–7. "I don't want to patch!"

In terms of patching failures, many parents find it difficult to begin any type of amblyopia treatment of school-aged children due to the difficulty functioning in school with a poorly seeing eye. Often, the occlusion therapy begins at a time that children are learning to read. They have enough difficulty seeing the blackboard and text with their preferred eye without the added difficulty of a nonseeing eye. Children should be given front row seats and be placed in an optimal position (without patch) for standardized testing. The teachers should be informed so that they understand their important role in this process. Their encouragement and participation in this process often help determine the outcome in school-aged children.

There are children who have a net difference of more than 7 to 8 diopters of spherical equivalent. In these children we know that it is quite rare for them, even in an optimal situation, to develop excellent acuity in this most often myopic eye. An attempt should be made to improve the acuity of all children and with great detailed explanation to the parents. However, the specific etiology of the amblyopia directly affects our realistic expectations and counseling of parents.

If, after many months, a child is unresponsive to occlusion therapy and a parent chooses to stop the treatment, it is important that a parent and a witness sign the chart, recording that there was a discussion between parent and physician as to the desired treatment, that the treatment was unable to be complied with, and that the parents understand the consequences of treatment cessation.

In the event that an examiner is treating a child for amblyopia and there is no change in the acuity despite the cooperation of the family, the examiner should rethink the diagnosis and at times consider a neurological examination in conjunction with a retinal specialist examination. An electroretinogram (ERG) and/or visual evoked potential in conjunction with other neuroradiologic testing, if deemed appropriate, might determine the presence of subnormal retinal functioning; a difficulty in the cortical region assumes a grossly normal intraocular examination and the absence of a refractive basis for the amblyopia. Visually significant oblique astigmatisms are often difficult to ascertain and are noted on repeat retinoscopy. Autorefraction can be very helpful in finding small yet significant oblique astigmatisms (Fig. 4–8).

■ Conclusion

Amblyopia forms the basis for many pediatric ophthalmic clinical diseases and the subsequent

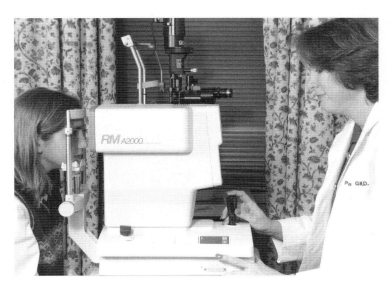

FIGURE 4–8. Autorefractor to help determine astigmatism.

visual rehabilitation. However, the treatment can be exceedingly daunting. Both parents and children need a great deal of moral support and cajoling. Often types of amblyopia treatment must be substituted to gain the compliance of these children.

REFERENCES

Doctors D.H. Hubel and T.N. Wiesel wrote multiple articles about their work in the *Journal of Physiology* between approximately 1959 and the early 1980s. For this work they won the Nobel Prize in medicine in 1981.

1. Duke-Elder S. *System of Ophthalmology*. St. Louis, MO: Mosby, 1958.
2. Wiesel TN, Hubel DH. Single-cell responses in striate cortex kittens deprived of vision in one eye. *J Neurophysiol*. 1963;26:1003–1017.
3. Hubel DH, Wiesel TN. Effects of mononuclear deprivation in kittens. *Arch exp Pharmak*. 1964;248:492–497.
4. Wiesel TN, Hubel DH. Comparison of the effects of unilateral and bilateral eye closure on cortical unit responses in kittens. *J Neurophysiol*. 1965;28:1029–1040.
5. Hubel DH, Wiesel TN. The period of susceptibility to the physiological effects of unilateral eye closure in kittens. *J Physiol*. 1970;206:419–436.
6. Dews PB, Wiesel TN. Consequences of monocular deprivation on visual behavior in kittens. *J Physiol*. 1970;206:436–455.
7. Hubel DH, Wiesel TN. Integrative action in the cat's lateral geniculate body. *J Physiol*. 1961;155:385–398.
8. Bangerter A. "Moderne Schelhandlung" Ther Umschau, Bern. 1957;14(1):8.
9. Repka MX, Gallin P, Scholz RT, Guyton DL. Determination of optical penalization by vectographic fixation reversal. *Ophtha*. 1985;92(11):1584–1586.
10. Aldestein AM, Scully J. Epidemiological aspects of squint. *Br Med J*. 1967;3:34–8.
11. Downing AA. Ocular defects in sixty thousand selectees. Medical Corps, Army of the United States, *Arch Ophtha*. February 1945; 33:137.

Pediatric Ophthalmology
Edited by P. F. Gallin
Thieme Medical Publishers, Inc.
New York © 2000

5

Prevention

LOUIS PIZZARELLO

Trauma remains among the three leading causes of unilateral blindness and vision loss in children.[1-3] **In particular, for children over 7 years of age, trauma is by far the leading cause of monocular vision loss**. If even half of these injuries were prevented, the savings in human suffering, medical costs, and shattered lives would be enormous. They would eclipse any gains that would be made from the eradication of retinoblastoma, congenital glaucoma, and rhabdomyosarcoma. No ophthalmologist will be able to claim the credit from such stupendous scientific advances, yet any ophthalmologist can assist in reducing the incidence of eye injury. Eye safety is the careful application of a few principles to the care of every child. It consists of a message for children, parents, teachers, and civic leaders. The message is simple, the execution complex, but the results are rewarding for patient and practitioner.

■ Epidemiology of Pediatric Eye Injury

There are 2.4 million eye injuries in the United States each year.[4] Ten percent of these—240,000—occur in children under 18. Annually, this means that *one in every 250 children will sustain an eye injury*. Several studies have described the nature and causes of these injuries. The setting is typically in the home for children under 5. A small number of eye injuries in this younger age group occurs as a result of automobile accidents. Children between 6 and 18 suffer about half the injuries at home, one quarter at school, one fifth in sports and recreation, and the remainder in miscellaneous settings.

Fortunately, most of the injuries are not vision threatening. They are superficial and heal rapidly, without sequelae. However, **it is estimated that 5%—or 14,000 injuries—are potentially blinding injuries.**[5] The goal of eye safety is to prevent these injuries. It has been proven that **up to 90% of such injuries can be prevented** with an effective safety program, meaning that **12,000 eyes can be saved each year.**

■ Eye Safety

The basic principle of eye safety is the use of appropriate, well-fitted, protective eyewear. The ophthalmologist can have little control over risk-taking behavior, but the use of protective eyewear can succeed in guarding the child from injury. This requires the ophthalmologist to have an understanding of the special needs that arise in prescribing such protective equipment for pediatric patients.

TABLE 5–1. Types of Lens Materials

Material	Strength (ft lb.)[7]	Advantages	Disadvantages
Heat-treated glass	1.03	Scratch resistant Widely available	Heaviest material Thickest lenses
Allyl resin	0.20	Lightweight Widely available	Scratches Poor safety performance
Polycarbonate	4.25	Thinnest, lightest material Strongest available	Can scratch Not available in all powers Difficult to fabricate

Fashion or dress eyewear comes in one of three materials: heat-treated glass, allyl resin (one brand called CR-39, a trademark of PPG industries), and polycarbonate. Each has advantages and disadvantages described in Table 5–1. In relation to trauma, the ability of the lens to withstand a blow without fracturing is crucial. This strength is measured by dropping a metal ball of fixed weight from varying heights until the lens fails. This is called the drop ball test, and the U.S. Food and Drug Administration (FDA) mandates that dress eyewear withstand up to 0.15 foot pounds of energy before fracturing. To give some sense of the magnitude of force involved, a tennis ball would strike the eye with at least 30 foot pounds of force. The lenses that are ground for street wear usually have a thickness at the center of 2 mm. By comparison, industrial safety lenses usually have a center thickness of 3 mm.

There is no question that polycarbonate lenses can withstand most blows and missiles, even a .22 caliber bullet. However, the use of polycarbonate in street eyewear for children on a routine basis is problematic, given its ease of scratching. Both heat-treated glass and allyl resin exceed the FDA standards for dress eyewear. When used appropriately, they will protect the eye from very low-velocity objects but are totally inappropriate in settings where the eye will be exposed to forces in excess of their fracture strength. **Any time there is need to protect the eye in specific high-risk circumstances, it is mandatory that polycarbonate be prescribed.** The practitioner who fails to indicate this on a lens prescription for those children who will be exposed to these risks can be successfully sued by the patient. In particular this is the case for one-eyed children, whose situation

will be described subsequently. In general, the community standard in most areas is to prescribe one of the three lens materials, unless extenuating circumstances are noted.

■ Sport Safety Eyewear

Children enjoy playing a range of sports in both organized and unsupervised leagues. Their frequent risk-taking behavior and athletic immaturity can expose them to even higher risks of injury than those seen in adults. Each sport is unique as to the risk of eye injury, and the necessary protective measures that should be taken. Table 5–2 lists the major sports by risk of injury and appropriate safety eyewear.

The use of eye protection can have a dramatic impact on the reduction of injuries. In Canada, a program to mandate face protection led to the complete elimination of blinding eye injuries.[6] This program was the creation of a group of dedicated ophthalmologists who worked with junior hockey leagues to require such equipment. The Hockey Eye Certification Council was formed to assure that equipment would continue to adhere to the standard. This program serves as a model of what can be accomplished in reduction of eye injuries.

■ School

Children and adolescents spend many hours in school. Risk of injury is particularly great during physical activity and laboratory work. Every lab is required to provide safety eyewear and instruction in its proper use. Goggles are the usual protection used because they can be

TABLE 5–2. Risk Factors and Protective Gear for Various Sports

Sport	Recommended Protector	Relative Risk Factor 1 (low); 10 (high)
Auto Racing	Helmet with separate eye protector	10
Baseball (catcher, umpire)	Full-face protector	7
Baseball (fielders)	Sports eye protector[a]	7
Baseball (hitters)	Helmet with face protector	7
Basketball	Sports eye protector	7
Boxing	Helmet only	10
Cycling	Helmet with separate eye protector	3
Fencing	Full-face protector	1
Fishing	Eye glasses	1
Football	Total head protector	5
Hockey	Certified face protector	10
Horseback riding/polo	Helmet with separate eye protector	5
Lacrosse (men's)	Total head protector	10
Lacrosse (women's)	Sport eye protector	10
Racquetball/squash	Sport eye protector, class II or III[b]	9
Ski racing	Helmet with separate eye protector	3
Snowmobiling	Helmet with separate eye protector	3
Soccer	Sport eye protector	3
Softball	Sport eye protector	7
Swimming	Tight-fitting goggles	1
Tennis	Sport eye protector	7
Water polo	Tight-fitting goggles	9

[a] Protective eyewear with strong frames comparable to ANSI Z87 industrial standards with polycarbonate lenses.
[b] Protective eyewear with wraparound frame design, which meets ASTM F803 for racquet sports.
Source: Adapted from Ellis GS in *Sports Ophthalmology.* Springfield, IL: Charles C Thomas; 1987.

worn over glasses as well as by children who do not wear glasses. The lenses are made of polycarbonate, and side shields guard against particulate and liquid matter. In sports, the appropriate safety eyewear should be required for all athletes.

■ Some Special Circumstances

Remember that contact lenses do not offer any protection for the eye. Children who wear them should wear safety glasses or goggles over them when exposed to increased risk. The same holds true for any children who may have had refractive surgery. Sunglasses are usually made of heat-treated glass or allyl resin and so have very limited fracture strength. There is a sunglass standard issued by the American National Standards Institute (ANSI Z80). This mandates the degree of transmittance that is acceptable. However, there is no standard for sunglasses to be used in sports. It is recommended that the frame used meets the standard set for industrial use (ANSI Z87) with lenses that transmit less than 1% of UVB and UVA less than 400 nm. Cost of sunglasses will not guarantee that they will meet these standards.

■ The One-Eyed Patient

Although all children must be protected from eye trauma, those with one functioning eye need particular protection. The definition of a poorly functioning eye is vision corrected to less than 20/40. This was chosen because many states deny driving licenses to those with worse vision.

The American Academies of Ophthalmology and Pediatrics have issued a joint statement for these children, which appears in Appendix 5–1.

■ Conclusions

Knowledge of eye safety is important for any practitioner who treats children. A common-sense approach that emphasizes appropriate protective eyewear for the needs of each patient can have potentially dramatic effects. Unique circumstances require specific care, such as for the one-eyed child or the specific athlete.

REFERENCES

1. Nelson LB, Wilson TW, Jeffers JB. Eye injuries in childhood: demography, etiology and prevention. *Pediatrics.* 1989;84:438–441.
2. Grin TB, Nelson LB, Jeffers, JB. Eye injuries in childhood. *Pediatrics.* 1987;80:13–17.
3. Prevent Blindness America. *1993 Sports and Recreational Eye Injuries.* Schaumburg, IL: Prevent Blindness America; 1994.
4. National Society to Prevent Blindness. Fact Sheet. New York: National Society to Prevent Blindness; 1978.
5. Schein OD, Hibberd PL, Shingleton BJ. The spectrum and burden of ocular injury. *Ophthalmol.* 1988;95:300–305.
6. Pashby TJ. Eye injuries in hockey. *Int Ophthalmol Clin.* 1981;21:41.

Pediatric Ophthalmology
Edited by P. F. Gallin
Thieme Medical Publishers, Inc.
New York © 2000

Appendix 5–1

■ ■ ■

Protective Eyewear for Young Athletes

AMERICAN ACADEMY OF PEDIATRICS COMMITTEE ON SPORTS MEDICINE AND FITNESS AND AMERICAN ACADEMY OF OPHTHALMOLOGY COMMITTEE ON EYE SAFETY AND SPORTS OPHTHALMOLOGY

The American Academy of Pediatrics and the American Academy of Ophthalmology recommend mandatory protective eyewear for all functionally one-eyed individuals and for athletes who have had eye surgery or trauma and whose ophthalmologists recommend eye protection. Protective eyewear is also strongly recommended for all other athletes.

■ Background

More than 41,000 sports-related and recreational eye injuries were treated in hospital emergency departments in 1993.[1] Seventy-one percent of the injuries occurred in individuals younger than 25 years; 41% occurred in individuals younger than 15 years; and 6% occurred in children younger than 5 years. Children and adolescents are particularly susceptible to injuries because of their fearless manner of play and their athletic immaturity.[2–4]

Ten sports or sports groupings are highlighted in this statement based on their popularity and the high incidence of eye injuries (see Table A–1).[1] Baseball and basketball are associated with the most eye injuries in athletes 5 to 24 years old.[5] Participation rates and information on the severity of the injuries are unavailable, however; therefore, the relative risk of significant injuries cannot be determined for various sports.

The high frequency of sports-related eye injuries in young athletes indicates the need for an awareness among athletes and their parents of the risks of participation and of the availability of a variety of approved sports eye protectors. When properly fitted, appropriate eye protectors have been found to reduce the risk of significant eye injury by at least 90%.[4,6,7]

■ Evaluation

It would be ideal if all children and adolescents wore appropriate eye protection for all sports and recreational activities. All youth involved in organized sports should be encouraged to wear appropriate eye protection.

Physicians must strongly recommend that athletes who are functionally one eyed wear appropriate eye protection during all sports and recreational activities. (Functionally one-eyed athletes are those with a best-corrected visual acuity of worse than 20/40 in the poorer-seeing eye, assuming that adequate amblyopia [lazy eye] therapy has been accomplished.)[4,5,8]

If the better eye is severely injured, functionally monocular athletes will be severely handicapped. In many states, they cannot obtain driver's licenses.[9]

Athletes who have had eye surgery or trauma to the eye may have weakened eye tissue that is more susceptible to injury.[10] These athletes may need eye protection and should be evaluated and counseled by an ophthalmologist.

TABLE A–1. Estimated Sports and Recreational Eye Injuries 1993[a]

Sport/Recreation Activity	Estimated Injuries	Age Group (y)		
		< 5	5–14	15–24
Basketball	8521	112	2241	3413
Baseball	6136	363	3150	1407
Swimming and pool sports	3439	43	1608	729
Racquet and court sports	3183	34	668	1064
Football	2197	0	1097	998
Ball sports (unspecified)	1749	194	743	320
Soccer	1319	0	731	365
Golf	969	43	486	112
Hockey (all types)	946	19	342	515
Volleyball	821	0	180	263
Total selected sports	29,280	808	11,246	9186
Other sports and recreational activities	11,751	1457	3483	2977
Total	41,031	2265	14,729	12,163

[a] Reprinted with permission from Prevent Blindness America (formerly National Society to Prevent Blindness), *1993 Sports and Recreational Eye Injuries.*[1]

Various kinds of eye protection are described below and in the glossary. Different brands of sports goggles vary significantly in the way they fit. An experienced ophthalmologist, optometrist, or optician can help an athlete select appropriate goggles that fit well.

Indigent athletes may have trouble affording eye evaluations or protective eyewear. Sports programs may have to assist these athletes in the evaluation process and in obtaining protective eyewear.

■ Recommendations

To implement the policy, we recommend the following specific interventions:

1. Appropriate protective eyewear for low–eye risk sports (see Table A–2) consists of an approved streetwear frame that meets American National Standards Institute (ANSI) standard Z87.1 with polycarbonate or CR-39 lenses. A strap must secure the frame to the head. These glasses must be fitted by an experienced ophthalmologist, optometrist, or optician.

2. Appropriate protective eyewear for high–eye risk sports is itemized in Table A–2. The sports goggles must have lenses made of polycarbonate, which is stronger than CR-39 plastic. An experienced ophthalmologist, optometrist, or optician must fit these goggles.

Because some children have narrow facial features, they may be unable to wear even the smallest sports goggles. These children must be fitted with approved streetwear frames described for low–eye risk sports.

Athletes with a high range of refractive error cannot use lenses made of polycarbonate. They may wear contact lenses (high power) protected by sports goggles with polycarbonate plano (nonprescription) lenses.

For sports in which face masks or helmets with eye protectors or shields must be worn, we strongly recommend that functionally one-eyed athletes also wear sports goggles with polycarbonate lenses to ensure protection. The helmet must fit properly and have a chin strap for optimal protection.

3. Contact lenses offer no protection; therefore, we strongly recommend that athletes who wear contact lenses also wear appropriate polycarbonate eye protection over the lenses. Polycarbonate (plano) nonprescription lenses should be used in streetwear frames for low–eye risk sports or in sports goggles for high–eye risk sports.

4. Athletes must replace sports eye protectors that are damaged or yellowed with age because they may have become weakened.

5. Functionally one-eyed athletes and those who have had eye injuries or surgery must not participate in boxing, wrestling, and full-contact martial arts. Eye protection is

TABLE A–2. Sports with Risk of Eye Injury with Appropriate Eye Protectors

Sport	Eye Protection[a]
Badminton	Sports goggles with polycarbonate lenses
Baseball	Polycarbonate face guard or other certified safe protection attached to helmet for batting and base running; sports goggles with polycarbonate lenses for fielding
Basketball	Sports goggles with polycarbonate lenses
Bicycling (LER)[b]	Sturdy streetwear frames with polycarbonate or CR-39 lenses
Boxing	None is available
Fencing	Full face cage
Field hockey (both sexes)	Goalie, full face mask; all others, sports goggles with polycarbonate lenses
Football	Polycarbonate shield on helmet
Full-contact martial arts	Not allowed
Handball[c]	Sports goggles with polycarbonate lenses
Ice hockey	Helmet and full face protection
Lacrosse (male)	Helmet and full face protection required
Lacrosse (female)	Should at least wear sports goggles with polycarbonate lenses and have option to wear helmet and full face protection
Racquetball[c]	Sports goggles with polycarbonate lenses
Soccer	Sports goggles with polycarbonate lenses
Softball	Polycarbonate face guard or other certified safe protection attached to helmet for batting and base running; sports goggles with polycarbonate lenses for fielding
Squash[c]	Sports goggles with polycarbonate lenses
Street hockey	Sports goggles with polycarbonate lenses; goalie, full face cage[d]
Swimming and pool sports	Swim goggles recommended
Tennis, doubles	Sports goggles with polycarbonate lenses
Tennis, singles	Sturdy streetwear frames with polycarbonate lenses
Track and field (LER)	Sturdy streetwear frames with polycarbonate or CR-39 lenses
Water polo	Swim goggles with polycarbonate lenses
Wrestling	None is available

[a] For sports in which face masks or helmets with eye protection are worn, functionally one-eyed athletes and those with previous eye trauma or surgery for whom their ophthalmologists recommend eye protection must also wear sports goggles with polycarbonate lenses to ensure protection.
[b] LER indicates low eye risk.
[c] Goggles without lenses are not effective.
[d] A street hockey ball can penetrate into a molded goalie mask and injure an eye.

not practical in boxing or wrestling and is not allowed in martial arts.

COMMITTEE ON SPORTS MEDICINE AND
  FITNESS, 1995 TO 1996
William L. Risser, MD, PhD, Chair
Steven J. Anderson, MD
Stephen P. Bolduc, MD
Elizabeth Coryllos, MD
Bernard Griesemer, MD
Larry McLain, MD
Suzanne M. Tanner, MD

LIAISON REPRESENTATIVES
Kathryn Keely, MD
  Canadian Paediatric Society
Richard Malacrea, ATC
  National Athletic Trainers Association
Judith C. Young, PhD
  National Association for Sport and
  Physical Education

AAP SECTION LIAISON
Reginald L. Washington, MD
  Section on Cardiology

CONSULTANTS
Oded Bar-Or, MD
Jack Jeffers, MD
Rainer Martens, PhD
Michael Nelson, MD

AMERICAN ACADEMY
  OF OPHTHALMOLOGY
Committee on Eye Safety and Sports
  Ophthalmology
John Jeffers, MD Chair
M. Bowes Hamill, MD
Francis G. La Piana, MD
Monica L. Monica, MD
John O'Neill, MD
William G. Squires, MD
C. Douglas Witherspoon, MD

GLOSSARY

CR-39 lenses. Lenses made of an allyl–resin plastic (CR-39 is a registered trademark of PPC Industrial) with a center thickness of 3 mm that meet or exceed ANSI standard Z87.1. They are used for strong prescriptions (above − 8.00 sphere and − 4.00 cylinder) for which polycarbonate is not suitable. Lenses made from this plastic are not as strong as those made with polycarbonate and should not be used in sports goggles for high–eye risk sports.

Polycarbonate lenses. Prescription or nonprescription lenses made of polycarbonate material with a center thickness of at least 2 mm that meet or exceed ANSI standard Z87.1. These are designed to fit in streetwear frames as well as sports goggles.

Polycarbonate shields and face guards. Molded protective shields and face guards designed to be a part of, or to be attached to, various sports helmets.

Sports goggles. Unhinged protective eyewear with a molded frame and temple with prescription or nonprescription polycarbonate lenses with a center thickness of 3 mm. An elastic band secures the goggles to the athlete's head.

Streetwear frames. Sturdy daily wear frames with a posterior lip to prevent inward displacement of the lenses. They should meet ANSI standard Z87.1.

RESOURCES

American Academy of Ophthalmology, Department ESC, Attention: Inquiry Clerk, PO Box 7424, San Francisco, CA 94120-7424 (*Eye Safety for Children* brochure, include a self-addressed, stamped, legal-size envelope with each request); and Prevent Blindness America (formerly National Society to Prevent Blindness), 500 E Remington Rd, Schaumburg, IL 60173.

Standards: American National Standards Institute, 11 West 42nd St, New York, NY 10036 (Practice for Occupational and Educational Eye Face Protection [ANSI standard Z87.1]); American Society for Testing and Materials, 100 Barr Harbour Dr, West Conshohoken, PA 19428 (Face Guards for Youth [ASTM standard F910-86] and Specifications for Eye Protectors for Use by Players of Racquet Sports [ASTM standard F803-88]; and American Hockey Association of the United States, Canadian Amateur Hockey Association, and Canadian Standards Association (Hockey Helmets and Face Guards).

REFERENCES

1. Prevent Blindness America. *1993 Sports and Recreational Eye Injuries.* Schaumburg, IL: Prevent Blindness America; 1994.
2. Nelson LB, Wilson TW, Jeffers JB. Eye injuries in childhood: demography, etiology, and prevention. *Pediatrics.* 1989;84:438–441.
3. Grin TR, Nelson LB, Jeffers JB. Eye injuries in childhood. *Pediatrics.* 1987;80:13–17.
4. Jeffers JB. An on-going tragedy: pediatric sports-related eye injuries. *Semin Ophthalmol.* 1990;5:216–223.
5. Erie JC. Eye injuries: prevention, evaluation, and treatment. *Phys Sports Med.* 1991;19:108–122.
6. Larrison WI, Hersh PS, Kunzweiler T, Shingleton BJ. Sport-related ocular trauma. *Ophthalmology.* 1990;97:1265–1269.
7. Strahlman E, Sommer A. The epidemiology of sports-related ocular trauma. *Int Ophthalmol Clin.* 1988;28:199–202.
8. Wichmann S, Martin DR. Single-organ patients: balancing sports with safety. *Phys Sports Med.* 1992;20(2):176–182.
9. Federal Highway Administration. *Manual on Uniform Traffic Control Devices for Streets and Highways*, Washington, DC: Department of Transportation; 1988.
10. Vinger PF. The eye and sports medicine. In: Tasman W, ed. *Duane's Clinical Ophthalmology.* 1994;5:chap 45.

Pediatric Ophthalmology
Edited by P. F. Gallin
Thieme Medical Publishers, Inc.
New York © 2000

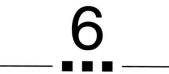

Learning Disabilities

DAREL M. BENAIM

I felt a cleavage in my head
As if my brain had split;
I tried to match it, seam by seam,
But could not make them fit.

The thought behind I strove to join
Unto the thought before,
But sequence ravelled out of reach,
Like balls upon the floor.

Emily Dickinson

We have all been intrigued by stories of great men and women throughout history who have overcome learning disabilities (LDs). Albert Einstein, Edgar Allen Poe, George Bernard Shaw, and Salvador Dali were expelled from school. Abe Lincoln, Thomas Edison, and Henry Ford were assumed to have limited promise by their teachers. What is the nature of this problem of the mind that produces individuals who may present at once as brilliant and quite the opposite? This chapter is intended to provide a broad overview of LDs, from both a conceptual and an empirical vantage point. The emergence of this field of inquiry as well as issues of definition, classification, and prevalence are considered. With regard to etiology, it is assumed that LDs are either the direct or indirect result of central nervous system dysfunction. Theory and data specifically pertaining to the neuropsychological underpinnings of these syndromes are briefly considered. The process of diagnosis is described from neurological, psychological, and educa-tional perspectives. Interventions and treatments are described, including educational remediation, medication, and psychotherapy.

The ophthalmologist is often the first professional consulted when a child is having difficulty learning, especially when reading is involved. The physician's task is to determine whether organic visual pathology is causing the learning problem. Can the patient see the target? This first visual arc is the domain of the ophthalmologist. The second arc involves the processing of visual information. This is the province of the LD specialists. The examining physician must deal with the thorny interaction between these domains when a child has no apparent visual pathology but is unable to correctly interpret the stimuli because of processing problems. The position of the American Academy of Pediatrics and Ophthalmology with regard to this interaction is unambiguous. For your convenience it has been reproduced at the end of this chapter (Appendix 6–1).

■ Problem of Definition

Although the problem of bright children who are unable to read was described in the medical literature a century ago,[1] attempts at precise definition have been relatively recent. Diagnosis is still primarily dependent upon psychometric assessment of significant discrepancy between academic performance or achievement in one or more aspects of learning and general intelligence. The disparity in early conceptualizations reflected our lack of understanding of the learning processs generally as well as the factors interfering with it. Along with the phenomenological description and differentiation of the concept, thorny issues include the theoretical, clinical, and even legal implications embedded in definitions of LDs, all of which guide our work with children. The practical significance of defining who is learning disabled is highlighted by the fact that federal legislation requires that children and adolescents with specific learning disorders be identified, evaluated, and provided with appropriate school services and academic provisions. Furthermore, the designation of those children eligible for specific educational programs impacts upon the selection of those schools receiving special funding. Currently, although definitions continue to reflect theoretical biases, the growing body of research pertaining to underlying deficits is leading to greater clarity and shared criteria for inclusion. This holds the promise of providing a common diagnostic reference point from which research populations of learning disabled children may be more accurately defined.

It became clear that a stable definition, acceptable to an interdisciplinary constituency, was needed. In response to the definitional confusion, The National Joint Committee for Learning Disabilities (NJCLD) proposed a comprehensive and research-based definition of learning disabilites. Their definition reads as follows:

> *Learning disabilities* is a general term that refers to a heterogeneous group of disorders manifested by significant difficulties in the acquisition and use of listening, speaking, reading, writing, reasoning, or mathematical abilities. These disorders are intrinsic to the individual, presumed to be due to central nervous system dysfunction, and ma occur across the life span. Problems in self-regulatory behaviors, social perception and social interaction may exist with learning disabilities but do not in themselves constitute a learning disability. Although learning disabilities may occur concomitantly with other handicapping conditions (for example, sensory impairment, mental retardation [MR], serious emotional disturbance [ED], or with extrinsic influences (such as cultural differences, insufficient or inappropriate instruction), they are not the result of the conditions or influences.[2]

Researchers found this vague and unspecific definition difficult to operationalize. The Association for Adults and Children with Learning Disabilities (ACLD) refined this definition, differentiating several characteristics of learning difficulty. This condition occurs in children who are typically of average or above average intelligence and is manifest in significant discrepancy between general level of intellectual functioning (or aptitude) and performance (or achievement) in one or more specific areas of learning and/or cognitive ability. LD may be expressed in either significant delay in acquisition or difficulty in mastering one or more areas of learning. The criteria for diagnosis are both clinical and statistical. LDs exist on a continuum varying from mild to severe. In addition to specific academic skills, other areas of learning that may be involved include organization, impulse control, attention, and coordination. The ACLD reiterates that LDs are generally believed to be neurologically based, with a genetic component. They are *not* due to intellectual inadequacy, socioeconomic disadvantage, or poor teaching. Over the course of development, LDs can affect self-esteem, education, vocation, socialization, and daily living activities. Three mandates were identified by this committee for presentation to Congress: (1) that prevalence and demographic studies of learning disabilities should be accurately undertaken, (2) that the literature on cause, diagnosis, treatment, and prevention be reviewed, and (3) that suggestions for legislation and administrative action be prioritized. Failure to reach agreement on definition and diagnostic criteria has been a crucial factor inhibiting research efforts.[3]

The *Diagnostic and Statistical Manual*[4] (DSM– IV) describes LDs as specific developmental disorders, distinguished by inadequate growth in isolated academic skill areas, such as reading, writing, and math, as well as in the underlying cognitive areas of language, speech, or motor skills. Diagnosis is based upon comparison of standardized achievement tests with tests of general intelligence, both verbal and nonverbal (visual–motor and spatial). The LD is inferred from patterns of performance on a standardized test of that academic area falling significantly below the level expected considering the child's education and intelligence as measured by a standardized IQ test. LD is diagnosed only when the disorder interferes with school achievement or activities of daily living. Skills vulnerable to specific developmental disorders include arithmetic, expressive writing, reading, expressive and receptive language, articulation, and coordination.

Although precise definition of LDs is still debated, enormous progress has been made in the understanding of the etiological and neuropsychological nature of the many syndromes included under the LD umbrella. As our understanding continues to deepen, it is likely that the universal relevance of this knowledge will be increasingly valuable.

■ Historical Background

In the 5th century B.C., Hippocrates speculated that language and thought as well as personality were products of the brain. Common knowledge of the time suggested that physical properties such as heat and moisture influenced mental processes such as reasoning. The antecedents of the LD field lie in the history of both educational practice and scientific research. Early definitions were inexact and frequently confusing, reflecting the lack of understanding of the learning process and the factors that interfere with it. It was not until the late 19th century that direct evidence became available confirming Hippocrates' notion, at least with regard to language.

Driven by their interest in the powerful relationship between brain and behavior, scientists including Wernicke and Broca studied acquired brain pathology, providing enduring observations central to later conceptualizations of the neurological substrate of LD. Their clinical and autopsy studies of adults after strokes or other brain injuries allowed them to localize specific cognitive abilities, such as language and spatial ability, to specific parts of the brain. They noted that aphasia resulted from injury to the left hemisphere, that language was localized in the second frontal convolution of the left hemisphere, and that this phenomenon was absolute in right-handed subjects.[5] These observations and the complex relationship between handedness and lateralized function continue to concern current investigators.

Dyslexia was the first specific LD described in the medical literature. In 1878, a German physician, Kussmaul, described a man of normal intelligence and perceptual ability who was unable to read. Kussmaul called this condition "congenital word blindness." The term *dyslexia* was coined 9 years later, and in the first years of the 20th century a series of clinical reports by other researchers appeared supporting the existence of a congenital syndrome characterized by a developmental inability to read.[6,7]

In the 1920s and 1930s, Orton advanced the notion that reading disabilities were independent of general intelligence. He differentiated acquired disorders from dyslexia, in which the impairment in reading sklls is assumed to be neurologically based and present at birth. He worked inferentially from acquired reading disabilities in adults unimpaired prior to brain injury. Orton speculated that reading problems in children with symptomatology similar to his adult subjects might be caused by a common neurological condition.[6] He popularized the idea that a delay or failure in the establishment of lateral dominance was causally central (i.e., lag in the left hemispheric central language processes). In the current literature, it is noteworthy that the elucidation of developmental disorders in childhood appears to illuminate the mechanisms of adult brain function more effectively than does the earlier tradition of extrapolation to the nature of the child from the analysis of acquired disorders in adults.

The complexity of developmental learning difficulties was powerfully highlighted by Gerstmann's 1940 description of an adult syndrome,[5] which included disorders in calculation. Gerstmann assumed interdependence among a tetrad of symptoms including dyscalculia, spelling difficulty, directional confusion, and difficulty with finger recognition. He believed this condition evolved from an acquired brain dysfunction involving the left parietal lobe. Studies of children presenting with this syndrome appeared in the literature shortly thereafter. In the reports, left-handedness was prevalent, as was family history of academic difficulty. Organic brain dysfunction was assumed to be the result of some acquired traumatic mechanism. The absence of hard evidence of brain injury in LD children as well as concern about the negative impact of labeling children as "brain injured" led researchers to drop this terminology while retaining the assumption of underlying neurological cause.

This early phase in the history of LD was thus characterized by studies of the relationship between brain and behavior and resulted in several theoretical formulations as to the essence and etiology of learning problems. From the 1940s until the mid-1960s, professional interest in LD was focused primarily on pragmatic issues of intervention rather than on refining our understanding of the essential nature of LD. This period was marked by the emergence of a variety of remedial systems for treating LDs.

Since the mid-1960s, the LD field has expanded rapidly. New remedial techniques, programs, and services have proliferated, and increasing numbers of professionals from several disciplines are involved. The term *learning disability* was introduced in 1963 to encompass these conditions, their manifestations, and assumed etiology. To enjoin educators to help those individuals manifesting selective academic underachievement, LD was presented as "special needs category" at a national conference addressing the provision of services by the public schools for reading- and language-impaired children. The resulting U.S. Public Law 94-142 made three pivotal assumptions that are shared by current conceptualizations as well: (1) the learning problem is specific to an articulated academic domain, (2) there is psychometric demonstration that achievement is not commensurate with intellectual ability, and (3) exclusionary criteria are met, demonstrating that the learning problem is not the result of a concomitant condition.

■ Epidemiology

Estimates of the prevalence of learning disabilities vary considerably across studies in the literature. In part, this is an artifact of research shortcomings, in that investigators do not always agree on criteria for identifying LD subjects. In addition, epidemiological studies are more complicated for behavioral syndromes than for physical syndromes, where classification is based on all-or-none criteria. Within the United States between 7 and 15% of the general school population is assumed to fall more than one standard deviation below average in nationally normed reading or math scores. **The literature estimates that between $2\frac{1}{2}$ and 5% of the school-aged population is identified as learning disabled. Although LD emerges as a diverse and variable phenomenon, at least one half of these children are dyslexic.**[8–10]

As for gender breakdown, it is commonly assumed that LD affects far more male than female children. **The most frequently reported 3:1 male:female ratio is consistent with ratios for other special education classifications.** Recent data suggest that these data be reconsidered to reflect variation in the ratios of difference from one dysfunction to another. Boys appear to outnumber girls in populations of children with receptive and expressive language problems as well as reading disorders. The more disruptive behavior of male pupils in classrooms may lead to their overreferral and subsequent more frequent diagnosis. These gender differences have led to the postulation of sex-linked mechanisms of genetic transmission of LD, although this theory is as yet unsubstantiated by hard data.[11] Curiously, family reports indicate an equal number of male and female learning disabled individuals.[6]

Within learning disabled populations, estimates of those who also have attentional deficits vary widely, ranging from one third to three quarters struggling with concomitant learning and attentional difficulties. Boys significantly outnumber girls with attention deficit disorder (ADD). At present, interest in learning and attentional problems is largely a phenomenon of the developed world, where academic success is valued, and unpredictable or unexplained failure is of great concern to parents, educators, and the child.

■ Etiology: Theory and Data

The data strongly support the assertion that many learning problems are the result of neurodevelopmental aberrations within the central nervous system, which interfere selectively with cognitive and academic functioning. Underlying this belief is the assumption that there is a lawful relationship between normal brain functioning and specific patterns of behavior. Indeed, neuropsychological assessment has consistently and systematically differentiated among children heterogeneously classified as learning disabled, relating hemisphere of impairment to specific nature of dysfunction.[7] Theoreticians and clinicians from a variety of perspectives have considered the causes of LDs. An extensive body of literature exists, focusing on underlying causal agents ranging from genetic factors to nutrition. Much of the literature suffers from a common problem. There are many unidimensional conceptualizations, narrowly focused on a circumscribed view of LD. Currently, those at the forefront of the LD field are working toward broader formulations that attempt to subsume and integrate the patchwork of extant data and theory.[10,12] At present, what may be described as a developmental-neuropsychological model appears to encompass and integrate much of the data in terms of explanatory and predictive power. Simply put, although the source of the problem in a specific LD is assumed to be embedded in the central nervous system (CNS), it is difficult to establish a direct link between the neurological impairment and academic difficulty. In addition, these correlational data explain little about the influences producing idiosyncratic brain function or what mediates between actual brain function and observable learning behavior. These relationships between brain and behavior are conceptually enhanced and logically strengthened by the inclusion of "intrinsic" genetic and "extrinsic" environmental factors as well as the imposition of those cognitive processing capacities that mediate between brain neurochemistry, or neurophysiology, and a child's ability to learn. The psychological processing of mental data, crucial to learning, suggests a more coherent group of capacities that are both essential to adequate learning experience and vulnerable to dysfunction. This model implies a complex, interactional approach to the investigation of LDs. Understanding of the neuropsychological underpinnings of LDs must always include examination of the genetic and/or environmental factors that may lead to brain malformation, dysfunction, or delayed development. These conditions in turn may contribute to deficits in the processing of mental data, which may ultimately be expressed in a specific LD. A brief description of these etiological factors that may interact in children with LDs will demonstrate the complexity of this group of syndromes and is likely to raise more questions than are answered!

The notion that some form of genetic transmission is involved in LDs is suggested by the finding that they seem to run in families. The literature estimates that up to 40% of children and adolesents with LD may have inherited this condition. The evidence includes family histories, often noting the presence of parents or siblings with similar difficulties. Compared to the general population, researchers have demonstrated statistically greater co-occurrence of LD in monozygotic and dyzygotic twins, with greater concordance in monozygotic pairs (71%) than their dyzygotic counterparts (49%). In addition, the likelihood that LDs persist over a lifetime supports the hypothesis that there is a genetic component. Comorbidity with other disorders has also stimulated investigation of the heritability of LD. For example, a linkage was postulated and confirmed among dyslexia, left-handedness, and autoimmune and allergic disorders, based on a theory of prenatal testosterone exposure in utero.[3] The authors warned, however, that it would be premature to assume that testosterone is a central etiological substrate of either dyslexia or left-handedness. The genetic basis of handedness has also been associated with LD. Although equivocal, the literature suggests a greater prevalence of left- or mixed-handedness among LD individuals than among their non-LD peers. The specific mechanism of inheritance remains a matter of speculation.

Both pre- and perinatal stress factors may set the stage for injury to or abnormalities in the maturation of the brain, subsequently expressed in the form of LDs. Many variables have been investigated to varying degrees. Autopsy reports have indicated both asymmetries in the planum temporale area and anomolies in the convolutional patterns of the parietal lobes of dyslexics. These data provided evidence for the "faulty wiring" concept of LD. Sociocultural factors, extrinsic to the LD child, can also have a negative effect on the developing brain. These may include poor maternal nutrition, inadequate prenatal care, metabolic or toxic factors, infections, and stress. There is evidence that the presence of pregnancy and birth complications (particularly anoxic episodes) as well as prematurity and low birth weight are statistically correlated with later speech and/or reading difficulty. Recent studies of substance abuse during pregnancy are distressing. The data confirm increased incidence of hyperactivity, distractability, and irritability in these babies, and of LD as they enter school. The investigators stress that the occurrence of such complications is neither a necessary nor a sufficient explanation for the existence of an LD.

Two contrasting explanatory models have been proposed to account for the neurodevelopmental aspects of learning problems. One focuses on cerebrally based, neuropsychological deficit that may take the form of faulty hemispheric organization, brain asymmetry, or abnormal development of neural cells and transmitters. The second is a neurodevelopmental delay model, which is based on several explanations, including a lag in the establishment of cerebral dominance or laterality.

The deficit hypothesis, an outgrowth of the medical disease model, assumes that the academic dysfunction is the result of a CNS deficit intrinsic to the child. A number of deficit-based explanations of LD have garnered empirical support. A major difficulty is the number of possible deficits that may be involved, including encoding, decoding, attention, memory, sequencing, and so on. Many studies have speculated on the possible locus of neurological dysfunction, but none has received unequivocal support. For example, studies using computed tomography (CT) scans have posited reversed asymmetry in LD groups (i.e., right rather than left hemisphere language). A limited number of autopsy studies have attested to structural abnormalities in the cerebral hemispheres of individuals with severe LD. The data suggested cortical disorganization and clusters of displaced neurons. Comparative studies of normal brains are necessary to draw conclusions as to the generalizability of these findings. Several researchers have found LD to be associated with significant irregularities in electroencephalographic protocols (EEGs) when compared to normal children. These differences are difficult to interpret because of variations in populations sampled, experimental methodology, and statistical analysis.[10]

Delay hypotheses invoke the concept of a maturational lag in the neurological development of left-hemisphere specialization. It is assumed that delayed growth of cerebral centers results in this neurological immaturity. The defining characteristic of LD children is believed to be a less mature level of patterning in perceptual, motor, or other mental activity. Neither structure nor function is viewed as defective. Maturation is expected to continue, if slowly, and may even accelerate after puberty. This approach thus implies that some of these children will eventually catch up with their peers, acquiring the neural circuitry necessary for learn normally. In fact, there is little convincing evidence of systematic changes in brain lateralization with age.[14] Proponents of the delay model have had to modify this line of reasoning, positing that learning difficulties may persist into adolesence and adulthood because the learning experience and attitude of the child are negatively affected.

Like the nature versus nurture controversy, the issue of deficit versus delay may most constructively be conceptualized interactionally rather than in opposition, as both factors may powerfully influence the development of LDs. Although a deficit or brain trauma in a child can result in developmental delay, a significant maturational delay could result in neurological organization that remains deviant.[13]

■ Clinical Presentation

LDs may present singly or in combination with other LDs. Both verbal and nonverbal functions are essential to school success, and both areas are vulnerable to developmental deficiency with fairly predictable dysfunctional manifestations. This section describes the clinical phenomenology likely to be encountered in children with specific LDs.

Differential Diagnosis

As noted in relation to the exclusionary criteria for defining LD, LD may occur concomitantly with other handicapping conditions. However, it must not be caused by or the result of these conditions or influences. Factors that must be considered for etiological elimination include mental retardation, physical disability (cerebral palsy), brain damage from trauma or infection, sensory impairments (auditory or visual), environmental deprivation (including inadequate instruction), emotional disturbances, and medication effects.

Classification

Two trends in the classification of LD syndromes prevail in the current literature, one focusing on the cognitive process underlying the dysfunction and the second describing their symptomatic manifestation. In the first, LDs are conceptualized by the cognitive processes centrally involved. Levine, for example, a foremost current researcher and clinician, differentiates among difficulties in the processes of attention, mental processing, and output.[12] More frequently, however, the specific academic subject area affected defines the diagnostic category or subtype of LD. Researchers concur that failure to differentiate among the various subtypes of LDs can lead to false conclusions or predictions

as to patterns of performance. For example, although it has been found that reading disabled children have problems with processing certain aspects of syntax, those with mathematically based disorders do not.[7] Both the clinical-inferential and process-based research models have yielded important contributions. Both neuropsychological and intervention studies are central to the validation of LD subtypes. For the purposes of the present discussion, the academic area affected comprises the diagnostic category.

Verbally Based Learning Disabilities

Language Disorders

Children with developmental or acquired language disorders are handicapped in comprehending and/or producing language from early childhood. A myriad of factors are involved in spoken and written language. These include the ability to retrieve words from short- and long-term memory, the organization of these words in keeping with the rules of syntax and grammar, the articulation of a sequence of ideas, and the execution of the complex motor act of speech.[12] In school settings, verbal and written language are of paramount importance to success. Beyond their increasing centrality in academic work, these skills are essential for self-monitoring, social interaction, and demonstrating competence in the outside world.

Both expressive and receptive features of a child's communication skills may be impaired. The linguistic aspects of expressive language vulnerable to disorder vary depending upon the severity of the disorder and the age of the child. They may include voice quality and resonance (i.e., monotonous intonation) as well as lack of fluency and/or poor articulation. The child may have problems manipulating and expressing linguistic symbols. The development of a working vocabulary and the internalization of syntax facilitate meaningful communication. Word finding problems and difficulty with narrative organization are common expressive language deficits. In addition, there may be difficulty in the composition of written text evidenced by grammar or punctuation errors or poor paragraph construction.

Receptive language skills include the capacities involved in understanding words, sentences, or specific categories of words or statements (i.e., spatial terms or subjunctive formulations). These abilities draw upon interpretation of auditory stimuli and the understanding of spoken language and/or verbal symbols (verbal dyspraxia). The capacity to decode language enhances a child's mastery of his or her environment. Because the development of expressive language in childhood is inextricably interwoven with the acquisition of receptive skills, a pure receptive language disorder is virtually never seen.[4] In keeping with the notion of delayed or deficient hemispheric lateralization, there is neuroimaging and EEG evidence that suggests that LD expressed in processing receptive language is localized in the left hemisphere.

Reading Disabilities (Dyslexia, or Word Blindness)

Dyslexia is defined as the inability to read at a level appropriate to one's general intelligence. There is great variability in the extent to which reading disorders may interfere with functioning. Their presence is inferred from a discrepancy between one's IQ score and reading performance. It is suggested that data from more than one context be compiled to substantiate and validate this diagnosis (i.e., from school and home reports). There are numerous patterns of difficulties in reading that have led to the differentiation of several types of dyslexias in the current literature. The symptoms of dyslexia often include lateness in acquisition of reading skills. Reading may be slow and halting, with a lack of fluidity in silent or oral reading. Any combination of several processes may be implicated in dyslexia, including difficulty with semantic decoding, phoneme segmentation and recombination, and comprehension. Both visual processing and visual memory may be involved. For example, letter reversals are common, including confusion in the perception of b and d, p and q, and E and 3.

Spelling Disabilities (Dysorthographia)

Spelling problems are typically part of a broader developmental dysfunction and can result from a variety of deficits. Accurate spelling involves the integration of visual memory, sequencing, and retention. In addition, sound–symbol or phoneme–grapheme correspondences or phonics must be understood. Children may struggle to break words into their component sounds (segmentation) and put these components together (blending). Spelling is vulnerable to problems in visual recall as well, reflected in errors involving the substitution of words that sound the same, although they are spelled and written differently (e.g., *grate* in place of *great*).

Nonverbal Learning Disabilities

Like the verbal LDs, this is a heterogeneous group of disorders. Several domains of functioning are clustered in this subset of LDs, including conceptual problems; organization, attention, and memory functions; and visual–motor integration. Some researchers claim that the lack of understanding of social convention often observed in these children may be an LD as well. Besides the ADDs, this area is somewhat less well studied by educators and neuropsychologists than the verbally based problems in reading. The data suggest that these syndromes may occur singly but most often present in combination and/or interaction with each other. For example, problems in visual memory processing may be implicated in difficulty in calculation, underlying failure to recognize or remember mathematical symbols. Delay or dysfunction primarily in the development of right hemisphere structures or processes of the brain is assumed to impede learning. However, many of the identified deficits including memory, symbolic relationships, attention, and organization are central elements in literacy as well as nonverbal capacities. The concurrence and causal relationships among these factors are not yet fully understood.

Attention Deficit Disorders

ADDs are presently the most frequently diagnosed childhood psychiatric disorder. Conservative estimates suggest that this syndrome may affect as many as 4 or 5% of American children. This places at least one child with ADD in every classroom. It is estimated that most children with attentional deficits experience difficulties in learning, whereas **25% of the**

children with LD are assumed to have attention deficits as well. Research suggests that symptoms persist into adulthood in modified form. **Nearly 90% of those children diagnosed with ADD are boys**, although some studies suggest the disorder may be equally common in both sexes in adulthood.[15]

Distractability, impulsivity, and sometimes hyperactivity are the hallmark traits. These are people on the go, action oriented. They seem to be always busy, with lots of projects going, although they procrastinate and have trouble finishing things. Affectively, they can be moody or irritable, especially when interrupted or making transitions, or when a situation taps directly into their limitation. Although all need not be present for the diagnosis to be made, the symptoms are always inextricably interwoven with specific difficulties in the modulation or consistency of attention. Experts do not agree as to which symptom is fundamental. These characteristics are often expressed in the most significant domains of the child's life: thought, activity, and interpersonal relations.

In the current DSM IV, the disorder is divided into three classes, depending upon whether it involves mainly inattentiveness, mainly hyperactivity and impulsivity, or both. Inconsistency of symptom expression makes ADD particularly difficult to diagnose. Children with ADD may concentrate effectively in a novel situation or when intensely interested in something. Thus, DSM IV requires that ADD symptoms be present in at least two settings, such as school and home. As some may mimic symptoms of other physical conditions, differential diagnosis is crucial to effective intervention. For example, lapses in visual attention or discrimination may masquerade as visual pathology.

In ADD, three categories of underlying attentional processes vulnerable to dysfunction have been differentiated by Levine,[12] any or all of which may be involved. They include inconsistent control or regulation of (1) mental energy, (2) cognitive processing, and (3) production. Each has a somewhat different developmental trajectory.

Inconsistency in mental energy refers to inconsistent alertness and mental effort. This is associated with fidgetiness, boredom, reduced work capacity, and extreme motivational dependency upon others for help.

With regard to cognitive processing, several aspects of thought are apparently affected by this inconsistency in the regulation of attention. It is clear that children with ADD struggle with a fluctuating attention span, typically shorter than those of their peers, especially when they are not particularly interested by the material at hand. We may find both superficial and/or excessively deep processing. The superficial is reflected in underorganized, unelaborated work. In another context, the same child may be capable of tunnel-visioned "hyperfocus." In this mode we infer uncontrolled activation, or "mind tripping." There is an intolerance of boredom, a craving for extreme stimulation that mirrors the whirlwind inside. Although distractability is a central feature of ADD, the literature is equivocal as to its impact upon cognition. Distractability may be reflected in a child's inability to sustain attention until a task is completed (e.g., an eye examination), in trouble filtering out irrelevant stimuli, in discriminating significance, or in prioritizing.

Inconsistent production control is a third aspect of attentional dysfunction. Impulsivity may underlie poor previewing, failure to anticipate the consequences of one's behavior, and the absence of a reflective pause between thought and word or action. Motor hyperactivity is often expressed in an overflow of movement that seems to have a driven quality. Poor regulation of pacing may lead to frenetic rhythms or perseverative stuckness. It may be difficult for these children to listen to, read, or follow instructions. The poignant consequences of these difficulties often include a chronic sense of underachievement or not meeting one's goals.

Mathematics Disabilities (Dyscalculia)

As in the case of language-based LD, mathematically based disabilities are inferred from scores on standardized tests that fall substantially below those expected for the child's chronological age, general intelligence, and education. In children with mathematics disabilities, language impairments may or may not present concurrently. LD children with dyscalculia may experience difficulty with any of the numerous steps, rules, and facts required to solve even simple mathematical problems. The most frequently observed symptoms include the use of immature arithmetical strategies with frequent procedural errors and difficulty with retrieval of arithmetical facts from long-term memory. Their slowness and/or struggle may reflect problems in the understanding of or lack of proficiency in one or more of the following conceptual areas: concreteness of thought, abstraction, selection of operation, computational ability, directionality, and sequencing. Thus difficulties can be logical, organizational, or computational or can enter into any combination of these domains. Symptoms of this condition may appear as early as kindergarten, in confusion of number concepts or the inability to count accurately. However, it is seldom detected before the end of first grade, when sufficient formal mathematics instruction has occurred.

There is evidence that both right and left hemisphere delay or deficit may be involved, depending upon the specific ability impaired. For example, spatially based problems, alignment of numbers, and directionality are assumed to be right hemisphere based, whereas the reading and writing of numbers tap into symbolic functioning, associated with left hemisphere activity.[11] Indeed, so many complex processes may be involved in mathematical problem solving that it is difficult to imagine such diverse functions as all located in one side of the brain.[16]

Memory Disabilities

Among the basic cognitive processes, memory processes are most frequently implicated in the LD child's impaired ability to learn and, when learning occurs, to retrieve previously learned concepts. Both short- and long-term memory may be deficient in LD individuals compared to their non-LD peers. The implications of this are monumental when we consider that learning is a cumulative process, relying on the storage of data, experience, and acquired skills. Children must be able to selectively store, retain, and retrieve information appropriately. Significant clinical distinctions have been made between recognition and recall as well as auditory and visual memory. Reviewing the literature, Brainerd and Reyna conclude that, over the course of childhood, LD children may have increasing deficits in

the rate at which information is stored in long-term memory when compared to non-LD peers.[7] Poor memory performance has been variously attributed by different researchers to difficulty in phonological encoding, the use of rehearsal strategies and retrieval cues, and organizational and evaluative strategies.[6]

Visual–Motor Integration and Coordination

Both gross and fine motor coordination are aspects of CNS functioning that are vulnerable to developmental dysfunction. Manifestations of this disorder vary with age and development. Gross motor delay may be expressed in younger children in clumsiness. Difficulty in the coordination and use of specific muscle groups may be reflected in delays in achieving developmental motor milestones, including sitting, crawling, walking, tying shoelaces, and dealing with buttons and zippers. Older children may struggle to assemble puzzles, build models, or coordinate ballplaying. Reluctance to participate in physical activities such as sports is not an uncommon result in school-aged children.

Over the course of development, children become increasingly capable of fine motor activities as distal precision is gradually achieved. For the school-aged child effective fine motor coordination is essential to many manipulative activities. Disorders of movement under visual control, particularly affecting the spatial component of the task, are called dyspraxias. Attention, experience, motor sequencing, and visual–motor integration are all called upon to successfully utilize a pencil to write.

Emotional and Social Development in Children with Learning Disabilities

Poor Social Adaptation

There is a widespread assumption that social and emotional difficulties frequently coexist with academic learning and attentional disabilities. The behavioral difficulty frequently observed in children with learning problems may arise from the same central nervous system substrate. On the other hand, such personality changes may be secondary to chronic frustration or failure or may represent unconscious or conscious defensive maneuvers designed to avoid humiliation. Interestingly, the empirically based literature is equivocal as to the co-occurrence of psychiatric disturbance in LD children. The inconsistency in these data may well be a function of incomparable subject pools rather than poorly conducted research.[17] Stronger statistical links have been documented between the ADDs and poor emotional and social adjustment. Although direct causal links are difficult to document experimentally, the literature consistently suggests complex interactions between learning and psychiatric disturbances.[7] Research designed to address these associations may shed light on those phenotypes associated with genetic transmission.

It is as yet controversial whether impairment of social skills may itself constitute a form of nonverbal LD, reflecting difficulty understanding social convention, or whether these conditions are secondary to a more basic cognitive dysfunction. Although the mechanisms thought to underlie the nonverbal LDs have been lateralized to the right hemisphere, these phenomena have been observed in a wide variety of contexts, including closed head injury, intracranial surgery, and radiation to the brain.[16] Other aspects of social adaptation may be intrinsic to or secondary to LD as well. Poor recognition of faces and/or affective expression may result in awkwardness or inappropriateness. Children with poor social skills frequently have trouble adapting to new situations. Specifically, they may have difficulty forming and maintaining friendships and are often unpopular with their peers. Referring to children with ADD, Hallowell and Ratey[18] succinctly state this dilemma: "To make friends you have to be able to pay attention. To get along in a group you have to be able to follow what is being said. ... Social cues are often subtle, the narrowing of eyes ... a slight change in tone of voice. ... Often the person with ADD doesn't pick up on these cues. ..." In addition to insensitivity to social cues, poor social judgment may be manifest in failure to predict the consequences of their actions, inappropriate disinhibition, and insatiability in their activities. Either shy, withdrawn behavior or aggressive, disruptive behavior may result. Aggressivity, disruptiveness, and impulsivity may thwart the LD child's awareness of his or her impact upon others. The shy, withdrawn child may be anxious in the presence of others and behave passively, taking little initiative.

The complex diagnostic profile of each learning disabled child includes the co-occurrence of one or many learning difficulties within a context of varying extrinsic influences, including socioeconomic, educational, and family conditions. Robust support for interactions or causal relationships between LD and psychological well-being must rest upon research differentiating subtypes of LD, addressing the comorbidities involved, and the complex interactions of subtypes with emotional and interpersonal adaptation. Longitudinal data on LD populations that include emotional and behavioral adjustment measures would greatly enhance our understanding.

Emotional Problems Secondary to Learning Disabilities
Anxiety

Heightened anxiety states and/or panic attacks are not uncommon in those with learning difficulties. The extent to which these are biologically based rather than reactive to a situation or life experience remains to be determined. Difficulty in school is commonly cited as a contributor to anxiety in LD children. Anxiety may be diffuse, or pervasive across situations, or it may be targeted around the area of academic weakness. A danger of chronically heightened anxiety is that it may become generalized in a cycle involving failure and negative feedback, which in turn heightens anxiety, etc. School phobia is diagnosed when an overwhelming fear of going to school overtakes the child. Anxiety about being intact or defective may be displaced into somatic concerns and bodily preoccupations in the LD child. These in turn can affect school adjustment and performance significantly.[12]

Depression and Aggression

Many investigators have documented an increased incidence of depression in LD children and adolescents. Low self-esteem and motivational loss are frequent complications of school-based frustration. A sense of hopelessness ensues when a child feels academic effort is futile and success is unattainable or would require heroic effort. Aggressive or noncompliant behavior may reflect a response to the child's frustration or a defense against underlying feelings of failure. Others may respond by withdrawing socially, thereby avoiding contact with those outside the family. School and/or homework phobia may result from distress around academic or social difficulties. Symptoms of depression may include feelings of sadness, futility, and hopelessness, self-deprecation, loss of appetite, and sleep disturbances. Sometimes angry feelings may be turned inward against the self and result in self-destructive or suicidal thoughts and behaviors. If the depression is prolonged or intense, or suicidality is present in any form, professional assistance should be sought at once.

■ Assessment, Evaluation, and Diagnosis

Assessment

The comprehensive evaluation and subsequent treatment of a child with LDs must reflect both its developmental nature and its complexity. Assessment of genetic, neurological, psychoeducational, medical, behavioral, and social factors may be involved. Observations and interviews as well as formal psychological and neurological testing comprise the data, collected from multiple observers including educators, psychologists, and physicians. As performance may be inconsistent in an LD child across various contexts, it is necessary to corroborate findings both within and outside the school setting. The presence of chronic or acute stressors in the child's life that may be interfering with academic performance must be considered, along with any idiocyncratic characteristics of the child or the child's family. Clinical assessment using a variety of methods assures a more thorough understanding and valid picture of the child's current level of adaptation as well as cognitive functioning. The aim of this evaluation is to arrive at recommendations for the provision of well-targeted assistance for the child.

Data gathering usually begins with informal but informed observation by a parent or teacher of a pattern of difficulty in learning.

Not every child with learning difficulty requires thorough evaluation. There are many levels of assessment. When the problem is not overwhelming and the school and parents feel they understand the student's needs, teachers and parents may be able to develop management and tutorial strategies to deal with the difficulty.

In-depth interviews with the children as well as their parents and teachers form an essential part of the evaluative workup. Although not necessarily statistically reliable, they provide a wealth of data useful to differential diagnosis and treatment planning. Awareness of the emotional climate within the family is crucial, as is sensitivity to the potential for anxiety, shame, humiliation, or guilt that can be aroused by evaluation. A clear and detailed description of the manifestations of the learning difficulty is essential. A developmental history from the parents will shed light on how well the child has adapted to developmental challenges and recommendations for both assessment and intervention. For example, a history of delayed milestones including language acquisition suggests some hypotheses as to the origins of the problems that may be tested in the evaluation. It is of interest to note whether the family history includes incidence of learning problems in the child's siblings, parents, and extended family.

Teacher reports are typically illuminating, in that teachers are typically able to evaluate the child's performance in relation to his or her peers. Often teachers are aware of the specific situations in which problems are apparent, and of the child's ability to focus and attend as well as of the general behavioral adjustment of the child.

Psychometric and Psychoeducational Testing

Generally, psychoeducational evaluation must cover academic achievement as well as the main factors constituting intelligence, including the language-based skills, visual–spatial and motor integration, and attention and memory. Therefore both general intelligence and academic achievement must be thoroughly assessed using well-standardized tests to demonstrate and confirm the significant discrepancy between a child's mental abilities and performance from which we infer the presence of an LD. It is assumed that the discrepancy between IQ and achievement test scores documented in LD children is not apparent in normally achieving children or those with other disabilities. Although an integral part of the defined construct, discrepancy definitions have been criticized as inadequate to differentiate the cognitive processes in those students with low IQ scores from those with high IQ scores, and although necessary this may not be sufficient to infer the presence of LD. Other critics discredit the aptitude versus achievement formula as identifying a result, not a causal relationship.[17]

The identified prevalence of LDs can obviously vary greatly as a function of one's criteria for significant difference. Researchers do not all agree on the formula to be used to calculate significant variation. The interpretation of the discrepancy between the tests can be based on the standard error of both tests or more commonly on the differences between them in standard deviations. Thus a 15-point difference, or 1 standard deviation, is typically deemed significant, when both tests have a mean of 100 and a standard deviation of 15. LD has also been diagnosed by comparing individual performance to standardized group norms. A score more than 1.5 standard deviations below the norm on an individually administered test suggests the likely presence of LD. A third approach being used in some current research combines both the discrepancy and normative criteria, thereby limiting some of the overinclusiveness of each of these two diagnostic guidelines when utilized individually. This approach yields data in relation to frequency in the population that are more consistent with large-scale epidemiological studies.[19]

Intelligence Tests

IQ tests are an efficient way to gather a differentiated view of a child's relative intellectual strengths and weaknesses. In addition, a great deal can be learned about the child's cognitive style, or approach to thinking and reasoning.

This in turn can provide insight into a child's difficulty learning in a classroom. **Standardized for children between the ages of 6 and 16 years, the Wechsler Intelligence Scale for Children (WISC) is the most commonly used overall measure of intelligence.** This test consists of 10 main subtests and 2 supplementary tests to be utilized at the evaluator's discretion. The 10 subtests are divided into verbal or performance measures. The verbal tests assess vocabulary, comprehension of social convention, functional and abstract concept formation, mental arithmetic, and general knowledge, or information. The performance tests measure the child's ability to pick out essential missing details from a drawing; analyze, synthesize, and reproduce patterns made from colored blocks; construct an object from jigsaw puzzle pieces; rapidly transcribe coded signs; and sequentially organize a series of drawings into a story that makes sense. One of the supplementary tests assesses auditory memory, requiring the child to repeat series of digits forward and backward from memory. The other requires the child to navigate a series of paper and pencil mazes. These are supplementary as they have been found to correlate less well than the other subtests with general intelligence. From the scaled scores within each group a verbal IQ and performance IQ are calculated, from which the full-scale IQ is derived. As an average, the full-scale IQ fails to convey the possible dramatic discrepancies in capacities exhibited by a learning disabled child. A nuanced profile of the child's functioning is provided by an examination of the patterning of the data from this test. Certain specific patterns of score "scatter" are associated with different learning problems. However, the significance of the scatter remains a matter of debate, particularly if attentional deficit is present, as impaired concentration can obviously reduce scores on any of the subtests.

Academic Achievement Tests

Once a profile of abilities has been obtained, systematic evaluation of academic achievement is in order, zeroing in on reading, writing, and mathematical skills. **The Wide Range Achieve-**

ment Test (WRAT-III) and the Peabody Individual Achievement Test (PIAT) are both frequently used measures for the screening of LD.
The WRAT, normed for children 5 years old
and beyond, is especially useful as an initial
measure, as it assesses single word reading as
well as written spelling and arithmetic in a test
taking under an hour. An advantage of the
Peabody is that it uses many multiple choice
items, for some of which the child just has to
point at the correct answer. Thus, it may be useful with language-impaired or extremely anxious children. The subtests in the PIAT include
reading recognition, reading comprehension,
mathematics, spelling, and general information. If LDs are suggested or identified by these
academic achievement tests, the findings may
then be followed up with with more differentiated cognitive abilities testing of the specific
functions involved, including but not limited to
visual, auditory, memory, and retrieval abilities.

Hopefully, it is evident that further progress in
the understanding of LDs requires a multidisciplinary effort involving a diverse group of schol-
ars and practitioners, including geneticists,
neurologists, psychologists, psychiatrists, and
educators. Clearly, the diagnosis of an LD
requires the interpretation and integration of a
great deal of data. Operational definitions
appear to be most useful to the diagnostic
process. For example, although definitions of
reading disability are most effectively based on
measures of phonological processing, mathematical disabilities must be inferred from measures of computational skills that are not
confounded by a reading element.

Neurological and Medical Evaluation

Clinical acumen in diagnosis is predicated on a
precise, unambiguous definition. In reality, however, it has been noted that an exclusionary definition is often used to infer the presence of an
LD by ruling out other potentially applicable disorders. Medical and neurological examinations
seek to identify and eliminate physical factors
that might interfere with a child's learning. Factors in sensory perception, including vision and
hearing pathology, must be considered (i.e., the
anatomical substrate of visual perception).

Recent research developments related to
both the neurophysiological and neuropsychological underpinnings of learning and attentional difficulties have yielded a wealth of data
with profound implications for our understanding of the biological substrate of these syndromes. Although still primarily a research tool,
the data provided by brain imaging will impact
assessment, diagnosis, and treatment of children with LDs. Functional imaging now makes
it possible for neurologists and neuropsychologists to demonstrate where specific cognitive
processes are ongoing in the brain by precise
mapping as well as quantification of brain activity. This documentation of neurological systems
implicated in childhood LDs is significant in
providing more direct evidence of neurological
involvement than is represented by the volumes
of correlative data. Over the last 2 decades,
advances in imaging the brain through CT, and
magnetic resonance imaging (MRI) have provided evidence of structural variation. Other
imaging techniques shed light on disordered
metabolic or electrophysiological systems
rather than structure. These include procedures such as positron emmission tomography
(PET), multichannel topographic brain electrical activity mapping (BEAM), and measures of
regional cerebral blood flow (rCBF). This
remarkable technology has confirmed that the
functional organization of the brain for phonological processing differs in men and women.
Although women demonstrate activation bilaterally, men are highly lateralized to the left
inferior frontal gyrus. The ability to pinpoint
specific neural pathways in activation provides a
quantum leap forward in our understanding of
LD. These data will be used as markers in the
comparative study of LD and non-LD individuals. In addition, it is now possible to do exact
and quantitative analysis of how cerebral functioning and learning are affected by significant
biological events that affect every child over the
course of maturation (i.e., adolescence). Studies of cognitive, hormonal, and brain organizational changes over childhood would add
significantly to our understanding of human
development as well as insight into developmental triggers for variations in brain development, which might eventually make prevention
a reasonable goal.[7]

Learning Disabilities in the Ophthalmologist's Office

The ophthalmologist is frequently the first specialist outside of school who is consulted in response to a child's academic difficulty. Obviously, a complex relationship exists between vision and learning. The mission is to establish whether visual pathology contributes to the child's struggle to learn. Although the presence of a visual defect may not cause a learning difficulty, there is general agreement that visual dysfunction may create fatigue and discomfort that may lead to inconsistency and slowness in processing the printed page and anxious resistance to or avoidance of learning involving reading. If the child has healthy eyes, good visual acuity both near and far, and normal binocular vision, it is unlikely that the eyes are contributing to a reading problem. Treatable ocular conditions such as refractive errors, focusing problems, and strabismus should obviously be identified and treated as early as possible by the ophthalmologist. Indeed, research has demonstrated that the majority of childhood and adult neurologically based learning difficulties do not stem from altered visual function. If no visual defect is apparent, the child should be referred for further evaluation, often coordinated by the pediatrician.

There are patterns of behavior and performance in the ophthalmologist's examining room that might suggest the presence of an LD. The various LDs would manifest themselves differentially. Diagnosis is at best a thorny problem, as some visual processing problems may mimic physical pathology of the eye, making differential diagnosis crucial to effective intervention. For example, performance on a test may be compromised by problems in visual discrimination, figure-ground discrimination, or deficits in visual memory. Language encoding or decoding difficulty might be manifest in a child's inability to name a letter on a chart or an object in an array. The conventional practice of assessing the eye must concern itself with the confounding fact that our data include the brain's interpretation of what we see.

Letter reversals provide a case in point. This rubric includes mirror images, inversions, and rotations. When learning to write, most children occasionally reverse letters, particularly those that are mirror images of each other. The proverbial admonition to children to "mind their p's and q's" highlights the commonness of this phenomenon that typically disappears by third grade. In LD, especially dyslexic children, this confusion persists with greater frequency than is observed in their non-LD peers. It is clear that visual defects do not systematically cause reversals of letters, words, or numbers. Dyslexia does. Directional and sequencing confusion may be symptomatic of LDs as well.

Inconsistencies in mental energy, fluctuation in visual attention or discrimination, distractibility, and impulsivity may interfere with performance on tests of visual acuity and thereby masquerade as visual pathology. All part of the ADD symptom cluster, behaviorally these deficits may be reflected in unusual restlessness, fidgeting, and an overflow of gross motor activity. A comparative study by Barkley[20] highlights this style. Monitoring physical activity, he found that children with ADD moved around the room nearly eight times more than controls, were three times more restless watching TV, and more than four times as fidgety during psychological testing. Thus, in an examining room, one might see finger or foot tapping as well as a need to pace or take frequent breaks. Any strategy or materials that increase the novelty, stimulation, or interest in the task at hand may be facilitating.

Consultation and Recommendations

Once the data have been collected, interpreted, and integrated by the collaborative team, diagnostic impressions and recommendations are reported to parent and child (when age appropriate). A good assessment should result in a thorough report, describing a child's strengths, weaknesses, and psychological health. Specific suggestions to parents and educators should be included. The therapeutic process begins with the demystification of the problem at hand. A pivotal part of the counseling process, this is done by explaining the symptoms in understandable terms that contribute to a sense of mastery rather than further bewilderment. Complicated terminology, professional jargon, and excessive abstraction are thus not facilitative. A thorough understanding of the issues informs the treatment process.

■ Interventions and Treatment

Conventional Management and Treatments

The assumption underlying the following treatment modalities for learning and attentional difficulties in childhood is that these are neurologically based developmental disorders interfering with the capacity to learn and to control attentional processes. As in the case of diagnosis, the implementation of good management may involve parents, teachers, psychologists, and physicians. The goal is to enable the child to be increasingly engaged and successful in school. This requires tangible evidence of improvement as well as the development of hopefulness about his or her potential to learn.

Medication

The use of medication to treat learning, attentional, and behavior disorders has become widespread. The medications are basically utilized to help the individual to focus. Drug therapies are best conceived as one aspect of a management program, which may also include academic remediation and counseling. Several factors influence decisions about the clinical use of psychopharmacology in the treatment of attentional deficits and LDs. These include professionals' knowledge of and amenability to medication, the availability of other management resources, the education and socioeconomic level of parents, and the severity of the problem at the time of referral. The stimulants and antidepressants work on that part of the brain that regulates attention, impulse control, and mood. When effective, they can reduce the inner turmoil and anxiety so common with attentional deficits. Used judiciously, they can provide profound relief and improve the efficacy of other interventions by allowing the child to respond to the environment more adaptively. Drug therapies must be closely monitored by a physician or psychologist with expertise in psychopharmacology to continually evaluate progress and monitor adverse side effects as well as the ongoing growth and development of the child.

Stimulant medications are most frequently prescribed to treat attentional deficits. Methylphenidate (Ritalin), dextroamphetamine (Dexadrine), and pemoline (Cylert) are all used extensively. In children 4 years of age and older, methylphenidate is usuallly the first choice of medication because there is more research documentation of its efficacy, dosage, and titration. There is abundant empirical evidence that these drugs often improve a child's ability to mobilize mental effort, concentrate, and behave less impulsively. Although reducing extreme motor hyperactivity, they may enhance memory functions. The dosage, schedule of administration, and decision to use short- or long-acting forms of the drugs must be considered by the physician managing the child's medication. In many cases regularly scheduled "drug holidays" are recommended, during which the child takes no medication. Thus, if medication is used primarily for classroom management, it may be discontinued on weekends, holidays, and summer vacations. This provides an opportunity to assess the child's current ability to control attention, behavior, and learning activities.

These psychostimulants may cause a myriad of side effects, including loss of appetite, insomnia, growth delay, and personality change. The likelihood of behavioral tolerance developing with chronic administration of stimulant compounds remains a matter of research controversy. As a significant percentage of children with attentional deficits continues to be symptomatic into adulthood, Pemoline, assumed to have less abuse potential than the others, may be a better first choice. However, it has been demonstrated that pemoline may disrupt liver enzyme elevations, and therefore it requires close monitoring. Investigators have further indicated that it is slower in achieving its peak effectiveness and in washing out of the body than the other stimulants.[21] Although all three stimulants can adversely affect physical growth during active treatment, most follow-up studies report catch-up growth when the medication is stopped. Extreme caution must be exercised when LD is diagnosed along with other neurological conditions, such as a seizure disorder or migraine, as stimulant medications are associated with decreased seizure threshold.

Other types of medication are used when the effectiveness of the stimulant therapy proves to be inadequate or variable in a child with an attentional deficit. These less frequently prescribed drugs include tricyclic antidepressants and α-adrenergic agonists, which inhibit the release of norepinephrine at the synapse, decreasing sympathetic responses. These medications are used to treat psychological conditions accompanying LDs and attentional disabilities, including anxiety, depression, and obsessive-compulsive disorder. The potential for complicated drug effects with comorbid diagnoses must be considered. For example, although reducing anxiety and depression, serotonin reuptake inhibitors such as fluoxetine (Prozac) may exacerbate attention deficits and result in oversedation.

Although drug treatments have proved to be helpful to many children with ADD, they are not a panacea. Further investigation is required to fully understand their precise dosages, short- and long-term side effects, and potential interaction effects in use in combination with other medications. Medications do not teach the child anything. They merely influence the likelihood of behaviors in the child's repertoire. Other interventions focusing on the educational, psychological, and social problems these children present are essential to enhance their skills. Thus, a conservative approach to the inclusion of medication in a child's treatment program is strongly recommended.[12,18]

Educational Remediation

School placement for the LD child is among the first concerns of the interdisciplinary evaluation or management team. Depending upon the severity of the problem at hand, recommendations may vary from inclusion in a regular, mainstream class, with little or special support services, to a full-time special class or school. A compromise between these is frequently advocated, in which the child may spend part of each day in both LD and regular classrooms, or a resource program, where the child is enrolled in the mainstream class but regularly attends a resource room for special education.

It is both possible and desirable to intervene directly to enhance weak cognitive skills or functions. Tutoring in reading, math, and writing is most common. If the tutor is knowledgeable about the child's relative strengths and weaknesses, remediation in the specific deficit area also allows the LD child to strengthen the development of compensatory strategies. The data do not systematically indicate that one type of remediation program is superior to another. Several pedagogical models are utilized in the instruction of LD and ADD children. Approaches to teaching reading and spelling are dichotomized into two methods. One emphasizes whole word methods, or language experience, and the other works from the bottom up, training in phonics, syllables, and intraword units. Recent studies are unanimous in supporting the efficacy of phonics training to either prevent or treat reading and spelling disabilities in children.[21] Other methods used include programmed learning systems, multisensory methods, computer-assisted programs, and cognitive behavioral modification interventions. With ADD, tutoring and coaching aid in the establishment of structure and organization, which can greatly reduce chaos and improve productivity and the child's sense of mastery and control.

Longitudinal data confirm the conclusion that LD tends to be chronic and persistent. More favorable outcomes tend to be related to both higher socioeconomic status and higher IQ. Remediation programs are particularly successful when they are intensive, last at least 2 years, and are followed by supportive assistance to maintain the rate of growth attained. Although symptoms may improve, a residual will remain that is likely to interfere with optimal performance over the life span. Under optimal conditions, severely dyslexic students usually do not catch up with their peers in reading ability. In fact, they may do worse over time if they acquire negative attitudes about reading. The core constellation of problems in LD are not easily overcome, as evidenced by their stubborn resistance to complete amelioration.

Psychotherapies

To date, studies of the relationship between LD and ADD and psychopathology have yielded inconsistent findings. However, it is assumed that academic underachievement related to LD or ADD increases a child's risk of developing emotional or behavior problems. There is in fact a great deal of data that correlate different psychopathologies with LDs or ADD. LD and ADD have been significantly associated with conduct disorders, juvenile delinquency, external locus of control, anxiety, and depression. Longitudinal studies suggest that many children with attentional deficits will continue to manifest dysfunctional symptoms into adulthood, including poorer educational and occupational outcomes and significantly higher rates of substance abuse, especially when hyperactivity persists.

There are several areas in which the adjunctive role of psychotherapy warrants consideration in assisting the child with LD or ADD. The goals of such treatment might include alleviation of problems with self-esteem, relationships, depression, anxiety, organization, and interpersonal skills. The literature suggests that the therapist be actively and directively involved in helping the individual to better manage time and develop strategies to organize his or her life.

In summary, the most promising approach to the management of LDs is one in which the interdisciplinary professional team attends to the psychological, educational, and pharmacological needs of the individual child. There is evidence that the effects of behavioral, psychological, and chemical interventions are complementary and synergistic. Whether treatment modalities are utilized singly or in combination, there is enormous variation both within and between individuals in response to treatments of any kind. This reflects the heterogeneity of this cluster of syndromes.

Controversial Treatment Modalities

Most educators and researchers currently accept the notion of neurological dysfunction underlying LDs. However, different notions as to the origins of the neural dysfunction have led to a variety of causal hypotheses and theories as well as controversial proposals for treatment. These therapies may be grouped by their main conceptual foundation either in neurophysiological retraining or in orthomolecular medicine. The neurophysiological retraining approaches assume that by stimulating specific sensory input or exercising specific motor patterns, one can retrain or reroute the CNS. Orthomolecular approaches treat mental disorders by providing optimum doses of substances normally present in the human body. The foci of these theories have included unstable eye movement control, ocular lock syndrome, cerebellar/vestibular dysfunction, sensory integration, dietary allergies, vitamin deficiencies, and lack of cerebral dominance. Not surprisingly, each hypothesis leads to the recommendation of a different treatment modality. In various remedial programs, children with LDs have been asked to learn how to crawl correctly, walk balance beams, be retrained in proper eye movements in reading including tracking, or eliminate additives or sugars from their diets. There is little evidence that any of these approaches has yielded the desired effect on cognitive skill acquisition.

In 1984 and 1992, The American Academy of Ophthalmology issued policy statements contending that children with LDs have the same ocular health statistically as those without such conditions and **that there is no peripheral eye defect that produces dyslexia or other LDs.** They warn that there is *no* substantiated evidence supporting the claim that LD children benefit from treatment based on visual training, tracking practice, glasses, muscle exercise, or laterality training. In fact, such training may lead to a false sense of security, thereby delaying or preventing adequate instruction and remediation. Effective thus far are more conservative approaches including the use of educational remediation and medication when indicated.

■ Conclusions

Current interdisciplinary efforts to improve the lives of children and adults with LD are directed toward maximizing and harnessing the extraordinary power of neurology, psychology, and education. Greater understanding of the biologically based variations within and among learners will enable us to anticipate the response that various learning environments might provoke. This in turn might empower clinicians, practitioners, and educators to set realistic goals and to adjust the setting to maximize their realization. In addition to facilitating school success, this may also enhance emotional and social well-being. The thorough exploration of these learning processes will hopefully lead to a deepened understanding of the brain in relation to the behavior it produces. Scientific discoveries illuminate our path on a course directed toward unlocking the potential of the LD child, allowing that child to participate in and contribute to society.

■ Resources

There are several organizations that address the specific needs and problems of the LD population. Assistance is available pertaining to assessment, treatment, and placement (see Reference 6 for an extensive listing of available resources and services). The National Joint Committee for Learning Disabilities (NJCLD) is a consortium of organizations serving LD individuals. In addition, The Orton Dyslexia Society (ODS) and The Learning Disabilities Association of America (LDA) provide remediation counseling. The National Center for Learning Disabilities offers a free information and referral service, as well as educational programs and advocacy for improved legislation. Universities are currently generating an enormous amount of research on both diagnosis and intervention. The addresses of these organizations are listed here as a starting point. Databases spanning available human services are currently available and can be searched in many university and public libraries as well as over the Internet.

The Learning Disabilities Association
of America (LDA)
4156 Library Road
Pittsburgh, PA 15234
Tel: (888) 300-6710
Web: www.I danat.org

The National Joint Committee for Learning Disabilities (NJCLD) & The Orton Dyslexia Society (ODS)
74 York Road
Baltimore, Maryland 21204
Tel: (410) 296-0232
Web: http://interdys.org

National Center for Learning Disabilities, Inc.
381 Park Avenue South, Suite 1401
New York, New York 10016 - 8806
Tel: (212) 545 - 7510
Web: www.ncld.org

REFERENCES

1. Silver AA, Hagin RA. *Disorders of Learning in Childhood.* New York: John Wiley & Sons; 1990.
2. National Joint Committee on Learning Disabilities. A Position Paper of the National Trust Committee on Learning Disabilities (letter to NJCLD member organizations). *J Learn Disab.* 1981;1:53–55.
3. Roswell F, Natchez G. *Reading Disability.* New York: Basic Books; 1989.
4. *Diagnostic and Statistical Manual of Mental Disorders,* 4th ed. Washington, DC: American Psychiatric Association; 1994.
5. Duane DD. Biological foundations of learning disabilities. In: Obrzut JE and Hynd GW. *Neuropsychological Foundations of Learning Disabilities.* San Diego: Academic Press; 1991.
6. Spafford CS, Grosser G. *Dyslexia: Research and Guide.* Needham Heights, MA: Allyn & Bacon; 1996.
7. Obrzut JE, Hynd GW. *Neuropsychological Foundations of Learning Disabilities.* San Diego: Academic Press; 1991.
8. United States Department of Education, Sixteenth Annual Report to Congress on the Implementation of the Individuals with Disabilities Education Act. Washington, DC: U.S. Government Printing Office; 1995.
9. Gaddes WH, Egdell D. *Learning Disability and Brain Function: A Neuropsychological Approach.* New York: Springer-Verlag; 1994.

10. Kavale KA, Forness SR. *The Nature of Learning Disabilities.* New Jersey: Lawrence Erlbaum; 1995.

11. Prior MR. *Understanding Specific Learning Disabilities.* East Sussex, UK: Psychology Press; 1996.

12. Levine M. *Educational Care.* Cambridge, MA: Educators Publishing Service; 1994.

13. Spreen OR, Anthony H, Edgell D. *Developmental Neuropsychology.* New York: Oxford University Press; 1995.

14. Molfese DL, Segalowitz SJ. *Brain Lateralization in Children.* New York: Guilford Press; 1988.

15. Lerner JW, Lowenthal B, Lerner SR. *Attention Deficit Disorders: Assessment and Teaching.* Boston: Brooks/Cole; 1995.

16. Rourke BP, Del Dotto JE. *Learning Disabilities: A Neuropsychological Perspective.* California: Sage Publications; 1994.

17. Dickman GE. The link between learning disabilities and behavior. In: Cramer SC, Ellis W, eds. *Learning Disabilities: Lifelong Issues.* Baltimore, MD: Paul H. Brookes; 1996.

18. Hallowell E, Ratey J. *Driven to Distraction: Recognizing and Coping with Attention Deficit Disorder from Childhood through Adulthood.* New York: Pantheon Books; 1994.

19. Barkley RA. *Attention Deficit Hyperactivity Disorder: A Handbook for Diagnosis and Treatment.* New York: Guilford Press; 1990.

20. Barkley RA. *Taking Charge of ADHD.* New York: Guilford Press; 1995.

21. Wolraich ML. *Disorders of Development and Learning.* St. Louis: Mosby; 1996.

22. American Academy of Pediatrics, American Association for Pediatric Ophthalmology and Strabismus, and American Academy of Ophthalmology. Learning Disabilities, Dyslexia, and Vision. Joint Statement. San Francisco; March 1992.

23. Cramer SC, Elli, W, eds. *Learning Disabilities: Lifelong Issues.* Baltimore, MD: Paul H. Brookes; 1996.

24. Farnham-Diggory S. *The Learning Disabled Child.* Cambridge, MA: Harvard University Press; 1992.

25. Selikowitz M. *Dyslexia and Other Learning Disabilities.* New York: Oxford University Press; 1993.

26. Silver LB. *The Misunderstood Child.* New York: McGraw-Hill; 1992.

27. Stevens SH. *The LD and ADHD Child.* Winston-Salem, NC: John F. Blair; 1996.

Pediatric Ophthalmology
Edited by P. F. Gallin
Thieme Medical Publishers, Inc.
New York © 2000

Appendix 6–1

■ ■ ■

Learning Disabilities, Dyslexia, and Vision

*A JOINT STATEMENT OF THE
AMERICAN ACADEMY OF PEDIATRICS,
AMERICAN ASSOCIATION FOR PEDIATRIC OPHTHALMOLOGY
AND STRABISMUS,
AND
AMERICAN ACADEMY OF OPHTHALMOLOGY*

■ Problem

The issue of learning disorders, including dyslexia, has become a matter of increasing personal and public concern. Inability to read and comprehend is a major obstacle to learning and may have far-reaching social and economic implications. Concern for the welfare of children with dyslexia and learning disabilities has led to a proliferation of diagnostic and remedial treatment procedures, many of which are controversial. This policy statement addresses these issues, which are of importance to affected individuals, their families, teachers, physicians, allied health personnel, and society.

■ Policy

A broad-based consensus of educators, psychologists, and medical specialists recommend that individuals with dyslexia or related learning disabilities should receive (1) early comprehensive educational, psychological, and medical assessment and (2) educational remediation combined with appropriate psychological and medical treatment.

■ Background

Reading is a complex function that involves integrating multiple factors related to an individual's experience, ability, and constitution. Although it is obvious some children do not read well because they have trouble seeing, research has shown that the majority of children and adults with reading difficulties experience a variety of language defects[1-3] that stem from complex, altered brain morphology and function and that the reading difficulty is not due to altered visual function per se.[4-6] In addition, a variety of secondary environmental factors may also have a detrimental effect on the learning process.

However, in spite of these facts, a certain number of children who experience reading difficulty may also experience a treatable visual difficulty in addition to their primary reading or learning dysfunction. Pediatricians can identify the majority of those who have reduced visual acuity. However, in a small percentage of children, a visual abnormality such as farsightedness may not be detected during pediatric office screening procedures. Therefore, pediatricians who evaluate children for reading difficulties should consider referral to an ophthalmologist familiar with children's eye problems.

■ Guidelines

1. **Early Detection.** Pediatricians and educational specialists may attempt to use screening techniques to detect children with learning disabilities in the preschool years. However, in many cases, the learning dis-

ability is discovered only after the child experiences academic failure in school. Learning disabilities can include dyslexia, a variety of language defects, and difficulty with mathematic computation. They are often complicated by attention deficits. A family history of learning disabilities is common in such conditions. Those considered to be at risk for these conditions should be thoroughly assessed by both educational and psychological specialists.

2. **Multidisciplinary Approach.** Learning disabilities, including dyslexia and other forms of reading or academic under-achievement, require a multidisciplinary approach to diagnosis and treatment, involving educators, psychologists, and physicians. Basic scientific research into the role the brain's structure and function play in learning disabilities has demonstrated that the basis of dyslexia and other specific learning disabilities is within the central nervous system and is multifactorial and complex.[4–6]

3. **The Role of the Eyes.** Decoding of retinal images occurs in the brain after visual signals are transmitted from the retina via the visual pathways. Unfortunately, however, it has become common practice among some to attribute reading difficulties to one or more subtle ocular or visual abnormalities. Although the eyes are obviously necessary for vision, the brain interprets visual symbols. Therefore, correcting subtle visual defects cannot alter the brain's processing of visual stimuli. Children with dyslexia or related learning disabilities have the same ocular health statistically as children without such conditions.[7] There is no peripheral eye defect that produces dyslexia or other learning disabilities,[8,9] and there is no eye treatment that can cure dyslexia or associated learning disabilities.

4. **The Role of the Physician.** Ocular defects should be identified as early as possible and when correctable, managed by the ophthalmologist. These treatable conditions include refractive errors, focusing deficiencies, eye muscle imbalances, and motor fusion deficiencies. The ophthalmologist may be consulted early, but, if no ocular defect is found, the child should be referred to a pediatrician to coordinate required multidisciplinary care.

5. **Controversies.** Eye defects, subtle or severe, do not cause reversal of letters, words, or numbers. No scientific evidence supports claims that the academic abilities of dyslexic or LD children can be improved with treatment based on (1) visual training, including muscle exercises, ocular pursuit, tracking exercises, or "training" glasses (with or without bifocals or prisms);[10–12] (2) neurological organizational training (laterality training, crawling, balance board, perceptual training);[13–15] or (3) tinted or colored lenses.[16,17] Some controversial methods of treatment result in a false sense of security that may delay or even prevent proper instruction or remediation. The expense of these methods is unwarranted, and they cannot be substituted for appropriate remedial educational measures. Claims of improved reading and learning after visual training, neurological organization training, or use of tinted or colored lenses are typically based upon poorly controlled studies that rely on anecdotal information or testimony. These studies are frequently carried out in combination with traditional educational remedial techniques.

6. **The Role of Education.** Teaching children, adolescents, and adults with dyslexia and learning disabilities is a challenge for educators because no single educational approach is applicable to all. The psychologist may help with educational diagnosis and classification. Physicians, including pediatricians, otolaryngologists, neurologists, ophthalmologists, and other appropriate medical specialists may assist in dealing with health problems. Because remediation may be more effective during the early years, early diagnosis is paramount.[18,19] The educator ultimately plays the key role in providing help for the LD or dyslexic child or adult.

■ Summary

Dyslexia and other related LDs are serious problems. The American Academy of Pediatrics, through its Committee on Children with Disabilities and the Section on Ophthalmology, The American Academy of Ophthalmology, and the American Association for Pediatric Ophthalmology and Strabismus strongly support the need for early diagnosis and educational remediation. There is no known eye or visual cause for dyslexia and learning disabilities and no effective visual treatment. Multidisciplinary evaluation and management must be based on proven procedures demonstrated by valid research.

REFERENCES

1. Mattis T, French JH, Rapin I. Dyslexia in children and young adults: three independent neuropsychological syndromes. *Dev Med Child Neurol* 1975; 17:150–163.
2. Vellutino FR. Dyslexia. *Scientific American* 1987; 256(3):34–41.
3. Council on Scientific Affairs. Dyslexia. *JAMA* 1989;261: 2236–2239.
4. Petersen SE, Fox PT, Posner MI, Mintun M, Raichle ME. Positron emission tomographic studies of the cortical anatomy of single-word processing. *Nature* 1988; 331:585–589.
5. Galaburda A. Ordinary and extraordinary brain development: anatomical variation in developmental dyslexia. *Ann of Dyslexia* 1989;39:67–80.
6. Hynd GW, Semrud-Clikeman M, Lorys AR, Novey ES, Eliopulos D. Brain morphology in developmental dyslexia and attention deficit disorder/hyperactivity. *Arch Neurol* 1990;47:919–926.
7. Metzger RL, Wemer DB. Use of visual training for reading disabilities: A review. *Pediatrics* 1984;73: 824–829.
8. American Academy of Pediatrics, Committee on Practice and Ambulatory Medicine and Section on Ophthalmology. Eye examination and vision screening in infants, children, and young adults. *Pediatrics* 1996;98:153–157
9. American Academy of Ophthalmology and American Association for Pediatric Ophthalmology and Strabismus. *Vision Screening for Infants and Children*. 1996.
10. Golberg HK, Drash PW. The disabled reader. *J Pediatr Ophthalmol* 1968;5:11–24.
11. Helveston EM, Weber JC, Miller K, et al. Visual function and academic performance. *Am J. Ophthalmol* 1985;99:346–355.
12. Levine MD. Reading disability: Do the eyes have it? *Pediatrics* 1984;73:869–870.
13. Keogh B, Pelland M. Vision training revisited. *J Learn Disabil* 1985;18:228–236.
14. Beauchamp GR. Optometric vision training. *Pediatrics* 1986;77:121–124.
15. Cohen HJ, Birch HG, Taft LT. Some considerations for evaluating the Doman-Delacato "patterning method." *Pediatrics* 1970;45:302–314.
16. Kavale K, Mattson PD. One jumped off the balance beam: meta-analysis of perceptual-motor training. *J Learn Disabil* 1983;16:165–173.
17. Black JL, Collins DWK, DeRoach JN, et al. A detailed study of sequential saccadic eye movements for normal and poor reading children. *Percept Mot Skills* 1984;59: 423–434.
18. Solan HA. An appraisal of the Irlen technique of correcting reading disorders using tinted overlays and tinted lenses. *J Learn Disabil* 1990;23:621–623.
19. Hoyt CS. Irlen lenses and reading difficulties. *J Learn Disabit* 1990;23:624–626.
20. Sedun AA. Dyslexia at New York Times: (mis)understanding of parallel vision processing. *Arch of Ophth* 1992; 110:933–934.
21. Bradley L. Rhyme recognition and reading and spelling in young children. In: Masland RL, Masland MW, eds. *Preschool Prevention of Reading Failure*. Parkton, MD: York Press; 1988;143–162.
22. Ogden S, Hindman S, Turner SD. Multisensory programs in the public schools: a brighter future for LD children. *Annals of Dyslexia* 1989;39:247–267.
23. Romanchuk KG. Skepticism about Irlen filters to treat learning disabilities. *CMAJ*. 1995;153:397.
24. Silver LB. Controversial therapies. *J Child Neurol*. 1995; 10 Suppl 1: S96–100.

Approved by: American Academy of Pediatrics
January 1984
American Association for Pediatric
Ophthalmology and Strabismus
February 1984
American Academy of Ophthalmology
February 1984

Revised and Approved by: American Academy of Pediatrics
American Association for Pediatric
Ophthalmology and Strabismus
American Academy of Ophthalmology
September 1998

Pediatric Ophthalmology
Edited by P. F. Gallin
Thieme Medical Publishers, Inc.
New York © 2000

7

■■■

Child Maltreatment

JOHN FIGUEROA AND RENIE EIS-FIGUEROA

Child maltreatment is defined as any physical, sexual, or emotional abuse or neglect suffered by a child as inflicted by the primary caretaker (usually the parent, but not always). Child abuse and neglect cases that are inflicted by adults other than the primary caretaker are considered criminal cases and are not covered under the social service laws that protect children from parents and caretakers in all of the 50 states.

Child maltreatment is a medical and social condition that affects not only the child victim and the entire family but also, to a certain extent, society as a whole. Child maltreatment causes a crisis that has short- and long-term consequences. In the short term, it causes a family crisis, separating the child from the parent and extended family members. In the long term, it has a dynamic impact on society in increased cost of mental health treatment, loss of employment, and most importantly the possibility of perpetuating the cycle of adult and child maltreatment.

The medical provider may face the issues of child maltreatment at any given time while providing medical care to a child or an adult. Child maltreatment may be discovered accidentally through statements from someone other than the child. The disclosure may come during a physical examination when the provider discovers injuries consistent with child maltreatment, and, when the child is asked, he may make dis-

closure of maltreatment and request help.

Child maltreatment creates challenging dilemmas for the provider. For example, what actions can be taken during an office visit to protect the child and any siblings when a disclosure of child maltreatment surfaces? How can the medical provider diagnose child maltreatment? What are the medical and psychosocial indicators for child maltreatment? Should the provider advocate for the family with Child Protective Services, and what form should this take? Should the provider advocate for the nonoffending parent to have that parent maintain custody of the child and keep the family together? Does the extended family have a role during the process of disclosure and thereafter? What are the mandated reporting requirements? Are there liabilities for reporting or failure to report? Once a case is reported to Child Protective Services for investigation, what action can the provider expect from that system? These are some of the difficult questions that will be explored in this chapter.

■ Scope of the Problem

Child maltreatment reports have continued to rise over the years. For example, in 1990 there were 2.5 million reports to Child Protective Services nationwide, a 100% increase over 1980. Deaths resulting from child maltreatment have also increased during this period. In addition, recently the criteria for reporting of deaths of children secondary to child maltreatment are being reevaluated. A standard method to classify a child's death as caused by either maltreatment or accident is being studied in New York City.

■ The Study of Child Maltreatment

We study child abuse and neglect for a very simple reason. These children need our help, and the alternative to not acting could result in the death of a child. The long-term sequellae of years of maltreatment are somewhat more difficult to quantify. Children who are maltreated do not do well in school. These children have poor peer relationships, do not form adequate attachments later in life, and often develop antisocial and criminal behaviors. In addition, children who have been maltreated may often abuse their own children, perpetuating the cycle of maltreatment from generation to generation.

■ Risk Factors

There are several risk factors, which should serve as red flags and prompt the provider to screen more closely for the presence of child abuse or neglect. The single most common thread tying many of these cases together is the presence or threat of domestic violence. Children are often caught in the middle of violent domestic disputes or may become the passive victims of their parents' actions. Additionally, later in life these children act out what they have learned, namely, that violence is the method for solving their marital problems. In addition, child abuse is very common in families where there is a history of drug or alcohol abuse. In many of these chaotic homes, the children's needs are not a priority due to their parents' addiction. Financial issues resulting from substance abuse not only cause strain in the family but also impact the child's ability to thrive in a healthy environment. Unemployment can add to the financial difficulties but

more important it can create a loss of parental self-esteem. Families where there is a history of mental illness must also be carefully screened for the potential for maltreatment. Due to the current economic crises in our country, we are rapidly creating a society of latchkey children who come from school and are forced to take care of themselves and younger siblings until their parents return home from work. In extreme cases, children have been left alone for days at a time, leading to reports of neglect to Child Protective Services.

With the increase of female head-of-household families, we also see young boys forced into roles that traditionally have been the responsibilities of the absent father, again creating an increased risk. Children learn how to become parents based on the way they have been parented. If they have been abused, there is a good chance that, without adequate prevention programs, such as home visitation to teach and support young parents, the cycle of child abuse will continue, and the young parent may abuse his or her own children. With teenage pregnancy, children are having children, usually without the necessary family supports or role models for parenting; this can lead to child maltreatment. Additionally, the young teenager now in a new role of parent without support becomes isolated at a time when family support is most needed. Overwhelmed and unable to manage the young infant, the teen has the potential of harming or neglecting the infant.

Although these risk factors in and of themselves do not serve as indicators of child maltreatment, they need to be considered and carefully probed when they are elicited in a family's history. These risk factors rarely exist in isolation, and, with a careful medical and psychosocial assessment, a more complete picture of child maltreatment, abuse, or neglect may be uncovered.

■ Indicators

Physical Indicators of Child Maltreatment, Abuse, and Neglect

There are many indicators of physical maltreatment, abuse, and neglect, but perhaps the most important consideration is the injury that cannot be explained by the parent or caretaker at the time of the medical examination. Also, any injury that is not consistent with the history provided by the parent or caretaker at the time of the medical examination should cause concern and raise the provider's level of suspicion for the possibility of child maltreatment. In cases of physical abuse the history often changes with repeated questioning by professionals. This occurs when the parent, in an effort to make the pieces fit, changes the history to conform to the injury being evaluated. The working parent is not present and not aware of the abuse and therefore develops a history that is not consistent with the injury and draws suspicion by the provider. Additionally, the parent may force the child to change the original account and recant his cry of child maltreatment. The changes in history should never be taken to mean that the story is false, and all of the histories should be followed to their conclusion, particularly the child's, as often the child is testing the provider to see if he·or she can be trusted and is willing to protect the child.

Unexplained bruises, welts, and bite marks on areas of the body that are usually protected are considered significant and probably inflicted. These include the face, lips, neck, wrists, ankles, back, inner thighs, and torso. Injuries that are bilaterally symmetrical, such as to both eyes, or that are circumferential are usually inflicted. The classic history of the child with two black eyes that "walked into a doorknob" is just one example of a history that gives you reasonable cause to suspect abuse. The likelihood of this type of injury would not be consistent with the physical examination. When bruises are in various stages of healing, the provider's level of suspicion should increase, leading to further assessment of the situation. These injuries include fresh purple or red marks as well as older healing green, yellow, or brown marks; this is called the "garden effect" because of all the colors. Clustered or repeated patterns of marks often in the shape of the article used to inflict the injury (belts or electric cord loop marks) are not uncommon in child physical abuse. Human bite marks need to be assessed carefully by a dentist to determine whether the bite marks were inflicted by an adult or a child. The dentist will usually mea-

sure the diameter of the lesion to reach a determination. Unexplained lacerations or abrasions are also indicative of abuse, especially when located on the lips, gums, eyes, or genitalia. Bald patches on the scalp should also be questioned and usually indicate that the child's hair was pulled out.

Unexplained burns from cigars or cigarettes that appear on the palms, soles, or genitalia are usually inflicted and significant for child abuse. The provider must be aware that burns are a product of both time and temperature, and it is instinctive for the child to pull away from a burning object unless held there. Patterned burns such as from curling or steam irons or rope burns of the arms, legs, or neck must also be considered suspicious for abuse and must be carefully assessed. Immersion burns from scalding water—"the dunking baby syndrome"—are suspicious for inflicted injuries due to symmetry of the burns as well as the absence of splash marks usually found in accidental scalding injuries.

Unexplained fractures or dislocations or any injuries where there is a delay in seeking medical attention must also be considered as potentially neglectful. Skull, nose, or other facial bone fractures or any fracture in various stages of healing are worrisome and require further investigation. Spiral fractures in the absence of a plausible history or bucket handle fractures are considered to be indicative of abuse.

Physical neglect or failure to thrive is somewhat less striking and difficult to assess to reach a diagnosis of child abuse. Children often demonstrate poor growth or weight gain, failure to thrive, poor hygiene, abdominal distention, or wasting of subcutaneous tissues. Children who present to the office hungry or inappropriately dressed for the season and whose medical needs are not being met or who are left alone or abandoned should be admitted to the hospital for medical evaluation and treatment in conjunction with a social service assessment and a report to Child Protective Services.

Specific Ophthalmologic Concerns

Any direct blow to the face from a fist or blunt instrument may result in bilateral periorbital swelling or ecchymoses. Also, small bruises under a child's eyes may be extremely significant as they are associated with other intracranial injuries.

Types of inflicted head injuries can include retinal hemorrhages and dislocated lenses, skull fractures, subdural hematomas, scalp bruises, and black eyes. Inflicted subdurals can be found with evidence of inflicted trauma such as fractures, scalp swelling, and bruises or without evidence of external trauma, as in the classic shaken baby syndrome or a whiplash injury, where there is no evidence of scalp swelling, skull fracture, or bruising. It is important to remember, however, that both types of subdurals can be associated with retinal hemorrhages and dislocated lenses. Subdural hematomas are rarely spontaneous in nature, and in the absence of a plausible history an inflicted injury must be considered.

Funduscopic examinations must be performed on all children under 2 years of age where there is a concern of inflicted injury or evidence of trauma, especially when head trauma is present. Retinal hemorrhages may be the only clue to the presence of subdural hematomas from a whiplash injury where there is no evidence of external trauma.

Specific discussions of ophthalmic child abuse pathology are woven throughout this text. They are also discussed in detail in Chapter 15.

Behavioral Indicators of Child Abuse and Neglect

During the medical examination, there is an opportunity to observe a child's behaviors. Children may exhibit extremes of behavior from being aggressive to overly compliant or submissive, from being wary of adult contact to feeling deserving of punishment. Children who appear frightened of their parents or who are afraid to go home must be protected. When children respond with a vacant stare or in monosyllables, it should be met with concern, and yet many abused children will exhibit manipulative or precocious behavior seeking affection indiscriminately. In advanced cases, children will resort to criminal behavior such as stealing, prostitution, drug use, truancy, and attempted suicide. Neglected children also can exhibit habit disorders such as rocking and biting and neurotic disorders such as sleep disorders, tics, and psychoses such as obsessions and phobias. These behaviors should raise the provider's index of suspicion especially when accompanied by an unexplained or inconsistent injury.

Indicators of Sexual Abuse

Sexual abuse is a specialized form of physical abuse. Unfortunately, most cases of sexual abuse do not have physical findings. In cases of sexual abuse where the injury is not acute, the exam is best done in a child-friendly space where the child can feel comfortable and will not be retraumatized. More recently, the child advocacy center and not the hospital's emergency room is the more appropriate location to evaluate a child's complaint of sexual abuse. In an acute presentation of child sexual abuse, there may be complaints of difficulty walking or sitting. The child may experience pain on urination or bleeding. The child may have some bruises or lacerations to the genitalia. There may also be a vaginal or penile discharge. Sexually transmitted venereal disease, pregnancy, presence of foreign bodies, or bruises to the hard or soft palate are all suspicious for child sexual abuse. Poor sphincter tone can be observed as a late but significant symptom as it may point to ongoing anal sexual abuse. Children who are sexually abused are often unwilling to change their clothes for gym or during a medical examination. Children may wear layers of clothing to make themselves unattractive or to hide marks or scars. Many sexually abused children exhibit either infantile behavior or provocative behavior. Children seen as perpetrators of sexual abuse on younger children have often been victims themselves and they need help as well. Overly sexualized behavior or sexual knowledge that is not age appropriate can be an indication of sexual abuse.

In acute cases of rape, the medical examination must be done with care to preserve any physical evidence found and to keep it free from contamination. However, sexual abuse is often a gradual increase in attention and fondling of a child, accompanied by promises of gifts and threats against the child or family members if the "secret" is not kept.

Indicators of Emotional Abuse

Children who suffer from emotional neglect often have very low self-esteem and feel they will not amount to much. Habit disorders, neuroses, and psychoses are common. Speech delays, hyperactivity, and emotional failure to thrive are also present in these cases. Any time a child is emotionally abused, an observant professional can find some indicators of stress in the child. Indeed, any of the behaviors previously elucidated can be evidence of emotional neglect.

■ The Interview

Because many cases of child maltreatment have no medical findings, the interview is the important method of diagnosing child maltreatment. Diagnosis of child maltreatment can best be accomplished by conducting a thorough, careful interview of the child that identifies the familial risk factor.

Although there are various accepted methods of interviewing a child, these methods require many sessions over several weeks and usually occur long after the initial incident or disclosure. During the office visit or the emergency room visit, the decision to mobilize the child protective system is critical and must be made prior to discharging and returning the child back to the home environment. It goes without saying that once confronted with the issue of child abuse the decision whether to activate the child protective system must be made by the provider. The provider's physical findings may fall short of a definitive diagnosis of child abuse as stated earlier. Therefore, the interview becomes the key factor in obtaining the necessary information to reach an informed determination as to whether child abuse might have occurred, and the matter requires a report to Child Protective Services. However, the provider must be prepared to devote great care from beginning to end as this effort requires time, patience, and a great deal of skill. Although it is always preferable to have the most skilled professional interview the child, it is not always possible. Any provider must be will-

ing to begin the process in the best interest of the patient and his or her family.

Things to consider before the interview are the following: the interviewer, the location of the interview, the timing of the interview, and the follow-up plan. Will the area where the child is to be interviewed be free of interruptions by other staff? Is the room comfortable and free of distractions so that the child will feel safe, yet not be distracted from the interview? Is the room large enough to allow the child some personal space or to allow for some time out from the interview? Is the room in close proximity to the parent, allowing the child a break to be reassured that the parent has not abandoned the child during this time? The timing of the interview is important because a child who is tired or hungry may be unable to concentrate, and therefore the information gathered may not be accurate.

Additionally, if the interview schedule conflicts with an important activity that the child has been anticipating it may also influence the information gathered. The interview should also be conducted during a reasonable time and not in the middle of the night in the emergency room or in an office. It is critical that the interview be accomplished without the parent present, as having a parent in the room may contaminate the interview. Children looking for approval from adults may look to the parent for support and encouragement. The parent may sit in a position to offer a nod of the head or a smile of encouragement or may help the child finish sentences. All of these actions by the parent although innocent may lead the child into giving a distorted account of what happened. The parent may also offer a reward for telling the truth or for giving the "correct" answer. Finally, and most importantly, the parent may not be aware that anything happened to the child or may not have heard the details of what happened. This revelation may prove overwhelming for the parent, causing uneasiness accompanied by some form of bodily or facial motion, which could prove disruptive to the narrative the child is giving. The provider should discuss all aspects of the evaluation and interventions with the parent. If this is done the parent will have a better understanding of the process and a more favorable outcome may occur.

The interviewer must maintain a professional posture at all times. The interviewer should not offer any words of encouragement such as "that's a good child" or touch the child in a gesture of support or approval for what the child is saying. It is also best to be at eye level with the child so as not to give the appearance of towering over or intimidating the child. The interviewer should be culturally competent. The use of interpreters should be considered as a last resort when a native speaker is not available and if used at all should be limited in scope.

The three phases of the recommended interview process are the engagement-rapport building phase, the fact-finding phase, and the termination phase.

Engagement and Rapport Building Phase

A child who is brought to the office or to the emergency department for care needs to know that the provider will be an active listener to the complaints and history given by the child. It is therefore critical that the provider demonstrates this to the child by creating a safe environment, allowing the child to become comfortable with both the setting and the provider. It is during this phase that the interviewer makes an effort to put the child at ease. This can be accomplished by engaging the child in a general discussion of areas of interest that are familiar to the child. These areas may include discussion of school activities, the child's teacher, the classroom and seating assignments, the child's favorite school subject, the child's best friend at school, and a common activity that they share together. The interviewer's role here is one of listener and evaluator while the child is sharing information. The interviewer is also evaluating the child's developmental level and language.

Additionally, it is important to remember that the questions posed by the interviewer must be at the child's cognitive level; otherwise, the child may be confused by the question and provide an inaccurate account of the incident.

Another area that may be explored and usually will lead to further discussion is the child's home. The interviewer may ask the child to describe the home. For example, the number of bedrooms, where the child's room is in relation to the master bedroom, the kitchen, the bathroom, or siblings' rooms. Here the interviewer is again evaluating the child's language, memory, and descriptive ability regarding positioning and color of the furniture and the location of bedrooms. Additionally, if the child is involved in some form of day care arrangements after school, the interviewer would also explore this home, and the child should be able to give information about this home. The interviewer however must be careful not to confuse the child when asking questions related to this day care home versus the natural home. Having the child identify who lives in the home as well as who sleeps in the home can provide important information later in the interview. The interviewer must keep in mind that at times adults that sleep in the home may be different from those who visit the home during the day or spend time in the home when the child is in the home. Any home activities such as watching television programs or participating in after-school activities allow the child to give the interviewer an idea of where the child is socially and where he or she is ranked within the family. It allows the interviewer to gauge what happens to the child in the home environment as well as who cares for the child when the parents are absent. The interviewer may want to explore a recent family event such as a birthday party, a holiday, or another special event. These initial exploratory questions help to engage the child in a nonthreatening manner and at the same time allow the child to become comfortable with the interviewer.

The Fact-Finding Phase

During this phase the interviewer has already determined the child's development level, knows the child's level of vocabulary and use of descriptive words and ability to give time frames, and understands the cognitive ability of the child. It is important in the initial stages of the evaluation that the child be given the opportunity to share the history in a free-flowing narrative, without interrupting questions from the interviewer, allowing the child to give an account of what if anything occurred. The interviewer must remain neutral and refrain from any verbal, facial, or body changes when hearing the child's history, whether or not there is a disclosure, remembering that the goal is to obtain the facts from the child.

One method to begin the fact-finding phase, although elementary, is to ask the child, "Why are you here?" With this question, the interviewer hopes to elicit the child's understanding of why he or she was brought to the medical provider's office and why a medical examination is necessary.

The questions should be open ended such as, "Can you tell me what happened?" To have the child continue the narrative the interviewer may use the phrases "and then what happened?" and "after that what happened?" The interviewer must be mindful not to introduce anyone's name or any type of descriptive information that would lead the child and contaminate the interview. Introduction of characters may cause the child to think that the interviewer is aware of what happened and cause the child either to take a shortcut in describing the incident or to assume that the interviewer already knows what happened. Additionally, it leads the child into providing information that may not be accurate. If the opened-question approach fails, a more directive and leading approach could be used, as long as the approach is documented in the child's chart. Documentation is important, particularly when the case is heard in the court system and the interviewer is questioned as to the methods used to obtain the disclosure.

When exploring the abusive incident use the child's own terminology based on the child's developmental and cognitive level that were assessed earlier. It is also important to document the information gathered by the child. In an attempt to draw the child out but remain within his or her developmental capabilities the interviewer should try to explore the duration and frequency of the incidents and location and whatever tastes, touches, and smells the child might remember. The child might also remember other people being at home or possibly participating in the incident. The child should describe the presence or absence of clothing and describe it if possible as well as identifying any force, coercion, or threats made. Try not to interrupt or interpret the child's statements or put them into acceptable adult terms. Allow the child to stop the interview or decline to answer a specific question. The child may need a break during the interview to visit with parents and be reassured that he or she has not been abandoned. Interviewing a child in a medical setting can be a challenging experience and should be approached with a great deal of care and sensitivity to the child, the siblings, and the family.

The Termination Phase

The termination phase allows the child to explore his or her feelings about the disclosure and to gain answers to questions or address fears about what happens next. The child must be reassured that the abuse was not his or her fault, and, if the parent is unaware of the incident, the interviewer should offer to serve as the liaison to discuss the incident with the parent. Explain the next steps to the child and the family, including reporting and investigation processes.

Arrange for medical and social service follow-up at an appropriate site, may include a follow-up visit at the local child advocacy center. Additionally, it is important to coordinate the follow-up visit with other agencies to ensure the child's safety and ongoing protection.

Additional Interviews

An interview with the family members, the extended family, teachers, primary care provider, and so forth should be conducted if possible to corroborate or enhance the child's description of the family, the setting, and even the incident if possible.

■ The Report

Professionals report their suspicion of child maltreatment because it is the law in the United States. After Kemp's article in 1962, which introduced the "battered child syndrome," all 50 states established statutory reporting requirements that mandate professionals to report cases of child abuse to the authorities. The professional who fails to report a case to the authorities may face both criminal and civil liabilities. More importantly, reporting child maltreatment to the authorities assists in stopping the cycle of maltreatment by securing support services for the family and may prevent the death of a child. In New York State, for example, the provider is required to report a suspicion of child maltreatment through the New York State Central Registry, which is staffed 24 hours a day, 7 days a week. The telephone number is 1-800-635-1522. Other states have their own hotline, and the provider should be familiar with the state's procedure and protocol in advance of confronting a child abuse case. Additionally, states also have area or regional child advocacy centers, where the issues of child abuse are addressed and could prove of some assistance to the provider in the initial stages and the follow-up management of these cases.

Hospitals are required by the Joint Commission on Accreditation of Hospitals to have a staff person designated to function as a child protection specialist. This person acts as the hospital's consultant in the identification and reporting of child abuse cases; monitors, coordinates, and manages these cases; and acts as the liaison among agencies mandated to investigate child abuse reports by hospital staff.

The child protective service agency and the caseworker are required to contact the source of the report within 24 hours of the report. This can happen by either visiting the provider at the office or by discussing the case on the telephone. Also, the caseworker must visit the child within 72 hours of receiving the report. This can be accomplished either at school, if the child is of school age, or at the child's home.

Once the provider files the report of child maltreatment to the authorities, it is up to the child protective agency to investigate and provide the appropriate interventions ensuring the protection of the child. Additionally, the child protective agency is required to complete a safety assessment of the child's home. If the child's home environment is determined to be unsafe, the child may be removed and placed in a safe environment such as through foster care placement. Then the case must be brought to the family court for disposition. The court process can be a lengthy one and may require that the provider maintain ongoing contact with the child protective caseworker and the court until the case reaches a final disposition. If, however, child protective services determines that the child's home environment is safe and removing the child is not necessary, the family court is not involved, and the agency provides the necessary services to the family, such as parent skills training, counseling, or help at home.

In New York State, one option the provider has is to admit the child to the hospital for protective custody involving the child protective agency directly. If admission to the hospital is not an option, the provider must advocate to have the child protective agency take appropriate action to ensure the child's safety. At no time should a provider discharge a child to an unsafe environment.

■ Conclusion

The concept that a parent has the right to raise children as he or she sees fit must be balanced against the child's right to grow up in a relatively safe and healthy environment. Interventions by health professionals and child protection agencies should not be regarded as for the child and against the parents, but rather for the family as a whole.

■ Resources

1. American Humane Association (Denver, CO): tel. (303) 695-0811.
2. C. Henry Kemp National Center for Prevention of Child Abuse/Neglect (Denver, CO): tel. (303) 321-3963.
3. Child Welfare League of America (Washington, DC): tel. (202) 638-2952.

4. Children's Defense Fund (Washington, DC): tel. (202) 628-8787.

5. Family Resource Coalition (Chicago, IL): tel. (312) 726-4750.

6. National Center of Child Abuse/Neglect (Washington, DC): tel. (202) 245-0616.

7. National Coalition Against Domestic Violence (Washington, DC): tel. (202) 638-6385.

8. National Committee for Prevention of Child Abuse (Chicago, IL): tel. (312) 663-3520.

9. National Network of Child Advocacy Centers (Washington, DC): tel. (202) 639-0597.

10. National Resource Center for Child Maltreatment (Baltimore, MD): tel. (800) 628-9944.

11. NY State Mandated Reporters-Central Registry Hotline: tel. (800) 635-1522.

SUGGESTED READINGS

American Academy of Pediatric Dentistry. Child abuse and neglect. *Pediatr Dentist.* 1986; 8:65–121. Special issue.

Anderson CL. Assessing parental potential for child abuse risk. *Pediatr Nursing.* 1987;13(5):323–332.

Asen, K et al. A systems approach to child abuse: management and treatment issues. *Child Abuse Neglect.* 1989;13:45–47.

Behanan N, Kiblinsky S. Child sexual abuse: the educator's role in prevention, detection, and intervention. *Young Childr.* September 1984.

Brassard M et al, eds. *The Psychological Maltreatment of Children and Youth.* Elmsford, NY: Pergamon Press; 1986.

Broadhurst D. *Educators, Schools, and Abuse.* Chicago: National Committee for the Prevention of Child Abuse; 1986.

Council on Scientific Affairs. AMA diagnostic and treatment guidelines concerning child abuse and neglect. *JAMA.* 1985; 254:796–800.

Cupoli M. Piecing together the pattern of child abuse. *Contemp Pediatr.* 1987; 4:12–30.

De Young M. A conceptual model for judging the truthfulness of a young child's allegation of sexual abuse. *Am J Orthopsychiatry.* 1986; 564:550–559.

Doxiadis SA. Children, society, and ethics. *Child Abuse Neglect.* 1989;13:11–17.

Dukes RL, Kean RB. An experimental study of gender and situation in the perception and reportage of child abuse. *Child Abuse Neglect.* 1989; 13:351–360.

Epstein MA, Markowitz RL, Gallor DM, et al. Munchausen syndrome by proxy: considerations in the diagnosis and confirmation by video surveillance. *Pediatrics.* 1987; 80(2):220–224.

Fallar KC. Characteristics of a clinical sample of sexually abused children: how boy and girl victims differ. *Child Abuse Neglect.* 1989;13:281–291.

Fallar KC. *Child Sexual Abuse.* New York: Columbia University; 1988.

Fallar KC. Decision-making in cases of intrafamilial child sexual abuse. *Am J Orthopsychiatry.* 1988; 58(1):121–128.

Feldman KW. Child abuse by burning. In: Helfer RE, Kempe RS, eds. *The Battered Child.* 4th ed. Chicago: University of Chicago Press; 1988:197–213.

Ferleger N, et al. Identifying correlates of reabuse in maltreating parents. *Child Abuse Neglect.* 1988;12:4–19.

Finkelhor D. What's wrong with sex between adults and children? Ethics and the problem of sexual abuse. *Am J Orthopsychiatry.* 1979; 49(4):692–697.

Finkelhor D, Browne A. The traumatic impact of child sexual abuse: a conceptualization. *Am J Orthopsychiatry.* 1985; 55(4):530–541.

Finkelhor D, Hotaling GT. Sexual abuse in the National Incidence Study of Child Sexual Abuse and Neglect: an appraisal. *Child Abuse Neglect.* 1984;8:23–33.

Gale J. et al. Sexual abuse in young children: its clinical presentation and characteristics patterns. *Child Abuse Neglect.* 1988;12:163–170.

Gammon JA. Ophthalmic manifestations of child abuse. In: Ellerstein NS, ed. *Child Abuse and Neglect: A Medical Reference.* New York: John Wiley & Sons; 1981:73–93.

Garbarino J, et al. *The Psychologically Battered Child.* San Francisco: Jossey-Bass; 1987.

Helfer RE, Kempe CH. *The Battered Child.* 4th ed. Chicago, IL: University of Chicago Press; 1988.

Hibbard RA, et al. Genitalia in children's drawings: an association with sexual abuse. *Pediatrics.* 1987;79(1):129–137.

Kelley SJ. Interviewing the sexually abused child. *J Emerg. Nurs.* 1985;11(5):224–234.

Kelley SJ. Sexual abuse of children. In: *Pediatric Emergency Nursing.* Norwalk, CT: Appleton and Lange; 1988:27–51.

Kempe CH. Cross cultural perspectives in child abuse. *Pediatrics.* 1982; 497–498.

Kempe CH, Goldbloom RB. Malnutrition and growth retardation ("failure to thrive") in the context of child abuse and neglect. In: Helfer RE, Kempe CH, eds. *The Battered Child.* 4th ed. Chicago, IL: University of Chicago Press; 1988:312–336.

Kempe CH, et al. The battered-child syndrome. *JAMA.* 1962; 181(1):17–24.

Klein DM. Central nervous system injuries. In: Ellerstein NS, ed. *Child Abuse and Neglect: A Medical Reference.* New York, NY: John Wiley & Sons; 1981.

Korbin J. Child abuse and neglect: the cultural context. In: Helfer RE, Kempe CH, eds. *The Battered Child.* Chicago: University of Chicago Press; 1988:23–41.

Ludwig S. Child abuse. In: Fleisher G, Ludwig S, eds. *Textbook of Pediatric Emergency Medicine.* 2nd ed. Baltimore, MD: Williams & Wilkins; 1988.

Money J. Munchausen's syndrome by proxy. *J Pediatr Psychol.* 1986;11(4):583–584.

Paradise JE. Predictive accuracy and the diagnosis of sexual abuse: a big issue about a little tissue. *Child Abuse Neglect.* 1989; 13:169–176.

Parker H, Parker S. Father-daughter sexual abuse: an emerging perspective. *Am J Orthopsychiatry.* 1986; 56(4):631–649.

Payne MA. Use and abuse of corporal punishment: a Caribbean view. *Child Abuse Neglect.* 1989;13:389–401.

Reece RN, Groden MA. Recognition of non-accidental injury. *Pediatr. Clin North Am.* 1985; 32(1):41–60.

Sgori SM. *Handbook of Clinical Intervention in Child Sexual Abuse.* Lexington, MA: Lexington Books; 1982.

Study of National Incidence and Relevance of Child Abuse and Neglect: Study Findings. National Center on Child Abuse and Neglect, U.S. Children's Bureau, Administration for Children, Youth and Families, Office of Human Development Services, USDHHS (Contract 105-85-1702); 1988.

Summit RC. (1983). The child sexual abuse accommodation syndrome. *Child Abuse Neglect.* 1983; 7:177–193.

Tower CC. *Child Abuse and Neglect: A Teacher's Handbook for Detection, Reporting, and Classroom Management.* Washington, DC: National Education Association; 1984.

U.S. Department of Health and Human Services. *Sexual Abuse of Children: Selected Readings.* USDHHS Publications (No. OHDS 78-30161).

Vander Mey BJ. The sexual victimization of male children: a review of previous research. *Child Abuse Neglect.* 1988;12:61–72.

Wolverton LM. *What's A Teacher To Do? Child Abuse Education for the Classroom.* ESCAPE, Family Life Development Center, Ithaca, NY: Cornell University; 1987.

Wohl A, Kaufman B. *Silent Screams and Hidden Cries.* New York: Brunner and Mazel; 1985.

Worlock P, et al. Patterns of fractures in accidental and non-accidental injury in children. *Br Med J.* 1986; 293:100–103.

Pediatric Ophthalmology
Edited by P. F. Gallin
Thieme Medical Publishers, Inc.
New York © 2000

8

Ocular Genetics

CHRISTINA BUTERA, JAMES PLOTNIK, J. BRONWYN BATEMAN, DEBORAH ALCORN, AND IRENE MAUMENEE

As the prevalence of communicable diseases capable of causing intrauterine embryopathies decreases worldwide, the relative importance of genetic bases for congenital malformations has increased. The identification, evaluation, and treatment of such disorders is multidisciplinary and, with few exceptions, should include the ophthalmologist. The key initial step is the establishment of a diagnosis to determine organ involvement, the spectrum of prognosis, affected status of relatives if desired, and recurrence risks for future offspring. About one half of visually impaired children have a heritable condition.

Historical information is useful and includes detailed prenatal, developmental, and family information. The prenatal history should include the ages of both mother and father and consanguinity as increased paternal age is associated with single gene mutations and increased maternal age is associated with chromosomal rearrangements. Review of previous pregnancies for miscarriages, stillbirths, and spontaneous abortions is useful, including prenatal testing; questions should be carefully phrased so as not to convey blame. Delivery information, birth weight, and Apgar scores can be very helpful in elucidating the state of the newborn infant. Known abnormalities at birth and details of initial hospitalization are helpful, for example, intracerebral bleeds, retinopathy of prematurity, surgery, and hospi-

talizations. Key questions include assessment of developmental milestones; the physician should distinguish between developmental delay and regression. The family history should delineate ocular disorders as well as other diseases such as seizures and developmental delay; for some disorders such as neurofibromatosis, cataracts, nystagmus, colobomata, and tuberous sclerosis, both parents should undergo an eye examination to determine the genetic basis. If one or more congenital abnormalities are present with delayed development and a diagnosis is not readily identifiable, chromosomal analysis should be obtained. A comprehensive eye exam should be performed on the patient. All families of patients with a genetic disease or the possibility of a genetic disease should undergo formal genetic evaluation by a geneticist to ensure understanding of the condition and reproductive alternatives; such referrals will minimize medical–legal risk for unexpected recurrence in future offspring.

Although there are many congenital/infantile abnormalities, we will limit our discussion to case studies of a few selected entities. The ocular findings of isolated ocular and periocular monogenic disorders (Table 8–1), ocular findings in multisystem syndromes (Table 8–2), ocular findings in metabolic disorders (Table 8–3), and ocular findings in selected chromosomal syndromes (Table 8–4) are summarized.

TABLE 8–1. Isolated Ocular and Periocular Monogenic Disorders

Achromatopsia (rod monochromatism)	Congenital absence of cone photoreceptors	AR, XLR
Aniridia	Absent iris tissue, glaucoma, foveal hypoplasia, cataracts	AD
Anterior megalocornea	Bilateral megalocornea, subluxed lenses	XLR
Axenfeld-Rieger anomaly	Posterior embryotoxin, iris strands, iris abnormalities	AD
Best disease	Bilateral retinal macular dystrophy	AD
Blepharophimosis-ptosis syndrome	Bilateral ptosis, epicanthus inversus, telecanthus	AD
Blue cone monochromatism	Nonprogressive disorder of cones, nystagmus, poor vision	XLR
Choroideremia	Progressive choriocapillaris and RPE degeneration	XLR
Congenital cataracts	Opacities of the crystalline lens	AD, AR, XLR
Congenital color blindness	Red-green color blindness or confusion	XLR
	Blue-yellow confusion	AD
Congenital hereditary endothelial bilateral dystrophy	Corneal haze, thickened cornea	AR > AD
Congenital-infantile glaucoma	Elevated intraocular pressure	AR
Congenital ocular fibrosis syndrome	Fibrosis of extraocular muscles, strabismus	AD > AR
Congenital stationary night blindness	Nonprogressive nyctalopia, variable visual acuity associated with poor vision, nystagmus, myopia	AD, AR XLR
Cornea plana	Flat corneal curvature	AR, AD
Cryptophthalmos	Fusion of eyelids, brow abnormalities, microphthalmia	AR
Degenerative myopia	High myopia, lacquer cracks, RPE atrophy	AR
Distichiasis	Extra row of abnormal lashes along lid margin	AD
Duane syndrome	Abnormal ocular motility associated with lid elevation	AD
Ectopia lentis et pupillae	Bilateral eccentric pupils, subluxed lenses, miosis	AR
Epithelial basement membrane dystrophy	Cortical epithelial and basement membrane abnormalities	AD
Familial exudative vitreoretinopathy	Peripheral retinal vascular abnormalities, RD	AD, XLR
Fleck corneal dystrophy	Corneal stromal opacities	AD
Fundus albipunctatus	Nonprogressive nyctalopia, midperipheral white dots	AR
Gelatinous droplike dystrophy	Localized corneal amyloidosis	AR
Goldmann-Favre syndrome	Bilateral vitreoretinal degeneration, nyctalopia	AR
Granular corneal dystrophy	Corneal stromal opacities	AD
Hereditary optic atrophy	Bilateral vision loss, optic nerve pallor	AD, AR
Jansen disease	Similar to Wagner disease, however RD common	AD
Keratoglobus	Corneal thinning, Descemet's breaks, astigmatism	AR
Lattice corneal dystrophy	Corneal stromal opacities	AD
Leber congenital amaurosis	Generalized tapetoretinal degeneration, abnormal ERG	AR (AD rare)
Macular corneal dystrophy	Corneal stromal opacities	AR
Meesmann corneal dystrophy	Corneal intraepithelial cysts	AD
Megalocornea	Enlarged corneal diameter	AD
Microcornea	Decreased corneal diameter	AD, AR
Microphthalmia	Congenital reduction of ocular volume	AD
Ocular albinism	Nystagmus, iris transillumination, macular hypoplasia	AR, XLR
Oguchi disease	Nonprogressive nyctalopia	AR
Optic nerve drusen	Hyaline and/or calcium deposits in the optic disc	AD
Peters anomaly	Corneal opacification, lenticulocorneal adhesions	AR, AD
Posterior embryotoxin	Anteriorly displaced ring of Schwalbe	AD
Posterior polymorphous dystrophy	Opacities on posterior corneal surface	AD
Progressive cone dystrophy	Progressive cone dysfunction	AD
Reis-Buckler corneal dystrophy	Corneal dystrophy affecting Bowman's layer	AD
Retinitis pigmentosa	Progressive degeneration of the photoreceptors	AD, AR, XL
Retinitis punctata albescens	White dots across retina, nyctalopia	AR
Schnyder crystalline dystrophy	Corneal stromal opacities	AD
Simple ectopia lentis	Subluxed lens	AD
Stargardt's disease; fundus flavmaculatus	Bilateral retinal macular dystrophy	AR, AD
Uveal coloboma	Incomplete closure of embryonic fissure	AD, AR, XLR
Wagner disease	Vitreoretinal degeneration, myopia, cataracts, glaucoma	AD
X-linked retinoschisis	Stellate maculopathy, peripheral retinoschisis	XLR

AD = autosomal dominant, AR = autosomal recessive, XLR = X-linked recessive, RD = retinal detachment, ERG = electroretinogram, RPE = retinal pigment epithelium.

TABLE 8–2. Ocular Findings in Multisystem Syndromes

Disease	Ocular Manifestations	Inheritance
Osteogenesis imperfecta congenita	Corneal arcus, keratoconus, glaucoma, megalocornea blue sclera, cataracts	AR
van der Hoeve	Blue sclera	AD
Osteopetrosis	Cranial nerve palsies; optic atrophy	AR, AD
Robert	Congenital cataracts	AR
Schwartz-Jampel	Blepharophimosis	AR
Spondyloepiphyseal dysplasia congenita	High myopia, vitreous syneresis, lattice degeneration of retina	AD
Stickler	High myopia, retinal detachments	AD
Weill-Marchesani	Ectopia lentis, shallow anterior chamber	AD
Wildervanck	Duane syndrome	??
Neurologic		
Aicardi	Chorioretinal lacunar lesions	XD
Alpers diffusecerebral degeneration	Cortical blindness	AR
Ataxia-telangectasia	Tortuosity of conjunctival vessels	AR
Behr	Optic atrophy	AR
Caravan	Optic atrophy, nystagmus	AR
Charcot-Marie-Tooth	Optic atrophy, tonic pupils	AR, AD, XR
Familial dysautonomia (Riley-Day)	Decreased tear production, corneal hypesthesia, corneal breakdown with scarring, optic atrophy, corneal ulcers	
Infantile subacute necrotizing encephalomyelopathy	Optic atrophy, nystagmus	AR
Marinesco-Sjogren	Congenital cataracts	AR
Meckel-Gruber	Colobomatous microphthalmia	AR
Olivopontocerebellar (OPCAIII)	Retinal degeneration	AD
Sjogren	Congenital cataracts	AR
Sjogren-Larrson	Colobomatous microphthalmia	AR
Warburg	Microphthalmia, congenital retinal detachment	AR
Dermatologic Syndromes		
Basal cell nevus	Colobomatous microphthalmia, cataract	AD
Cockayne	Juvenile cataracts, retinitis pigmentosa	AR
Cross	Microphthalmia	AR
Dyskeratosis congenita	Blepharitis, nasalacrimal duct obstruction	
Ectodermal dysplasia (anhidrotic)	Alacrima or decreased tear production	XR, AR
Ehlers-Danlos		
Type I, II, III	Retinal detachment	AD
Type VI	Blue sclera, retinal detachment, scleral rupture, keratoconus, ectopia lentis	AR
Focal dermal hypoplasia (Goltz-Gorlin)	Conjunctival papillomas, colobomatous microphthalmia	XD

TABLE 8–2. *(continued)*   Ocular Findings in Multisystem Syndromes

Disease	Ocular Manifestations	Inheritance
Hereditary benign intraepithelial dyskeratosis	Conjunctival gelatinous plaques, corneal dyskeratosis	AD
Histiocytic dermato-arthritis Ichthyosis	Glaucoma, uveitis, cataracts	AD
Congenital ichthyosis (harlequin fetus)	Ectropion, congenital cataracts	AR
Lamellar ichthyosis	Ectropion	AR
Ichthyosis vulgaris	Blepharitis, corneal erosions	AD
Bullous ichthyosiform erythroderma	Blepharitis	AD
X-linked, ichthyosis	Blepharitis, corneal erosions	XR
Incontinentia pigmenti	Infantile retinal detachment cataracts	XD
Lipoid proteinosis (Urbach-Wiethe)	Hyalinized deposition in mucous membrane and lids,corectopia	AR
Marfan syndrome	Ectopia lentis, glaucoma retinal detachment, myopia	AD
Melkersson-Rosenthal	VII nerve palsy and corneal exposure	AD
Pachyonychia congenita	Corneal dyskeratosis, cataracts	AD
Pseudoxanthoma elasticum	Blue sclera, angioid streaks, myopia, drusen	AR, AD
Rothmund-Tompson	Acquired cataracts	AR
Waardenburg	Lateral displacement of lacrimal punctae, heterochromia of irides, pigmentary, variability within or between fundi, strabismus	AD
Xeroderma pigmentosa	Lid telangectases, photophobia, conjunctivitis	AR
Craniofacial Syndromes		
Cerebro-oculo-facial-skeletal	Microphthalmia, infantile Cataracts	AR
Cornelia de Lange	Long eyelashes, synophrys, optic atrophy	??
Cryptophthalmia	Fusion of eyelids, brow abnormalities, microphthalmia	AR
Goldenhar-Gorlin (oculoauriculo vertebral-dysplasia)	Epibulbar choristomas, strabismus, blepharoptosis, eyelid defects, optic nerve hypoplasia, tortuous retinal vessels, macular hypoplasia, microphthalmia, anophthalmia, lacrimal drainage system anomalies, colobomas	??
Hallermann-Streiff	Congenital cataracts, microphthalmia	??
Lenz microphthalmia	Microphthalmia, colobomatous or noncolobomatous	AR
Moebius	Congenital VI and VII nerve palsy, corneal exposure	AD
Reiger	Iris hypoplasia, pseudopolycoria, glaucoma	AD
Rubinstein-Taybi	Coloboma, glaucoma, cataract, strabismus, optic atrophy	??

continued on next page

TABLE 8–2. *(continued)* Ocular Findings in Multisystem Syndromes

Disease	Ocular Manifestations	Inheritance
Smith-Lemli-Opitz	Congenital cataracts	AR
Treacher Collins (Franceschetti)	Lid defects, antimongoloid slant to lids	AD
Whistling face (Freeman-Sheldon)	Ptosis	AD
William	Stellate pattern of iris, strabismus abnormalities of retinal vessels	
Hematologic Syndromes		
Granulomatous disease (chronic) of childhood	Chorioretinal lesions, blepharitis	XR
Fanconi	Noncolobomatous microphthalmia	AR
Diamond-Blackfin	Noncolobomatous microphthalmia	AR
Hemoglobin SS	Venous tortuosity, vascular occlusion, comma-shaped conjunctival capillaries	AR
Hemoglobin SC	Sea-fan arteriovenous shunts, vascular occlusion	
Phakomatoses		
Sturge-Weber	Glaucoma, choroidal hemangioma, choroidal effusion	??
Neurofibromatosis	Neurofibromas, congenital glaucoma, optic nerve glioma, Lisch nodules	AD
Tuberous sclerosis	Retinal hamartomas, punched-out chorioretinal defects, iris depigmentation, angiofibromas of lids, poliosis	AD
von Hippel-Lindau	Retinal hemangioma	AD
Wyburn-Mason malformations	Retinal arteriovenous, optic atrophy	??
Multisystem		
Alstrom	Retinal degeneration, optic atrophy	XR
Bloom	Conjunctivitis; conjunctivial telangectasia	
Jeune	Retinal degeneration	AR
Joubert	Retinal degeneration	
Mulibrey nanism	Retinal hypopigmentation, retinal pigment epithelial clumping	AR
Multiple endocrine neoplasia IIB	Conjunctival and eyelid neuromas, keratoconjunctivitis sicca	AD
III (mucosal neuromata)	Conjunctival neuroma	AD
Multiple endocrine deficiency	Keratitis, anterior stromal vascularization autoimmune disease, candidiasis, and keratitis	AR
Noonan (Turner phenotype)	Cataract, ptosis, coloboma	??
Saldino-Mainzer	Retinal degeneration	AR
Werner	Cataracts, retinal degeneration	AR
Wolfram	Optic atrophy	AR

AD = autosomal dominant, AR = autosomal recessive, XR = X-linked recessive, XD = X-linked dominant, ?? = unknown.

TABLE 8–3. Ocular Findings in Metabolic Disorders

Disease	*Ocular Manifestations*	*Inheritance*
Lysosomal storage disorders		
Sphingolipid storage		
Niemann-Pick A	Corneal clouding, anterior lens capsule clouding, macular grayness or cherry red spot, optic atrophy	AR
B	Macular granularity	AR
C(D,E)	Not affected	AR
Gaucher	Strabismus, brown pingueculas, macular grayness, white retinal deposits	AR
Fabry	Cornea verticillata, spoke-like cataract, saccular conjunctival and retinal vessels	XR
GM1-I gangliosidosis	Cherry-red spot, optic atrophy, variable corneal clouding	AR
Juvenile gangliosidosis (GM1-II)	Cherry-red spot	AR
Tay-Sachs (GM2-I)	Cherry-red spot, optic atrophy	AR
Sandhoff (GM2-II)	Cherry-red spot, optic atrophy	AR
Juvenile GM2 gangliosidosis (GM2-III)	Cherry-red spot, optic atrophy	AR
Pelizaeus-Merzbacher (diffuse cerebral sclerosis)	Optic atrophy	XR
Krabbe	Optic atrophy	AR
Metachromatic leukodystrophy		
Infantile	Possible cherry-red spot, optic atrophy	AR
Juvenile	Optic atrophy	AR
Adult	Optic atrophy	AR
Multiple sulfatase deficiency	Cherry-red spot, cataracts retinal degeneration	AR
Fucosidosis	Conjunctival and retinal vessels tortuosity	AR
Sialidosis (Mucolipidosis I)	Variable cherry-red spot	AR
Mannosidosis	Cataract, corneal clouding	AR
Mucopolysaccharidoses		
Hurler (I-H)	Corneal clouding, peripheral retinal degeneration, optic atrophy	AR
Scheie (I-S)	Corneal clouding, peripheral retinal degeneration, optic atrophy	
Hunter (II) (2 types)	Peripheral retinal degeneration, optic atrophy	XR
San Filippo (III) (4 types)	Peripheral retinal degeneration, optic atrophy	AR
Morquio (IV)	Corneal clouding, optic atrophy	AR

continued on next page

TABLE 8–3.   *(continued)*   Ocular Findings in Metabolic Disorders

Disease	Ocular Manifestations	Inheritance
Maroteaux-Lamy (VI) (2 types)	Corneal clouding, optic atrophy	AR
Sly (MPS VII)	Corneal clouding,	AR
Wolman	Peripheral retinal degeneration, optic atrophy	AR

Secondary Lysosomal Storage Disorders

Mucolipidoses

Disease	Ocular Manifestations	Inheritance
Mucolipidosis II (I-cell)	Corneal clouding, cataract	AR
Mucolipidosis III (pseudo-Hurler polydystrophy)	Corneal clouding	AR
Mucolipidosis IV	Corneal clouding, peripheral retinal degeneration	AR
Neuronal ceroid lipofuscinosis	Optic atrophy, peripheral retinal degeneration, maculopathy	
Santavuori-Haltia	Peripheral retinal degeneration, optic atrophy	AR
Jansky-Bielschowsky	Optic atrophy	AR
Spielmeyer-Voyt	Peripheral retinal degeneration, optic atrophy	AR
Kufs	Peripheral retinal degeneration, optic atrophy	AR

Amino acid metabolism

Disease	Ocular Manifestations	Inheritance
Cystinosis	Corneal clouding, peripheral retinal degeneration, crystals at all levels	AR
Gyrate atrophy (hyperornithinemia)	Gyrate chorioretinal atrophy, cataract, myopia	AR
Homocystinuria	Ectopia lentis, myopia peripheral retinal degeneration	AR
Hyperlysinemia	Ectopia lentis, spherophakia	AR
Methylmalonic aciduria	Corneal clouding	AR
Molybdenum cofactor deficiency	Cataract	AR
Sulfite oxidase deficiency	Ectopia lentis, optic atrophy	AR
Tyrosinemia	Corneal crystals and ulcers	AR

Peroxisomal disorders

Disease	Ocular Manifestations	Inheritance
Zellweger	Corneal clouding, cataract	AR
Neonatal adrenoleukodystrophy	Peripheral retinal degeneration, optic atrophy	AR
Refsum disease	Pigmentary retinopathy, cataract, optic atrophy, microphthalmia	AR
X-linked adrenoleukodystrophy	Optic atrophy	XR
Infantile Refsum disease	Peripheral retinal degeneration, optic atrophy	AR

Porphyria

Disease	Ocular Manifestations	Inheritance
Congenital erythropoietic	Corneal clouding	AR
Acute, intermittent	Cataract, peripheral retinal degeneration, optic atrophy	AD

Lipoprotein/lipid Metabolism

Disease	Ocular Manifestations	Inheritance
Abetalipoproteinemia	Peripheral retinal degeneration, angioid streaks	AR
Lecithin-cholesterol acytransferase (LCAT) deficiency	Corneal arcus and opacities	AR

TABLE 8–3. *(continued)*   Ocular Findings in Metabolic Disorders

Disease	Ocular Manifestations	Inheritance
Lipod proteinosis (Urbach-Wiethe)	Corneal opacities	
Tangier disease	Corneal clouding	AR
Carbohydrate Metabolism		
Galactose-1-phosphate uridyl transferase deficiency	Cataract	AR
Galactokinase	Cataract	AR
Metal Metabolism		
Acrodermatitis enteropathica	Corneal clouding, cataract, peripheral retinal degeneration, optic atrophy	AR
Wilson disease	Kayser-Fleischer ring, peripheral retinal degeneration, chalcosis lentis with cataract	AR
Ceramidase Deficiency		
Farber lipogranulomatosis	Corneal clouding, peripheral retinal degeneration	AR

AD = autosomal dominant, AR = autosomal recessive, XR = X-linked recessive, XD = X-linked dominant.

TABLE 8–4. Ocular Findings in Selected Chromosomal Syndromes

Trisomy Syndromes

Trisomy 8	Hypertelorism, downward slanting of palpebral fissures, strabismus, blepharoptosis, blepharophimosis, corneal opacities, cataract, iris heterochromia, colobomatous microphthalmia, megalocornea, retinal vessel tortuosity
Trisomy 9	Up- or downslanting of the palpebral fissures, narrow palpebral fissures, hypertelorism, epibulbar dermoid, corneal opacities, enophthalmos, microphthalmia
Trisomy 13 (Patau Syndrome)	Colobomatous microphthalmia, cyclopia, cataracts, corneal opacities, glaucoma, persistent hyperplastic primary vitreous, intraocular cartilage and retinal dysplasia, anophthalmia, microcornea, optic nerve hypoplasia, epicanthus, hypertelorism
Trisomy 14	Hypo- and hypertelorism, downslanting of the palpebral fissures, blepharoptosis, deep-set eyes, eversion of the eyelids, microphthalmia
Trisomy 18 (Edwards Syndrome)	Epicanthus, hypoplastic supraorbital ridges, corneal opacities, congenital glaucoma, cataract, microcornea, retinal pigment epithelial alterations, cyclopia, colobomatous microphthalmia, blepharoptosis, hypertelorism, strabismus
Trisomy 21 (Down Syndrome)	Epicanthus, upward slanting of the palpebral fissures, refractive errors (especially high myopia), strabismus, nystagmus, blepharitis, eyelid ectropion, keratoconus, Brushfield iris spots, glaucoma, congenital or acquired cataracts, abnormal retinal blood vessels
Trisomy 22	Epicanthus, hypertelorism, upward or downward slanting of palpebral fissures, colobomatous microphthalmia, strabismus, blepharoptosis, synophrys, cataract, dislocated lenses, optic nerve hypoplasia, persistent hyperplastic primary vitreous, myopia

Monosomy Syndromes

Monosomy 21	Epicanthus, downward slanting of the palpebral fissures, Peters' anomaly of the anterior segment, cataracts, microphthalmia
Monosomy 22	Epicanthus, hypertelorism, upward slanting of the palpebral fissures, blepharoptosis

Sex-Determining Chromosomes

Turner syndrome	Ptosis, strabismus, cataracts, refractive errors, corneal scars, blue sclera, color blindness hypertelorism, epicanthus, antimongoloid slant, abnormalities of retinal blood vessels, nystagmus
Klinefelter syndrome	Epicanthal folds, hypertelorism, upward slant of palpebral fissures, strabismus, Brushfield spots, myopia, choroidal atrophy, colobomatous microphthalmia

■ Leukocoria

A young infant is referred because of asymmetry of the pupillary reflexes in a photograph; the right eye appears to have a red reflex, whereas the left eye has white; the parents have noted a left esotropia. Otherwise, the parents believe their 20-month-old child is healthy and developing normally. The child fixates the right eye and demonstrates a left esotopia. There is a large creamy-colored intraocular mass with a "cottage cheese" appearance to the mass. The retinal vessels are not "stretched," and there are no vitreoretinal changes. The right eye is completely normal. Both parents are examined, and no abnormalities are present.

After reviewing your differential diagnosis for leukocoria (Table 8–5), include retinoblastoma, Coat's disease, ocular toxocariasis, retinal hamartomata, and persistent hyperplastic primary vitreous in the differential diagnosis. A diagnosis of retinoblastoma (Rb) is made based on the appearance.

Rb, a malignancy, may come to the attention of the parents, the primary care physician, and/or the ophthalmologist in a wide variety of clinical presentations (Table 8–6). The risk for the disease may be inherited in an autosomal dominant pattern; if the patient is the only member of the family with the disease, the term "sporadic" is used. The gene, on chromosome 13p14, was originally cloned in 1986 and is a nuclear protein that regulates cellular growth. Normally, an individual has two normal copies (alleles) of the gene in each cell; if an individual has only one normal copy, he or she is at increased risk for the development of Rb. Both hereditary and nonhereditary forms arise as a result of mutations in both alleles at the cellular level; this cancer confirmed the "two-hit" theory of tumorigenesis proposed by Knudson and established the concept that a malignancy could be caused by an autosomal recessive mechanism at the cellular level. Approximately 60% of Rbs are unilateral and unifocal. Forty percent of affected individuals have the heritable (germinal mutation) form and usually have large multifocal and bilateral tumors; patients with the hereditary form usually present at an earlier age. Two thirds of heritable forms are the result of new mutations in germ cells; patients with sporadic unilateral tumors have a 20% risk of developing Rb in the second eye. The risk of additional tumors decreases with time and is small after the age of 2 years; second nonocular tumors may develop in those patients with germinal mutations of the Rb gene and include osteosarcoma, Ewing sarcoma, malignant melanoma, fibrosarcoma, and medulloblastoma.

Formal genetic counseling should be documented for recurrence risk of the tumor in subsequent siblings of the affected child and, later, for the patient's offspring. All patients with bilateral Rb or a positive family history and 10 to 15% of those with a unilateral Rb have a germinal mutation; the risk for transmitting the mutated gene to an embryo is 50%. If two affected children are born to the same apparently normal parents, one of the parents has a mutated Rb gene, and the risk of transmission of the mutated Rb gene is 50%. Because the Rb gene has been cloned and sequenced, it is theoretically possible to identify the mutation in the Rb gene; unfortunately, such testing is not commercially available because the gene is large and many different mutations have been identified. In those families in which a mutation has

TABLE 8–5. Differential Diagnosis of Leukocoria

Cataract
Retinoblastoma
Toxocariasis
Retinopathy of prematurity
Retinal detachment/dysplasia
Persistent hyperplastic primary vitreous
Norrie disease
Familial exudative vitroretinopathy
Coat disease
Vitreous hemorrhage
Uveitis
Astrocytic hamartoma
Myelinated nerve fibers
Morning glory syndrome
Coloboma

TABLE 8–6. Presenting Signs and Symptoms of Retinoblastoma

Leukocoria (white reflex)
Strabismus
Glaucoma
Cellulitis (preseptal or orbital)
Hyphema
Inflammation with hypopyon

been identified, it is possible to determine those individuals and/or embryos at risk.

Only approximately 4% of Rb patients have detectable deletions of the long arm of chromosome 13; such patients generally have microcephaly, developmental delay, broad prominent nasal bridge, malformed and low set ears, short stature, and congenital cardiac disease in addition to the Rb.

■ Ectopia Lentis

A young child is referred because of a failed school screening. Your exam is remarkable for an uncorrected visual acuity of 20/80 O.D. and 20/100 O.S. Slit lamp biomicroscopy following pupillary dilation reveals ectopia lentis bilaterally with both lenses being dislocated inferiorly. By current nomenclature, any displacement of the lens from its normal position associated with intact zonules is termed subluxation, and total detachment of the zonular attachments and free movement of the lens is termed dislocation; ectopia lentis refers to either. Although pupillary dilation may be essential to identify lens subluxation or dislocation and to assess the status of the zonules, evaluation of the patient with an undilated pupil is useful to ascertain the effect on vision; the retinoscope is frequently useful. Posterior displacement of the lens may be assessed using the indirect ophthalmoscope with the patient's eye in infraduction or, more reliably, by measurement of the anterior chamber by ultrasonography.

Subluxation/dislocation may be an isolated ocular abnormality or associated with systemic features (Table 8–7). A careful history regarding trauma, developmental delay, cardiac or skeletal abnormalities, or other associated eye problems is useful. Both parents should undergo slit lamp biomicroscopy and dilation of pupils to determine the diagnosis and inheritance pattern. Careful assessment of the pupils may provide evidence for the diagnosis of autosomal recessive ectopia lentis et pupillae. It is useful to note if the zonules are stretched (as in Marfan syndrome) or if they are detached and/or scrolled onto the anterior surface of the lens (as occurs in homocystinuria). The lens may assume a notched or "flattened" edge (crenated) in the region of the absent or deficient zonules. In addition to the extent and direction of lens dislocation, the shape and size of the lens should be documented. If the majority of zonules are detached, the lens will assume a microspherophakic configuration and lenticular myopia develops; a tilted lens may be associated with significant astigmatism. The direction of the dislocation is important diagnostically and optically. In homocystinuria, the lens progressively dislocates and usually is displaced inferiorly into the vitreous by gravity or into the anterior chamber; in Marfan syndrome patients, the lenses may be displaced in any direction.

Body habitus may provide important diagnostic clues. Weill-Marchesani patients tend to be shorter and stockier and with broad hands and feet in contrast to the typical taller, lankier configuration of patients with homocystinuria and Marfan syndrome. Marfan syndrome patients may have chest wall deformities, and the wrist and thumb signs may be diagnostically useful. If the thumb overlaps the distal phalanx of the fifth digit when grasping the contralateral wrist it is considered a positive wrist sign; the thumb sign is positive when the entire nail of the thumb extends beyond the ulnar border (little finger) of the hand if the hand is folded over.

Marfan syndrome is the most common cause of subluxated lenses in childhood. It is an autosomal dominant multisystem disorder with cardiac, skeletal, and ocular manifestations. Cardiac abnormalities include dilation of the aorta, dissection of the aorta, or mitral valve prolapse. Chest wall deformities (pectus carinatum or excavatum), excessive height (in comparison to other family members), reduced upper to lower segment ratio (arm span to height ratio >1.05), wrist and thumb signs, joint

TABLE 8–7. Differential Diagnosis of Subluxated/Dislocated Lenses

Trauma
Isolated dislocated lenses
Etopia lentis et pupillae
Aniridia
Syphilis
Megalocornea (X-linked recessive)
Marfan syndrome
Homocystinuria
Weill-Marchesani
Sulfite oxidase deficiency
Hyperlysinemia

hypermobility, and a typical facial appearance (dolichocephaly, malar hypoplasia, enophthalmos, and retrognathia) may be evident. The diagnosis is established clinically if the patient fulfills the diagnostic criteria (having two of the three major organ systems involved).

In the Marfan syndrome, lens dislocation is present in 30 to 80% of patients. There may be slow progression of the lens dislocation, most noticeable between years 2 and 4 and again in early puberty. Although complete dislocation is much more common in homocystinuric patients, it may occur in Marfan syndrome patients; acute glaucoma with a red, painful eye may be the presenting problem for either. Microspherophakia is present in about 15% of patients with Marfan syndrome and contributes to myopia. Additionally, axial elongation of the globe (usually with high myopia) places the patient at increased risk for retinal detachment. The iris may appear smoother and more "velvety" with loss of crypts and furrows, and occasional transillumination defects may be evident. A relatively common finding is megalocornea. Treatment modalities vary from center to center, and lensectomy for a clear lens remains controversial; good vision can be obtained in these patients with meticulous refractions and aggressive treatment for amblyopia. Patients tend to develop "presenile" cataracts. Monitoring of their intraocular pressure is essential because of the higher incidence of glaucoma. Regular dilated fundus exams are required to search for retinal detachments, lattice degeneration, or holes.

The gene for Marfan syndrome is fibrillin (chromosome 15); not all patients with Marfan syndrome have a readily identifiable mutation, and molecular diagnostic testing is not yet commercially available. In families in whom linkage to fibrillin has been shown or where a specific mutation is present, linkage analysis or direct gene sequencing may allow diagnosis of individuals or embryos.

In contrast to Marfan syndrome, homocystinuria is an autosomal recessive disorder affecting methionine metabolism. Untreated affected individuals may develop progressive dislocation of the lenses, mental retardation, and thromboembolic complications. Thromboembolic

episodes are a result of homocysteine accumulation causing abnormal platelet adhesiveness and frequent cerebral thromboses. If surgery is necessary, local anesthesia is preferred. Classic homocystinuria is due to a deficiency of the enzyme cystathionine-β-synthetase with accumulation of homocystine and methionine in blood and other tissues. A less common form results from reduced activity of 5-methyltetrahydrofolate-homocysteine methyltransferase. Forty to 50% of patients with homocystinuria show biochemical improvement after treatment with high doses of pyridoxine (vitamin B6 acts as a cofactor with cystathione-β-synthetase). Mental deficiency occurs mostly in those B6 nonresponders.

In the absence of definitive trauma, all patients with subluxed or dislocated lenses should undergo quantification of urine or serum homocystine. Patients with the disease should be treated with oral supplementation of vitamin B6 (50 to 1000 mg/day). A high cystine and low methionine diet improves metabolic control and is especially important in the nonresponders. Early treatment with vitamin B6 and alterations in the diet may prevent or delay mental retardation.

■ Nystagmus

A 3-year-old boy is brought into your office by his parents because of "dancing eyes." While you are obtaining your complete history, you observe the child at play in the room to evaluate how well the child functions visually in a new environment and any head posturing or unusual movements. Your history should include a comprehensive review of the pregnancy, delivery, and development with particular attention to age of onset of nystagmus and any particular head or body movements. Specifically, you inquire as to the progression of the nystagmus and any variations, especially with lighting conditions; the parents should be queried regarding how the child watches TV (any particular position), if the symptoms are worse with any head movements or position, and if lighting affects visual functioning. Your family history includes any history of nystagmus and evidence for any ocular or neuro-ophthalmologic disorders; particular attention should be addressed to the maternal grandfather inquiring about the possibility of any signs, symptoms, or diagnoses suggestive of X-linked recessive conditions. Of note, the boy is otherwise healthy but has a similarly affected maternal grandfather.

On examination, you note the child is visually attentive in each eye and has moderate frequency, moderate amplitude horizontal nystagmus without an identifiable null point. Evaluation should include assessment for a paradoxical reaction in which the pupils dilate in light; this observation, rarely diagnostic, may be identified by comparing a Polaroid of the child in a fully lit room and again in a dark room. In this child, there was no evidence of any paradoxical pupils. Although the boy has brown eyes, he has extensive transillumination defects of the irides. A cycloplegic refraction is performed, and you find 6 diopters of against-the-rule astigmatism in each eye. On ophthalmoscopy, a diagnosis of macular hypoplasia is made because the foveal pit is not apparent, there is reduced foveal pigmentation, and a vessel traverses the macula. The optic nerve appears grayish, and the fundus is blonde with sparse retinal pigment epithelium and prominent choroidal vessels. Based on the ocular features, a diagnosis of ocular albinism is made.

Because of the history of the maternal grandfather having nystagmus, you conclude the boy has X-linked ocular albinism and evaluate the mother for carrier signs. She has iris transilluminations defects, and you note disturbances of hypopigmentation in the midperipheral retinal pigment epithelium on dilated retinal examination. The identification of carrier status in the mother confirms the diagnosis of X-linked ocular albinism. Each male child of a female carrier has a 50% chance of inheriting the disease, the gene for which is located at Xp22.

Although all forms of oculocutaneous albinism are autosomal recessive, ocular albinism can be transmitted in X-linked recessive or autosomal recessive patterns with the X-linked form being more common. A diagnosis of the X-linked recessive form of ocular albinism can be confirmed on the basis of cutaneous macromelanosomes by electron microscopy. There are many genetic types of oculocutaneous albinism, and most are inherited as an autosomal recessive trait. The easiest form of oculocutaneous albinism to diagnose is that of the tyrosinase-negative type. These individuals present with a prominent red reflux, pinkish-gray irides, pink-white skin, and snow-white hair, and visual acuity is usually 20/100 or worse. In contrast to tyrosinase-negative form, tyrosinase-positive ("incomplete") oculocutaneous albinism may be more difficult to diagnose. Depending upon the age and race of the individual, the color of skin and eyes varies in this type; unlike the tyrosinase-negative form, these individuals may have an increase in pigmentation with age; visual acuity ranges from near normal to 20/200. To date, two genes have been identified as the basis of oculocutaneous albinism, the tyrosinase and P genes; commercial testing is not available.

Oculocutaneous albinism is a component of two multisystem autosomal recessive syndromes. Hernansky-Pudlak syndrome is characterized by generalized albinism and easy bruisability or excessive bleeding from minor procedures; the bleeding diathesis is due to a platelet dysfunction with accumulation of ceroid-like pigment within leukocytes and bone marrow macrophages. Additionally, they may have pulmonary symptoms or abdominal pain secondary to an accumulation of abnormal reticulendothelial cells. The disease is relatively common in Puerto Rico. If one considers this diagnosis, bleeding times and platelet aggregation studies should be done in conjunction with a hematologist. In individuals with tyrosinase-positive oculocutaneous albinism and repeated infections, a diagnosis of Chediak-Higashi syndrome should be evaluated. In addition to generalized albinism, patients have a silvery tint to their hair and slate grey patches in their skin; they have an increased incidence of skin and/or respiratory tract infections, which may be life threatening. By adolescence, hepatosplenomegaly becomes evident; cranial nerve palsies, seizures, and peripheral neuropathies may occur. The pathogenesis is unknown.

In any patient with nystagmus, it is important to document the type of nystagmus, including amplitude, frequency, intensity, laterality, and the presence or absence of a null point (zone of least intensity). Most nystagmus is conjugate, and asymmetry suggests monocular vision loss, an intracranial lesion, or possibly spasmus nutans. The two major pediatric categories include sensory nystagmus and congenital idiopathic nystagmus, a diagnosis of exclusion. Sensory nystagmus is caused by an organic basis for visual loss; potentially genetic causes include foveal hypoplasia, maculopathy or macular scarring, optic nerve hypoplasia, optic atrophy, retinal dystrophy, colobomata, and corneal opacities. Regardless of color of the irides, it is essential to check for iris transillumination defects (using the iris transilluminator or retroillumination by slit lamp biomicroscopy) to evaluate nystagmus; in some children with oculocutaneous albinism, the irides are pink, and transillumination can be appreciated with the naked eye. Regardless of the clinical features, if the basis for the nystagmus cannot be identified readily, an electroretinogram (ERG) is essential even with an apparently normal ocular exam. Diagnoses such as congenital stationary night blindness, cone dystrophy, any form of achromatopsia, and Leber congenital amaurosis are only made on the basis of the ERG and, in some cases, formal color vision testing. Visual evoked potentials may show crossed asymmetry secondary to the misrouting of fibers in albinism with the most temporal retinal fibers crossed over to the contralateral side; it is not a useful diagnostic test.

Leber congenital amaurosis is an autosomal recessive rod-cone dystrophy; affected individuals are otherwise normal. In addition to nystagmus and a sluggish pupillary response, their fundi vary from being entirely normal to frankly dystrophic, and most will progress with time. Diagnosis is established on the basis of an extinguished ERG. Other diseases in which the ERG is extinguished include Joubert syndrome, an autosomal recessive disease; in addition to the ocular features, affected individuals have a characteristic breathing pattern and hypoplasia of their cerebellar vermis. Magnetic resonance imaging (MRI) is indicated in the evaluation of children with an abnormal ERG if other neurologic symptoms are evident.

Foveal hypoplasia may be isolated or associated with additional ocular pathology, such as albinism and aniridia; isolated forms may be autosomal dominant or of unknown etiology.

Optic nerve hypoplasia may be associated with young maternal age or maternal ingestion of antiseizure medications or alcohol. It may be associated with pituitary dysfunction; MRI to identify midline malformations and endocrine evaluation is warranted.

Optic atrophy associated with nystagmus may be caused by hydrocephalus or perinatal disease such as intraventricular hemorrhages; neuroimaging is indicated.

The differential diagnosis of nystagmus and/or significant visual impairment (Table 8–8) in an infant or young child includes a large group of inborn errors of metabolism such as the peroxisomal disorders (infantile Refum disease, neonatal adrenoleukodystrophy, and Zellweger syndrome) and the ceroid lipofuscinoses. The peroxosomal disorders are inherited in an autosomal recessive pattern. Nystagmus is not an isolated presenting symptom in this group of disorders, and developmental delay is evident; in all three, vessel attenuation and pigmentary changes develop in the retina, and the ERG becomes abnormal early in life. In infantile Refsum disease, neurosensory deafness and hepatomegaly are features; elevated plasma levels of phytanic acids are key to the diagnosis. Additional features of neonatal adrenoleukodystrophy include adrenal cortical atrophy and seizures. In the peroxisomal disorders, death usually occurs in childhood. The ceroid lipofuscinoses are a group of autosomal recessive diseases characterized by loss of intellectual and physical milestones; the age of onset varies, and seizures may occur. The diagnosis is made on the basis of electron microscopy of conjunctiva, skin, or leukocytes.

TABLE 8–8. Neonatal Visual Impairment

Cortical blindness
Corneal opacities
Cataract
Retinal dystrophy/degeneration
    Leber congenital amaurosis
    Achromatopsia
    Peroxisomal disorders
    Joubert syndrome
    Ceroid lipofuscinoses
Neonatal adrenoleukodystrophy
Optic nerve hypoplasia
Coloboma

Although there is no treatment for any form of nystagmus at this time, clinical management should include careful and repeated cycloplegic refractions to maximize visual potential and binocularity. In all forms of nystagmus, particularly albinism, astigmatism can be significant. In albinism, sun protection is important; some individuals prefer tinted glasses, and baseball caps or visors can be helpful.

SUGGESTED READINGS

Bateman JB. Microphthalmia. In: Kivlin J, ed. *Developmental Abnormalities of the Eye: International Ophthalmology Clinics.* Boston: Little, Brown; 1984;24:87–107.

Bateman JB, Lang GE, Maumenee IH. Genetic metabolic disorders associated with retinal dystrophies. In: Ryan SJ, Schachat AP, Murphy RB, Patz A, eds. *Retina.* 2nd ed. St. Louis: Mosby; 1994;467–491.

Bateman JB. Chromosomal anomalies and the eye. In: *Pediatric Ophthalmology and Strabismus.* St. Louis, MO: Mosby Year Book; 1995;533–615.

Heher KI, Traboulsi EI, Maumenee IH. The natural history of Leber's congenital amaurosis. Age related findings in 35 patients. *Ophthalmol.* 1992;99:241–245.

Maumenee IH. The eye in Marfan syndrome. *Tr Am Ophthalmol Soc.* 1981;79:696–733.

Muphree AL. Molecular Genetics of Retinoblastoma. In: Grossniklaus H, ed. *Ophthalmology Clinics of North America.* Philadelphia: WB Saunders; 1995.

Smith BJ, O'Brien JM. The genetics of retinoblastoma and current diagnostic testing. *J Pediatr Ophthalmol Strabismus.* 1996; 33:120–123.

Pediatric Ophthalmology
Edited by P. F. Gallin
Thieme Medical Publishers, Inc.
New York © 2000

9

Ocular Pharmacology in Children

KIM L. COOPER, KULDEV SINGH, AND THOM J. ZIMMERMAN

Adult medications considered innocuous may be potentially hazardous in children, especially neonates. Cycloplegic, mydriatic, antiaccommodative, antibiotic, antiinflammatory, and intraocular pressure-lowering medications all are commonly used in children. This chapter will address therapeutic issues pertaining to the use of these agents in children.

■ Pharmacological Considerations Unique to Infants and Children

Drugs that have been approved by the Food and Drug Administration for use in adults but not children should be used with caution. There is perhaps greater responsibility and vulnerability when a physician prescribes a drug not approved for use in children based on his or her own judgment. We must weigh potential benefits and risks of the medications. For this reason as well as the relative inability of children to describe side effects the ophthalmologist should be particularly careful in looking for untoward signs and symptoms of toxicity.

Multiple organs and organ systems may be adversely affected by topical ocular medications.[1] These effects may be allergic or dose related. Neonates, especially when premature, may be particularly vulnerable to dose-related side effects. The ophthalmologist should work in conjunction with the neonatologist or pediatrician to jointly assess the risk of ocular medications.

All topical ocular medications have the potential to be absorbed systemically through the nasolacrimal system. There is considerable variability in the drug levels found systematically in patients.[1] Nasolacrimal occlusion may be effective but is often difficult in uncooperative children.

■ Dilation

Cycloplegic Agents

This class of drugs plays an important role in the diagnosis and therapy of eye disorders in infants. Ocular cycloplegic agents block muscarinic receptors in the ciliary body, thereby paralyzing the ciliary muscle and relaxing accommodation. Because the constrictor muscles of the iris also are blocked, which allows the iris dilators to act unopposed, dilation is often another secondary effect of cycloplegic therapy. The antimuscarinic effect of cycloplegic agents is dose dependent.[1]

Cycloplegic agents are used routinely to relax accommodation when performing retinoscopy in children. Pupil dilation is often augmented by an additional mydriatic agent, which allows better visualization of the retina and optic nerve.

Darker pigmented irides dilate more slowly[2] and often require a second dose of medication.

Cycloplegic agents also are commonly used in inflammatory eye conditions. In addition to decreasing the potential risk of posterior synechiae, these agents may relieve ocular discomfort by diminishing ciliary body spasm.

The most commonly used cycloplegic agents in pediatric ophthalmology are tropicamide (Mydriacyl), cyclopentolate (Cyclogel), atropine, homatropine, and scopolamine.

Tropicamide (0.5 and 1.0%)

Tropicamide is a weak cycloplegic agent with rapid onset of action. Used alone, it is less reliable than cyclopentolate in relaxing accommodation for cycloplegic retinoscopy and refraction[3] and therefore is most often used in conjunction with cyclopentolate. Despite this, it continues to be commonly used in routine eye exams both to partially relax accommodation and to dilate the pupil. It is a relatively safe cycloplegic agent without reported serious adverse systemic side effects.

Cyclopentolate 0.5, 1, and 2%

Cyclopentolate remains the cycloplegic agent of choice in most routine pediatric eye exams, especially when cycloplegic refraction is necessary. It can be used in conjunction with tropicamide. The peak accommodative effect occurs in approximately 20 to 45 minutes in most eyes. Residual accommodative effects and pupil dilation may last from 24 to 36 hours, most often reversing between $1\frac{1}{2}$ and 3 hours.

Because of the possibility of severe dose-dependent systemic side effects with this agent, the use of 2% cyclopentolate has become obsolete. Although local or systemic allergic reactions to the drug may occur, they are rare.[4] Feeding intolerance and gastrointestinal discomfort are relatively common side effects.[5] Hyperthermia, hyperactivity, hallucinations, seizures, and delirium have also been described.[6]

Atropine (0.5 and 1.0%)

Atropine is the slowest in onset, longest acting, and likely the most completely paralyzing commercially available antiaccommodative agent. Because the duration of action is often 1 week or greater, atropine is rarely used for routine ophthalmic examinations unless complete or prolonged ciliary muscle paralysis is desired. It is often used in amblyopia therapy, following glaucoma procedures, and as a treatment adjunct for intraocular inflammation.

Ocular side effects of atropine include follicular conjunctivitis and contact dermatitis.[7] Hypotension, hyperthermia, respiratory depression, delirium, and death also have been reported. Other physicians, including intensivists and anesthesiologists, should be informed of the use of these medications, especially when administered only in one eye. Parents should be instructed that, in the event of head trauma or car accidents, medical personnel should be informed of the use of ocular dilating agents to prevent any misdiagnosis of compressive intracranial nerve injuries.

Homatropine (2 and 5%)

Homatropine has a shorter onset and duration of action but is otherwise quite similar to atropine. It is a useful alternative to atropine in inflammatory eye conditions when mild pupillary mobility is desired. It should not be used in patients who are allergic to atropine.

Scopolamine (0.25%)

Scopolamine is a rarely used cycloplegic agent that has the benefit of not being cross-reactive with atropine and thus can be used in atropine allergic patients.[6]

Mydriatic Agents

Although cycloplegic agents may dilate the pupil, and thus may be considered mydriatic agents, the mydriatic agents discussed in this section primarily dilate the pupil without significant antiaccommodative action.

All mydriatic agents have sympathomimetic activity in that they mimic the action of epinephrine and norepinephrine by affecting α- or β-catecholamine receptors. Both α and β receptors have two subtypes, α-1 and -2 and β-1 and -2.[1]

Phenylephrine hydrochloride (1.0, 2.5, and 10.0%) is a commonly used mydriatic agent that often is used in conjunction with a cycloplegic drug. It acts directly on catecholamine receptors with primarily α-1 activity. It has a rapid onset (less than 15 minutes) and a duration of action of approximately 6 hours. Although 10.0% phenylephrine is sometimes used prior to cataract surgery in adults, it is rarely used in children because of the potential for untoward cardiovascular and systemic side effects. Increased blood pressure and bradycardia are the most commonly encountered problems. The 1.0 and 2.5% concentrations are associated with fewer cardiovascular side effects and are thus the preferred dilating agents.

Other uses of phenylephrine hydrochloride include vasoconstriction of conjunctival blood vessels at the time of strabismus surgery and temporary blanching of blood vessels in eyes with allergic conjunctivitis[6–8] and episcleritis.

Both epinephrine and its prodrug dipivefrin are sympathomimetic drugs that lower intraocular pressure and secondarily dilate the pupil.

Apraclonidine and brimonidine are α-selective sympathomimetic drugs that lower intraocular pressure by decreasing aqueous humor production at the ciliary body but are not routinely used as mydriatics. The efficacy and side effect profiles of these drugs have not been well established in children.

Cocaine is a powerful topical anesthetic agent that is rarely used in children. Potential side effects, including tachycardia, hypertension, seizures, and arrhythmias, limit its use in pediatric ophthalmology.

Hydroxyamphetamine is a sympathomimetic agent used only to differentiate pre- and post-ganglionic lesions producing Horner's syndrome. In preganglionic lesions, hydroxyamphetamine induces the release of norepinephrine at the neuromuscular junction resulting in pupil dilation, whereas pupil dilation is not seen in postganglionic lesions.

■ Medical Antiaccommodative Therapy

Accommodative esotropia is one of the most common forms of acquired strabismus. Excessive hyperopia and a high accommodative convergence–accommodative ratio are both etiologic factors. Numerous reports and reviews have established miotics as adjuncts to the optical and surgical treatments for accommodative esotropia.[9,10]

Miotics constrict the pupil and act directly on the ciliary muscle. Cholinesterase inhibitors act indirectly by facilitating neuromuscular transmission, whereas parasympathomimetic agents directly cause accommodative spasm.[11,12] Because miotics effectively reduce accommodative effort, less accommodative convergence occurs. Conditions for the development of fusional amplitudes are encouraged.

Longer acting drugs such as echothiophate iodide [phospholine iodide (PI)] and demecarium bromide (humorsol) have largely replaced the shorter acting physostigmine and pilocarpine. Initially, low percentages of PI (0.3%) are used before bedtime. The dose is titrated upward on follow-up exams.[13,14]

Possible systemic complications include lowering cholinesterase in red blood cells, which may persist for several weeks. Potential risks for children on miotics undergoing general anesthesia include prolonged respiratory paralysis when used in conjunction with succinylcholine (SCH). SCH should be avoided in patients treated with PI within 6 weeks of surgery,[15] and some strabismologists issue a letter to the parents of children regarding anticholinesterase drops:

> Your child is receiving topical phospholine (echothiophate) iodide therapy. This drug may cause enhanced or prolonged action of muscle relaxants that are sometimes given during general anesthesia. If your child requires emergency surgery for whatever reason, the anesthesiologist must be advised of the use of this medicine.[16]

Transient blurry vision, darkening of the visual field, and iris cysts are among the ocular side effects of miotics. Iris cysts may begin 2 to 40 weeks after initiation of therapy and occur in 20 to 50% of patients. They may be prevented with the concurrent use of topical phenylephrine 2.5% qHs twice weekly.[17–19] Cysts usually disappear after treatment is discontinued.[19]

Cataractogenic action has been reported only in adults on glaucoma therapy,[20,21] except for a single isolated case of reversible lens opacities after 3 months of treatment in a child.[22] Retinal detachment has not been observed in children.

Shallowing of the anterior chamber and angle closure glaucoma are infrequent complications in children.[23]

■ Conjunctivitis

Principles in Treatment of Conjunctivitis

Conjunctivitis in children is most commonly associated with infections (viral or bacterial) or allergies. However, other ocular and systemic diseases can present as a "red eye." These include trauma, corneal abrasions, corneal or conjunctival foreign bodies (especially metallic), traumatic iritis, hyphema, perforating injuries, nasolacrimal duct obstruction, and lice (pubic and ocular) (Table 9–1).

The chronological and symptomatic history of the conjunctivitis is vital to the diagnosis (see Chapter 16).[24] Cultures, although not mandatory, are indicated in chronic or recurrent infections, severe acute infections, and follicular or atypical reactions. Hyperacute conjunctivitis, especially in neonates, must be cultured to rule out *Neisseria* sp. and chlamydia (see Chapter 16 for detailed explanation of neonatal conjunctivitis).[24]

Bacterial Conjunctivitis

The most common bacterial pathogens are *Haemophilus influenzae, Streptococcus pneumonia,* other streptococcus isolates, *Branhamella catarrhalis,* and *Moraxella.*[25,26] Because staphylococcus is considered normal lid flora, cultures have questionable significance. Acute bacterial conjunctivitis is usually self-limiting (10 to 14 days); however, antibiotic treatment shortens the clinical course.[27,28] Antibiotic choices are described subsequently.

Polytrim (trimethoprim sulfate and polymixin sulfate) solution is active against a wide variety of gram-positive and -negative ophthalmic

TABLE 9–1. Conjunctivitis: Differential Diagnosis

Etiology	Clinical Findings				
	Unilateral or Bilateral	Discharge	Lids	Onset/Course	Treatment
Viral* (usually adenovirus)	Bilateral	Thin, mucoid	Follicular	Gradual Upper respiratory tract infection? Preauricular adenopathy	Compresses
Herpes simplex	Unilateral	Thin, mucoid	Follicular	Gradual Keratitis Dendritic ulcer	Idoxuridine
Bacterial	Unilateral or bilateral	Purulent	Papillary, purulent	Gradual	Topical antibiotics
Gonococcal	Unilateral	Purulent	Edema, inflamed	Hyperacute	Systemic antibiotics
Chlamydial	Unilateral or bilateral	Thin, mucoid	Follicular	Indolent Persistent Neonate Sexually active	Oral erythromycin or tetracycline (>10 years of age)
Allergic	Bilateral	Watery	Papillary	Gradual Seasonal	Topical vasoconstrictors Systemic antihistamine Topical steroids
Vernal	Bilateral	Watery	Giant papillary	Adolescents Seasonal	Cromolyn?
Contact lens irritation	Bilateral	Watery	Giant papillary	Lenses	Adjust lens Change solution
Chemical	Unilateral or bilateral	Watery	Variable	Acute	Irrigate Remove irritant

*Undifferentiated viral conjunctivitis, not due to herpesvirus infection.
Source: From Kliegman RM, ed. *Practical Strategies in Pediatric Diagnosis and Therapy,* Philadelphia, PA: WB Saunders; 1996: 720.

pathogens, selectively interfering with bacterial biosynthesis of nucleic acids and proteins.

Polymixin B is bacteriocidal for a variety of gram-negative organisms. It increases the permeability of the cell membrane and is indicated for use in patients over 2 months of age.[29-31]

Sulfacetamide sodium solutions (AK-Sulf 10%, Bleph10 10%, isoptocetamide 15%, sulamyd sodium 10%, 30%, sulf 10 10%, generic 10%, 15%, 30%) are bacteriostatic and inhibit bacterial synthesis of dihydrofolic acid by competitive inhibition. They are active against *Escherichia coli*, *Staphylococcus aureus*, *S. pneumonia*, *Streptococcus* (viridans gp), *Haemophilus influenza*, *Klebsiella* sp., and *Enterobacter* sp.[29,30,32]

These drops are inexpensive but only have a bacteriostatic mechanism of action and sting on instillation. Their coverage is inadequate for *Neisseria* sp., *Serratia marcescens*, and *Pseudomonas aeruginosa*. A significant percentage of staphylococcal isolates are completely resistant to sulfa drugs.

Neosporin (polymixin B/neomycin/gramicidin) is an aminoglycoside antibiotic, available in drops and ointment, which inhibits protein synthesis, causing misreading of the bacterial genetic code. It is bacteriocidal for many grampositive and -negative organisms. There is a high incidence of sensitivity to neomycin, especially in children.

Gramicidin increases the permeability of the bacterial cell membrane and is bacteriocidal for a variety of gram-positive organisms.

Chloramphenicol (AK-Chlor, chloromycetin, Chloroptic, Ocuchlor) is a broad-spectrum primarily bacteriostatic antibiotic that acts by inhibiting protein synthesis. This drug is especially good for eliminating *Haemophilus* and *Moraxella* sp. but provides poor coverage for *Pseudomonas* and *Serratia* sp. Short-term use of topical chloramphenicol has not been reported with adverse systemic reactions; however, rare cases of bone marrow hypoplasia, aplastic anemia, and death have been reported with prolonged topical use (months to years).[29,30,33]

Aminoglycosides, including gentamicin and tobramycin (gentamicin sulfate 0.3%, Garamycin, Genoptic, Gentacidin, Gentak), is a class of bacteriocidal antibiotics that inhibits normal protein synthesis against a wide variety of microorganisms. The ophthalmologist should be aware that most species of streptococci, including *S. pneumonia* and anaerobic organisms such as *Bacteroides* sp. and *Clostridium* sp. are normally resistant to aminoglycosides. This antibiotic is considered as initial therapy in suspected or confirmed gram-negative infections. Anaerobic bacteria are not susceptible to aminoglycosides due to a lack of active transport mechanism for aminoglycoside uptake.[29,30,34,35]

Tobramycin sulfate (Tobrex 0.3%) is a bactericidal drug used against many microorganisms, mostly gram-negative rods. Bacterial susceptibility studies demonstrate that some cases resistant to gentamicin remain susceptible to tobramycin.

The bactericidal action of fluroquinolones (Ciprofloxacin, Ofloxacin, and Norfloxacin) is from their interference with the enzyme DNA gyrase, which is needed for synthesis of bacterial DNA.

Ciprofloxacin hydrochloride (Ciloxan 0.3%) is active against a broad spectrum of grampositive and -negative ocular pathogens. Some strains of *Pseudomonas* as well as most anaerobic bacteria are resistant to ciprofloxacin.[29,30,36] Frequent topical dosing with Ciloxan in the treatment of corneal ulcers can produce white crystalline precipitates. These do not appear to affect the efficacy of treatment. Ciloxan is approved for use in patients ages 1 year and older. Although oral administration of quinolones can cause arthropathy, topical administration does not, and there is no evidence that the ophthalmic dosage has any effect on weight-bearing joints. However, orally administered fluoroquinolones do appear to cross the placenta and are excreted in breast milk.

Ofloxacin (Ocuflox 0.3%) has a similar mechanism of action and bactericidal spectrum to ciprofloxacin, except it is less active against *P. aeruginosa* and *H. influenza* but more potent against *Xanthomonas maltophilia*.

Norfloxacin (Chibroxin 0.3%) is indicated for treatment of bacterial conjunctivitis caused by *Aeromonas hydrophila*, *Acinetobacter calcoaceticus*, *H. influenza*, *P. murabelis*, *S. marcescens*, *Staphylococcus aureus*, *S. epidermidis*, *S. warnerri*, and *Streptococcus pneumonias*.

Combination antibiotic and steroid ophthalmic preparations (tobradex; tobramycin and dexamethasone; blephamide: sulfacetamide sodium and prednisolone acetate) should be used cautiously for treating bacterial infections because they may predispose to secondary infections. Fungal infections can develop coincidentally with long-term steroid applications. Combination medications are contraindicated in viral conjunctivitis and keratitis. Prolonged use of corticosteroids also may result in ocular hypertension, glaucoma, and posterior subcapsular cataract formation. Safety and efficacy in patients under 6 years of age have not been established.

Ointments

Although ointments may be easier to administer and last longer, the vehicle may cause visual blurring, which is undesirable in children with amblyogenic potential.

Erythromycin (Ilotycin, EES) is a macrolidic antibiotic that binds to the 50S ribosomal subunit, inhibiting bacterial protein synthesis. Erythromycin is effective against a wide range of microorganisms, but it should not be used for *H. influenza*. Other organisms that have shown susceptibility include *Chlamydia trachomatis*, *Entamoeba histolytica*, *Listeria monocytogenes*, *Borrelia burgdorferi* (a causative agent of Lyme disease), *Mycoplasma pneumoniae*, *Treponema pallidum*, and *Ureaplasma urealyticum*. Always consult susceptibility data at your institution to determine any antimicrobial activity.[29,30,37] Oral erythromycin crosses the placenta and is distributed in breast milk.

Viral Conjunctivitis

Adenoviruses are the most important cause of pediatric conjunctivitis (Table 9–2). Clinical symptoms usually resolve in 1 week. Because antiviral therapies are ineffective, treatment is symptomatic with artificial tears and cool compresses. Secondary infections should be treated with antibiotic drops.

Primary herpes simplex can present as a conjunctivitis but usually will be associated with corneal dendrites and iritis. Treatment includes topical debridement and/or topical antivirals (trifluorothymidine—Viroptic, vidarabine—Vira-A, or idoxuridine).

Because of the high mortality rate (70%) associated with disseminated neonatal herpes simplex, all neonates less than 1 month of age with a herpes simplex infection should be treated with systemic acyclovir, and treatment should be coordinated with the patient's pediatrician. This is true even if involvement is initially limited to only cutaneous or ocular involvement.

Viroptic 1% (trifluridine) has activity against herpes simplex virus types 1 and 2 and vaccinia virus. Trifluridine interferes with DNA synthesis

TABLE 9–2. Clinical Features of Conjunctivitis

Sign	Bacterial	Viral	Allergic	Toxic	TRIC
Injection	Marked	Moderate	Mild to moderate	Mild to moderate	Moderate
Hemorrhage	+	+	−	−	−
Chemosis	+ +	±	+ +	±	±
Exudate	Purulent or mucopurulent	Scant, watery	Stringy, white	−	Scant
Pseudomembrane	± (*Streptococcus, Corynebacterium diphtheria*)	±	−	−	−
Papillae	±	−	+	−	±
Follicles	−	+	−	+ (medication)	+
Preauricular node	+ (purulent)	+ +	−	−	±
Pannus	−	−	− (except vernal)	−	+

TRIC = trachoma-inclusion conjunctivitis (group).
Key: + + = strongly positive, + = positive, ± = sometimes positive, − = negative.
Source: From Pavan D, Langston MD, eds. *Manual of Ocular Diagnosis and Therapy*, 2nd ed. Boston/Toronto: Little, Brown; 1986:74.

in cultured mammalian cells, but the exact antiviral mechanism of action is not completely known. Safety and efficacy in pediatric patients have not been established. Viroptic drops nine times per day or ointment five times a day is used in conjunction with cycloplegics, which relieve the ciliary spasm and photophobia of the associated iritis. Children resistant to the administration of topical medications may use adjunctive oral acyclovir (Zovirax). The dose should be calculated based on the child's age and weight, and treatment should be coordinated with the patient's pediatrician.

Vidarabine (Vira A) ointment has activity against herpes simplex types 1 and 2, varicella zoster virus, cytomegalovirus, vaccinia, and hepatitis B. Viral DNA synthesis is inhibited by intracellular phosphorylation, and it is also deaminated to an active metabolite, which may have synergistic effect.

Acyclovir (Zovirax) is an oral, parenteral, and topical antiviral. As a synthetic purine nucleoside analog, after phosphorylation it competes for position in the viral DNA and terminates DNA synthesis. It is effective only against actively replicating viruses. [29, 30, 38]

Allergic Conjunctivitis

Clinical symptoms—itching, tearing, watery red eyes, and boggy, chemotic conjunctivae with occasional lid edema—can provide a clue to an allergic etiology. Hay fever sufferers have associated rhinorrhea, and symptoms are usually recurrent and seasonal. Treatment includes withdrawal of inciting allergens, topical and/or systemic medications, and cold compresses.

Topical mast cell inhibitors/stabilizers such as cromolyn sodium (Crolom), olopatadine (Patanol), and lodoxamide (Alomide); selective H1 receptor antagonists such as levocabastine (Livostin); and topical antihistamines (Naphcon, Vasocon, AK-Con-A, and Opcon A) are typically used. Alomide appears to be superior to cromolyn sodium in alleviating the signs and symptoms of vernal keratoconjunctivitis.[39,40] Topical nonsteroidals, including ketorolac (Acular 0.5%), are indicated for the treatment of seasonal allergic conjunctivitis[41,42] and work by decreasing inflammation by inhibiting prostaglandin biosynthesis. No spe-

cific pediatric side effects have been noted, but usage in children has been limited to date.[29,30,38]

REFERENCES

1. Katzung BG, ed. *Basic and Clinical Pharmacology*. 6th ed. Norwalk, CT: Appleton & Lange; 1995:1046.
2. Salazar-Bookaman MM, Wainer I, Patil PN. Relevance of drug-melanin interactions to ocular pharmacology and toxicology. *J Ocul Pharmacol*. 1994;10(1):31–33.
3. Egashira SM, et al. Comparison of cyclopentolate versus tropicamide cycloplegia in children. *Optom Vis Sci*. 1993; 70(12):1019–1026.
4. Jones LW, Hodes DT. Possible allergic reactions to cyclopentolate hydrochloride: case reports with literature review of uses and adverse reactions. *Ophthalmic Physiol Opt*. 1991;11(1):16–21.
5. Hermansen MC, Sullivan LS. Feeding intolerance following ophthalmologic examination. *Am J Dis Child*. 1985;139(4):367–368.
6. Zimmerman TJ, et al. *Textbook of Ocular Pharmacology*. 1997:788.
7. Vadot E, Piasentin. Incidence of allergy to eyedrops. Results of a prospective survey in a hospital milieu. *J Fr Ophthalmol*. 1986;9(1):41–43.
8. *Physicians' Desk Reference for Ophthalmology*. 23rd ed. Montvale, NJ: Medical Economic Data Production Company; 1995.
9. Goldstein JH. The role of miotics in strabismus. *Surv Ophthalmol*. 1968;13:31.
10. Letson RD. The use of drugs in the management of strabismus. *Surv Ophthalmol*. 1970;14:428.
11. Ripps H, Breinin GM, Baum JD. Accommodation in the cat. *Trans Am Ophthalmol Soc*. 1961;59:176.
12. Abraham SV. The use of miotics in the treatment of convergent strabismus and anisometropia: a preliminary report. *Am J Ophthalmol*. 1949;32:233.
13. Haddad HM, Rivera H. Echophenyline B3 and phospholine (ecothiophate) iodide 0.03% in the management of esotropia. *J Pediatr Ophthalmol*. 1967;4:24.
14. von Noorden GK. *Binocular Vision and Ocular Motility*. 5th ed. St. Louis, MO: Mosby; 1966:508.
15. Kinyon GE. Anticholinesterase eyedrops: need for caution. *N Engl J Med*. 1969;280:53.
16. von Noorden GK. *Binocular Vision and Ocular Motility*. 5th ed. St. Louis, MO: Mosby; 1966:409.
17. Abraham SV. Intraepithelial cysts of the iris: their production in young persons and possible significance. *Am J Ophthalmol*. 1954;37:327.
18. Hill K, Stromberg A. Ecothiophate iodide in the management of esotropia. *Am J Ophthalmol*. 1962;53:88.
19. Miller JE. A comparison of miotics in accommodative esotropia. *Am J Ophthalmol*. 1960;49:1350.
20. Morton WR, Drance SM, Fairclough M. Prospective study of the effect of ecothiophate iodide on the lens. *Am J Ophthalmol*. 1969;68:1003.
21. Schaeffer RN, Hetherington, J. Anticholinesterase drugs in cataracts. *Trans Am Ophthalmol Soc*. 1966;64:204.

22. Harrison, R. Bilateral lens opacities associated with use of diisopropyl fluorophosphate eye drugs. *Am J Ophthalmol.* 1960;50:153.

23. Jones DP, Watson DM. Angle closure glaucoma precipitated by the use of phospholine iodide for esotropia in a Child. *Br J Ophthalmol.* 1967;51:783.

24. Jackson, WB. Differentiating conjunctivitis of diverse origins. *Surv Ophthalmol.* 1993;38:91–94.

25. Gigliotti F, Williams FT, Hayden FG, Hendley JO. Etiology of acute conjunctivitis in children. *J Pediatr.* 1981;98:531–536.

26. Weiss A, Brinser JH, Nazar-Stewart V. Acute conjunctivitis in childhood. *J Pediatr.* 1993;122:10–14.

27. Weiss, A. Acute Conjunctivitis. In: *Childhood, Decision Making in Pediatric Ophthalmology.* St. Louis, MO: Mosby; 1993:164–165.

28. Ogawa GSH, Hydriuk RA. *Textbook of Ocular Pharmacology.* Philadelphia, PA: Lippincott-Raven; 1997:543–544.

29. *Physicians' Desk Reference.* 52nd ed. Montvale, NJ: Medical Economic Data Production Company; 1998.

30. *Physicians' Desk Reference for Ophthalmology.* 26th ed. Montvale, NJ: Medical Economic Data Production Company; 1997.

31. DíAversa G, Stern GA. *Textbook of Ocular Pharmacology.* Philadelphia, PA: Lippincott-Raven; 1997:552–557.

32. Kelly, L. *Textbook of Ocular Pharmacology.* Philadelphia, PA: Lippincott-Raven; 1997:493–495.

33. Karp CL, Gussler JR, Alfonso, EC. *Textbook of Ocular Pharmacology.* Philadelphia, PA: Lippincott-Raven; 1997:528–529.

34. Meredith TA. *Textbook of Ocular Pharmacology.* Philadelphia, PA: Lippincott-Raven; 1997:374–376.

35. Patalano SM, Hyndriuk RA. *Textbook of Ocular Pharmacology.* Philadelphia, PA: Lippincott-Raven; 1997:531–535.

36. Ogawa GSH, Hyndriuk RA. *Textbook of Ocular Pharmacology.* Philadelphia, PA: Lippincott-Raven; 1997:537–548.

37. Leonard RE, Karp CL, Alfonso EC. *Textbook of Ocular Pharmacology.* Philadelphia, PA: Lippincott-Raven; 1997:515–523.

38. Hill JM, O'Callaghan RJ, Richard KP. *Texibook of Ocular Pharmacology.* Philadelphia, PA: Lippincott-Raven; 1997:575–586.

39. Santos CI, Hueng AJ, Abelson MB, Fosters CS, Friedlander M, McCulley JP. Efficacy of loxoxamide 0.1% ophthalmic solution in resolving corneal epitheliopathy associated with normal keratoconjunctivitis. *Am J Ophthalmol.* 1994;117:488–497.

40. Caldwell DR, Verin P, Hartwich-Young R, Meyer SM, Drake MM. Efficacy and safety of lodoxamide 0.1% vs cromolyn sodium 4% in patients with vernal keratoconjunctivitis. *Am J Ophthalmol.* 1992;113:632–637.

41. Tinkelman D, Rupp G, Kaufman H, et al. Ketoralae tromethamine 0.5% ophthalmic solution in the treatment of seasonal allergic conjunctivitis: a placebo controlled clinical trial. *Surv Ophthalmol.* 1993;38(suppl):133.

42. Ballae Z, Blumenthal N, Tinkelman D, et al. Clinical evaluation of ketoralae tromethamine 0.5% ophthalmic solution for treatment of seasonal allergic conjunctivitis. *Surv Ophthalmol.* 1993;38(suppl):141.

43. Abelson MB, McGarr PJ, Richard KP. *Textbook of Ocular Pharmacology.* Philadelphia, PA: Lippincott-Raven; 1997:609–633.

Pediatric Ophthalmology
Edited by P. F. Gallin
Thieme Medical Publishers, Inc.
New York © 2000

10

Neuro-Ophthalmology

DOUGLAS R. FREDRICK AND CREIG S. HOYT

In evaluating a child with neuro-ophthalmic symptoms and signs, it is useful to divide the involved neural systems into afferent and efferent pathways. However, it should be recognized that many disease processes do not limit themselves to one of these single pathways. In general, disorders of the afferent visual system in children present as visual loss or as the motor consequences of visual loss (i.e., nystagmus in bilateral congenital cataracts). Efferent disorders, on the other hand, present as misalignment of the ocular axis or as impairment of ocular movement. In young children efferent disorders may present without the obvious complaints of diplopia or oscillopsia as these symptoms are conspicuously absent until the age of 5 or 6 years. That children with neurological disorders rarely present with localizing symptoms makes the neuro-ophthalmic examination critically important in arriving at the correct diagnosis.

■ Pediatric Neuro-ophthalmic Examination

Because children usually cannot describe ocular symptomatology, accurate diagnosis depends on a thorough history obtained from the parent or caretaker and a neuro-ophthalmic exam-

ination tailored for children. The history of the illness should focus on onset, duration, variability, frequency, and progression of the ocular sign, whether it is decreased vision or abnormal eye movement. Associated symptoms such as headache, nausea, vomiting, sleep problems, polyuria, polydypsia, and clumsiness should be elicited. Medical history is vital, with obstetrical and birth history often providing clues to the diagnosis (i.e., congenital Horner's syndrome associated with brachial plexus injury). It must be emphasized to the parents that, although this information is important, most congenital anomalies cannot be attributed to the actions of the parents, and guilt is not being ascribed. The parents must be questioned about the child's physical, motor, and intellectual development. Delayed development or loss of motor milestones points to generalized neurological disorder. The examiner must be familiar with the norms for attainment of these milestones. A history of preceding or coexistent trauma or generalized illness should be elicited if present. Chronic medication use must be determined because medications can sometimes result in neuro-ophthalmic conditions (i.e., Dilantin toxicity and ethambutol neuropathy). The social and family history cannot be forgotten as there are autosomal dominant forms of optic atrophy, nystagmus, and neuropathy. The examiner must always consider psychogenic factors that may present as sudden loss of vision in children with no objective findings.

The neuro-ophthalmic examination of a child begins the moment the child enters the examination room. Is the child visually attentive to the new surroundings? Does the child interact with the caretaker appropriately and show motor skills that are age appropriate? Is the child's body or head position abnormal? Once these observations are made, formal examination can begin. The topical diagnosis of a neuro-ophthalmic disorder is made by knowing the visual acuity, visual fields, pupillary behavior, ocular movement, and optic nerve appearance.

Assessment of visual acuity must be conducted by using techniques that are age appropriate. In infants, visual fixation behavior can be assessed binocularly and monocularly. An infant with poor vision will object to occlusion of the sound eye. Acuity can be objectively recorded using visually evoked potential (VEP) or forced preferential-looking (FPL) tests, but both techniques require specialized equipment and well-trained interpreters. Verbal preliterate children can be tested using HOTV, Allen cards, Lea cards, or tumbling E. Older children should be tested with full-line Snellen acuity optotypes. Although subtle visual field changes cannot be quantitated in young children, hemianopias can readily be detected by a two-examiner technique. One examiner sits in front of the child, who is seated on the parent's lap. Fixation is maintained using an interesting toy. The second tester stands behind the child and introduces a brightly colored toy into the child's peripheral field. A child with normal peripheral vision will turn toward the second object, and a child with a hemianopia will ignore the object.

Examination of the pupils can be difficult in children because they will not often maintain fixation for prolonged periods of time. Anisocoria is easy to determine in light-colored eyes, and pupil size should be noted in both dim and full light. Fixation on the toy at distance should be assured when checking pupillary reaction to light and when looking for afferent pupillary defect. If fixation is not maintained, pupillary constriction associated with convergence may confound reaction to light. A normal pupillary response provides information about both efferent and afferent systems.

Assessment of the oculomotor system should include an evaluation for strabismus, ductions and versions, and abnormal ocular movements. When examining a child for strabismus, fixation must be maintained using a visually interesting accommodative target. The cover–uncover test is used to detect tropias, and the prism-cover test is used to quantitate the degree of deviation. In younger children, the Hirschberg corneal light reflex test should be used to detect strabismus. Ductions are evaluated by having the child follow a moving target. If a child is not visually attentive, it is still possible to test the efferent visual pathways by utilizing the vestibular ocular reflex. This can be performed by holding the infant facing the examiner and then rotating the child at arm's length. This will result in conjugate slow deviation with a quick phase refixation. By rotating the child in both directions, cranial nerves III and VI can be evaluated. This is particularly useful in infants with congenital esotropia with abduction deficit.

Although many neuro-ophthalmic conditions will be readily diagnosed and treated by the ophthalmologist, neurological disorders are often best treated using a multidisciplinary approach. A consultation with a pediatric neurologist, neuroradiologist, endocrinologist, neurosurgeon, oncologist, and developmental pediatrician should be obtained when indicated.

Approaching the Blind Infant

Obtaining an objective visual acuity measurement is difficult in children less than 2 years of age. Poor vision in this group can be caused by lesions anywhere in the visual pathway. However, depending on the etiology, visual prognosis can range from normal (delay of visual maturation) to complete blindness. Parents are the most important source of information regarding the visual function of their infant. Questions such as Can your baby see and respond to (smile or follow) your face? and Does your infant respond when you turn on or off the room lights? should be asked. Infants normally fixate on a face by eight weeks of age.

Visual function in infants can be measured in various ways. Because most of these techniques involve interpretation of motor responses, i.e., FPL, fix and follow "visual behavior," central steady maintained (CSM), the observer must consider and exclude abnormalities in the efferent motor pathways. Despite the dependence on motor pathways, assessing visual function in infants and toddlers primarily relies on the observation of behavior. Guidelines have been established to assess normal visual development. Preverbal children who fail to meet these visual milestones or present with nystagmoid ocular movements should undergo a complete

Milestones of Visual Behavior

Steady fixation on [mother's] face: days to 6 weeks
Fixation and following and reaction (smile)
  to mother's face: 2 months
Visually directed reaching: 4 months
Pointing to desired objects: 12 months

ophthalmic and neurological examination.

Optokinetic nystagmus (OKN) testing, which is also dependent on efferent pathways, may be helpful in determining an infant's visual function. To elicit a jerk nystagmus (which is the normal response to an OKN stimulus), the infant must have visual function. Normal vertical OKN responses in an infant with horizontal nystagmus is said to be predictive of visual function sufficient to attend regular schools.

Psychophysical tests such as FPL and VEP have been employed to quantify visual responses in preverbal children. Although these techniques have been useful in studying the visual development of normal infants, quantification of functional vision in the visual and neurologically handicapped infants has proved to be highly variable and should not be employed to predict vision.

Evaluation of the visually impaired infant begins with the general observation of the infant's tone, head control, and signs of dysmorphism. By 6 weeks of age, an infant should be able to lift the head when prone and smile. At 3 months, the infant should be able to hold objects with the hand and coo. At 6 to 8 months, an infant should be able to sit, roll over, and feed itself. By 12 months of age, the infant should be able to crawl, stand with an aid, and begin to walk.

A complete ophthalmic examination including cycloplegic refraction and ophthalmoscopy is then performed. The ophthalmic exam is geared toward (1) identifying clarity of the visual

axis (i.e., excluding anterior dysgenesis, cataract, persistent hyperplastic primary vitreous [PHPV], etc.), (2) assessing the status of the retina (i.e., degree of retinal pigment epithelium [RPE] pigmentation, foveal reflexes, colobomas, falciform folds, etc.), and (3) evaluating the size, morphology, and color of optic nerve (optic nerve hypoplasia, atrophy, or malformation).

Retinoscopy is not only critical to evaluate refractive status but is very sensitive in identifying media (clarity) problems. In the context of a normal ophthalmic examination, a significant refractive error may indicate a syndrome or retinal dystrophy.

Associations with Refractive Status

Myopia

Prematurity and retinopathy of prematurity

Vitreoretinal degeneration
  (Stickler's syndrome and Wagner's dystrophy)

Retinal syndromes
  (Bassen-Kornsweig syndrome and Laurence-Moon-Bardet-Biedl syndrome)

Albinism

Collagen disorders
  (Ehlers-Danlos syndrome and Marfan syndrome)

Other syndromes
  (Alport's syndrome, Alagille syndrome, Down syndrome, Fabray's disease, Flynn-Aird syndrome, and Marshall's syndrome)

Hyperopia

Albinism

Microphthalmic syndromes

Leber's congenital amaurosis

Retinitis pigmentosa (dominant)

Nystagmus in the visually impaired infant is an important clue to distinguishing anterior from posterior visual pathway pathology. Nystagmus manifests between 2 and 3 months of age in the congenitally blind infant or 1 month following acquired visual loss in an infant less than 2 years of age (nystagmus is not present at birth nor is it acquired as a consequence of visual loss after 2 years of age). Nystagmus in this age group (less than 2 years) almost always indicates a defect in the sensory visual system (even in the infant with a normal ophthalmic examination). Roving eye movement, a type of nystagmus, is characterized by slow, large amplitude "to and fro" eye movements, which are indicative of very poor visual function and prognosis.

As stated earlier, the presence of nystagmus in an apparently blind infant points to an afferent defect in the visual system. Opacities and malformations of ocular structures will be manifest. If optic atrophy or abnormal disc configuration is detected, neuroimaging should be performed. If the exam is normal, an electroretinogram (ERG) should be obtained to rule out Leber's congenital amaurosis or cone/rod dystrophy.

When nystagmus is absent, the blindness may be cortically mediated due to cortical visual impairment (CVI) or delayed visual maturation (DVM). Neuroimaging is useful in both of these conditions. It is important not to confuse congenital ocular motor apraxia with blindness because these patients cannot generate saccades voluntarily but do have excellent visual acuity despite the appearance of visual inattention.

■ Disorders of the Afferent Visual Pathway System

Congenital Optic Disc Anomalies

Many infants presenting with low vision and nystagmus will have bilateral optic disc abnormalities. Unilateral cases typically present later in life with strabismus (esotropia) and without nystagmus. Disc anomalies are important to recognize due to their association with central nervous system abnormalities. Visual acuity is highly variable and is typically much better than predicted based on optic disc appearance. Structural anomalies may coexist with amblyopia, and every attempt should be made to correct associated refractive errors and patch accordingly.[1]

Congenital Optic Disc Anomalies

Optic nerve hypoplasia
Morning glory disc
Optic disc coloboma
Peripapillary staphyloma
Optic disc pits
Optic nerve head drusen
Congenital tilted disc syndrome
Optic disc pigmentation
Myelinated nerve fiber layer

Optic Nerve Hypoplasia

Hypoplasia of the optic nerve is a developmental anomaly characterized by a diminished number of axons in the context of a structurally normal optic nerve (Fig. 10–1). Vision is highly variable and is dependent on the number of intact neurons. Visual acuity ranges from 20/20 to no light perception. There may also be generalized or segmental visual field loss.

Optic nerve hypoplasia is caused by a gestational central nervous system injury that results in transsynaptic degeneration and neuronal migration defects. The most common known etiologies are the maternal ingestion of drugs (neuroleptics, alcohol, cocaine, and LSD) during the first trimester and maternal diabetes, but in most cases no known cause can be identified. Optic nerve hypoplasia is also associated with young maternal age.[2]

Optic nerve hypoplasia is associated with a variety of midline central nervous system defects. In septooptic dysplasia (de Morsier syndrome), there is an associated thinning or absence of the septum pellucidum and corpus callosum. Forty-five percent of patients have cerebral hemispheric abnormalities caused by injury or migration defects (holoprosencephaly, schizencephaly, or periventricular leukomalacia), whereas 15% have posterior pituitary ectopia caused by maldevelopment of the pituitary infundibulum. Therefore, endocrine function must be monitored carefully. Neuroimaging should be performed on children who fall off the growth curve (growth hormone deficiency) or have a history of neonatal jaundice or neonatal hypoglycemia. Neonatal jaundice is associated with congenital hypothyroidism, whereas neonatal hypoglycemia is associated with generalized pituitary dysfunction.[3] Due to a suppressed

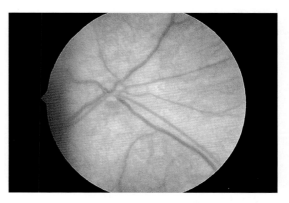

FIGURE 10–1. Optic nerve hypoplasia. Note small amount of nerve tissue surrounded by pigmented epithelium (double-ring sign).

pituitary–adrenal axis, these children are at risk for sudden death during febrile illnesses.[4]

Morning Glory Disc

The morning glory anomaly is usually unilateral and is characterized as a large, funnel-shaped optic nerve with multiple peripheral radial retinal vessels and a central glial tuft. Peripapillary RPE mottling is common and is related to associated serous retinal detachments, which may spontaneously resolve. Like other disk anomalies, visual acuity varies from 20/20 to no light perception, but low vision is the rule. Transspheniodal encephalocele should be suspected in children with morning glory and midfacial anomalies such as hypertelorism and clefting syndromes.[5]

Optic Disc Coloboma

Colobomas of the optic disc represent a defective closure of the fetal fissure and usually affect the inferior part of the retina and choroid. Mild forms are limited to an inferior excavation of an otherwise normal optic nerve. More profound defects extend into the inferior choroid (including the ciliary body and iris) and retina. In the extreme case, microphthalmos with or without cyst may result. Serous retinal detachments are common with high spontaneous reattachment rates. Colobomas are bilateral in 50% of cases and may be inherited in an autosomal dominant or sporadic fashion.[1] Unlike the morning glory anomaly, optic disc colobomas are associated with multisystem genetic disorders.

Systemic Conditions Associated with Optic Disc Colobomas

CHARGE association
 (coloboma, heart defects, atresia choane,
 mental retardation, genito–urinary abnormalities,
 ear defects/deafness)

Goltz syndrome
 (X-linked dominant, focal dermal hypoplasia)

Lenz microphthalmia syndrome
 (X-linked, microphthalmos with or without coloboma,
 mild mental retardation, large ears)

Meckel-Gruber syndrome
 (autosomal recessive, coloboma, renal abnormalities,
 occipital encephalocoele)

Walker-Warburg syndrome
 (autosomal recessive, hydrocephalus, encephalocoele,
 retinal dysplasia)

Goldenhar syndrome
 (lid coloboma, epibulbar dermoid, ear abnormalities)

Peripapillary Staphyloma

This very rare unilateral peripapillary excavation is associated with RPE changes. Despite a relatively normal appearing optic nerve, visual acuity is invariably depressed due to cecocentral scotomas.

Optic Disc Pits

Optic pits are unilateral ovoid depressions of the optic disc that are typically located on the temporal margin. Over half the pits have an associated cilioretinal artery arising at their base. Subretinal fluid accompanied by decreased vision (optic pit maculopathy) is common (50%). Spontaneous reattachment occurs in 25% of cases, and the remaining cases may benefit from vitrectomy followed by internal gas tamponade. Due to the schisis nature of the retinal defect, laser photocoagulation does not appear to improve the condition. In the absence of subretinal fluid, visual acuity is not affected. Visual field findings include an enlarged blind spot and arcuate scotomas. Optic pits may represent a mild optic disc coloboma; however, their temporal location and lack of associated genetic syndromes cast doubt on this relationship.

Optic Nerve Head Drusen

Optic nerve head drusen are relatively common (0.3%) and can be confused with papilledema (Fig. 10–2). They are bilateral (86%) and associated with cupless optic nerves, visual field defects, transient visual loss, peripapillary subretinal neovascular membranes (which are usu-

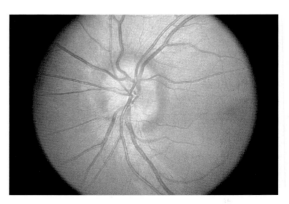

FIGURE 10–2. Optic nerve head drusen. Drusen in optic nerve cause elevation of disc but no edema or obscuration of capillaries.

ally self-limited), and peripapillary retinal and subretinal hemorrhage. Optic nerve head drusen can be differentiated from papilledema because (1) disc elevation is confined to disc, (2) there is a lack of venous congestion, (3) the peripapillary nerve fiber layer is not swollen and opaque (i.e., the peripapillary retinal vasculature is readily seen), and (4) ultrasound images show characteristic reflective images.[1]

Congenital Tilted Disc Syndrome

The congenital tilted disc is characterized as an oval disc with an elevated superonasal rim and depressed inferotemporal rim. The tilted disc is associated with situs inversus of the retinal vessels, high myopia with astigmatism, and bitemporal visual field defects that do not respect the vertical meridian.

Optic Disc Pigmentation

A dark disc may represent melanin deposition on the lamina cribosa characteristic of Aicardi's syndrome, RPE hyperplasia following papillitis, or neoplasm as seen in melanocytoma and RPE hamartomas. Aicardi's syndrome is an X-linked lethal condition (seen only in heterozygous girls) characterized by infantile spasms, severe mental retardation, agenesis of the corpus callosum, and typical fundus findings. The disc is often pigmented and dysmorphic with multiple peripapillary lacunae.[6]

Myelinated Nerve Fiber Layer

Myelination of the nerve fiber layer anterior to the lamina cribosa occurs in approximately 1% of the population. It is bilateral in 20% of cases. The white fluffy fibers usually radiate from the disc but discontinuous patches are not uncommon (Fig. 10–3). Extensive diffuse unilateral myelination has been associated with high myopia and amblyopia that is often refractive to occlusion therapy.[1]

Optic Atrophy

Optic nerve atrophy is most commonly caused by an injury to the anterior visual pathway with subsequent retinal ganglion cell and axon loss. Prior to birth, posterior visual pathway lesions have been implicated though the process of transsynaptic degeneration. The atrophic optic

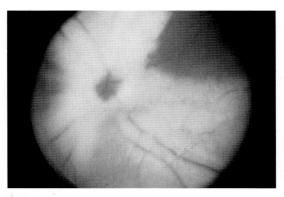

FIGURE 10–3. Myelinated nerve fiber layer. Myelin obscures detail of optic nerve head and retinal vasculature.

nerve is diffusely or segmentally pale with associated retinal nerve fiber layer loss. Approximately half the cases of optic atrophy are caused by tumors (29%) and inflammation-related insults (meningitis and optic neuritis) (17%). The remaining etiologies include trauma (11%), idiopathic causes (11%), hereditary causes (9%), perinatal problems (9%), hydrocephalus (6%), and neurodegenerative causes (5%). Rarely (1%), toxic or metabolic etiologies are identified. Hydrocephalus or anterior visual pathway tumors should be suspected in an otherwise normal child with optic atrophy and negative perinatal, medical, and family histories, whereas intracranial, genetic, and neurometabolic etiologies are common in children with associated neurological findings. Optic atrophy is a leading cause of low vision in these mentally handicapped children. Unilateral, asymmetric, and band optic atrophies are highly suggestive of compressive lesions.[7]

Based on etiology, optic atrophy can be divided into three categories: (1) hereditary and neurodegenerative, (2) compressive, and (3) noncompressive. Except for dominant optic atrophy, hereditary and neurodegenerative optic atrophies typically present to the ophthalmologist as part of a multisystem work-up. Children with compressive and noncompressive forms of optic atrophy may present directly to the ophthalmologist as a consequence of abnormal eye movements (nystagmus or strabismus) or failed vision screening exam.

Causes of Optic Atrophies

Hereditary Optic Atrophies

Dominant optic atrophy (Kjer optic atrophy)
Leber's hereditary optic neuropathy
Recessive optic atrophy
Behr optic atrophy
DIDMOAD

Compressive Optic Atrophies

Craniopharyngioma
Optic nerve and chiasmal gliomas
Pituitary adenoma
Meningioma
Sphenoid sinus mucocele
Osteopetrosis
Craniosystonosis
Fibrous dysplasia

Noncompressive Optic Atrophies

Hydrocephalus
Perinatal hypoxia/ischemia
Toxic/nutritional
Retinal degenerative

Hereditary and Neurodegenerative Optic Atrophies

Dominant Optic Atrophy

Dominant optic atrophy, or Kjer optic atrophy, has been localized to chromosome 3 and is the most common inherited optic atrophy with an incidence of 1:50,000 births. These children usually present between the ages of 4 and 8 years subsequent to a failed visual screening exam. Visual loss is insidious over the first decade with subsequent gradual deterioration. Children do not have nystagmus and typically have better than 20/80 visual acuity associated with blue–yellow dichromatopsias. Approximately 10% of affected children also have sensoral neural hearing deficits. By age 60 years, visual acuities are typically in the 20/800 range.[8,9]

Leber's Hereditary Optic Neuropathy

Patients with Leber's hereditary optic neuropathy (LHON) usually present in their second to third decades with asynchronous bilateral central loss of vision to the 20/200 level. LHON is a mitochondrial (maternally) inherited disease that primarily affects males. Prior to the acute phase, the retinal examination may reveal pseudoedema of the disc with surrounding telangiectatic microangiopathy. Several point mutations have been implicated, and genetic testing is available at several academic institutions.

Recessive Optic Atrophy

An isolated recessively inherited optic atrophy is very rare and is a diagnosis of exclusion. Neuroimaging and retinal electrophysiological testing must be performed to rule out more common conditions such as congenital retinal dystrophies and autosomal recessively inherited neurodegenerative disorders that are associated with optic atrophy.

Behr Optic Atrophy

Behr optic atrophy is characterized as an early-onset optic atrophy with serious central nervous system abnormalities. Children present between the ages of 1 and 8 years with nystagmus (>50%) and gross psychomotor retardation. The classic features of the syndrome include optic atrophy, mental retardation, spasticity, and pes cavus. Neuroimaging reveals diffuse white matter abnormalities.[10] Behr optic atrophy likely represents a genetically based neurodegenerative disorder that must be differentiated from other recessively transmitted metabolic neurodegenerative diseases. In particular, 3-methylglutaconic aciduria has recently been associated with the disorder, suggesting a defect in the mitochondrial respiratory chain.

DIDMOAD

Wolfram syndrome, or DIDMOAD, which stands for diabetes insipidus, diabetes mellitus, optic atrophy, and deafness, is an early-onset, rapidly progressive disorder that may represent another mitochondrial inherited disease. Diabetes mellitus is usually the first feature of the disorder. The remaining findings typically manifest before the age of 20 years. Other neurodegenerative disorders that feature diabetes mellitus and optic atrophy include Friedreich's ataxia, infantile Refsum's, and Alstrom syndrome. Sensorineural hearing loss is a common feature in neurodegenerative optic atrophy. Other rare neurodegenerative disorders associated with optic atrophy include the metabolic disorders such as Krabbe infantile leukodystrophy, Canavan disease, subacute necrotizing encephalopathy, Pelizaeus-Merzbacher disease, neonatal adrenoleukodystrophy, neuronal ceroid lipofuscinosis, and mucopolysaccharidosis.[11]

Compressive Optic Atrophies
Craniopharyngioma

Craniopharyngioma, a slow-growing benign suprasellar epithelial neoplasm, causes optic atrophy by direct compression on the chiasm or secondary to chronic papilledema. Children typically present between the ages of 4 and 10 years with reduced vision or symptoms associated with elevated intracranial pressure. Recurrence following total resection is approximately 25%.[12]

Optic Nerve and Chiasmal Gliomas

Optic nerve and chiasmal gliomas (juvenile pilocytic astrocytomas) in children are usually a benign-acting proliferation of astrocytes. Most children are diagnosed before the age of 10 years. Orbital gliomas frequently cause unilateral loss of vision associated with proptosis, disc swelling, or optic atrophy. Chiasmal lesions may cause hydrocephalus, endocrine dysfunction, and "bow-tie" optic nerve atrophy. Most gliomas are asymptomatic and are diagnosed following the screening neuroimaging studies of a child with cafe au lait spots presumed to have neurofibromatosis 1.[13] Children with gliomas should be followed by visual acuity, fields, and color vision tests; when visual loss is progressive radiation therapy or chemotherapy may be indicated.

Various Compressive Lesions

Other compressive lesions that cause optic atrophy include pituitary adenoma geminoma, meningioma, sphenoid sinus mucocele, osteopetrosis, craniosynostosis, and fibrous dysplasia. Neuroimaging will be diagnostic in these cases.

Noncompressive Optic Atrophy

Hydrocephalus

Hydrocephalus can cause optic nerve atrophy through (1) direct compression of the chiasm by the third ventricle, (2) chronic papilledema, or (3) traction on the optic nerves. Hydrocephalus associated optic atrophy is usually bilateral. Acute rises in intracranial pressure as seen in congenital hydrocephalus with shunt failure or hydrocephalus with intraventricular hemorrhage can cause optic atrophy without papilledema.[14]

Perinatal Hypoxia/Ischemia

Perinatal hypoxia/ischemia rarely causes optic atrophy in the absence of other profound neurological findings. More commonly, reduced vision is attributable to CVI because the anterior visual pathway is relatively resistant to hypoxic damage. However, 25% of children with CVI have coexisting optic atrophy.

Toxic/Nutritional

Traumatic Optic Atrophy

Blunt trauma can injure the optic nerve through a variety of mechanisms. Orbital and canalicular fractures and hematomas can cause compressive damage, whereas optic atrophy seen in traumatic chiasmal syndrome and shaken baby syndrome is tractional in nature. Optic atrophy typically appears 4 to 6 weeks following injury.

Retinal Degenerative Disease

Retinal degenerative disease is commonly associated with optic atrophy. Generally, optic nerve head pallor is a late finding that postdates retinal and RPE degenerative changes. Electrophysiological testing may be helpful in distinguishing primary retinal pathology with secondary optic atrophy from a primary optic atrophy. This is particularly true in neurological children with a congenital retinal dystrophy.[15]

Optic Nerve Head Swelling

Optic nerve head swelling is caused by an arrest of axonal transport across the optic nerve. Axonal transport can be disrupted by mechanical or metabolic forces. Mechanical conditions include neoplasm or masses that compress the optic nerve (optic nerve glioma or osteopetrosis) and cerebrospinal fluid pressure gradient across the lamina cribosa (intracranial hypertension or ocular hypotony). Because axonal transport is energy (adenosine triphosphate [ATP]) dependent, a disruption in oxidative metabolism will also cause optic nerve head swelling. This disruption can result from hereditary factors (Leber's hereditary optic neuropathy), toxins, or diminished cofactors that affect the electron transport chain (cyanide, methanol, or nutritional/vitamin B deficiency) or from lack of oxygen needed for the last step of oxidative metabolism (hypoxia, anoxia, and ischemia). A third mechanism for optic nerve swelling is inflammatory/infiltrative as is seen in optic neuritis, sarcoidosis, and leukemia.

Causes of Optic Nerve Swelling

Papilledema

Idiopathic intracranial hypertension (pseudotumor cerebri)
Hydrocephalus
Craniosynostosis
Intracranial tumors
Spinal cord tumors
Child abuse
Meningitis and subarachnoid hemorrhage

Compressive Optic Nerve Head Swelling

Optic nerve gliomas
Optic nerve sheath meningiomas
Also, see table Causes of Optic Atrophies (p. 106)

Metabolic Optic Nerve Head Swelling

Diabetic papillopathy
Malignant hypertension

Infiltrative/Inflammatory Optic Neuropathy

Leukemia
Optic neuritis
Leber's idiopathic stellate neuroretinitis

Papilledema

Papilledema is a term that implies optic nerve head swelling as a result of increased intracranial pressure. Papilledema appears 1 to 5 days following an acute rise in intracranial pressure. The key features of papilledema are (1) bilateral optic nerve swelling, particularly in children, (2) mild reduction of visual acuity, and (3) neurological symptoms, including headaches, transient visual obscurations, and nausea and vomiting with absence of localizing findings. The degree of visual function (visual acuity and color vision) retained is dependent on rate of progression and chronicity. An acute and severe rise in intracranial pressure, as is seen in shunt dysfunction or intracranial hemorrhage, and chronic low-grade papilledema will produce optic atrophy with profound dyschromatopsia and visual loss. Ophthalmoscopic signs of the more severe cases of papilledema include peripapillary subretinal and flame hemorrhages, cotton wool spots, and venous congestion.

Increased intracranial pressure can be caused by any restriction in cerebrospinal fluid outflow. This can occur in the ventricular system (obstructive hydrocephalus caused by mass lesions), arachnoid granulations (benign intracranial hypertension, meningitis, sub-arachnoid hemorrhage), or intracranial venous system (arteriovenous malformation, sinus thrombosis, and compressive mass).

Idiopathic Intracranial Hypertension

Idiopathic intracranial hypertension (IIH), or pseudotumor cerebri, is a diagnosis of exclusion. The affected child usually presents with nonlocalizing neurological signs characteristic of increased intracranial pressure and papilledema. Neuroimaging and cerebrospinal fluid studies are normal, except for elevated opening pressures on lumbar puncture. Clinical features in postpubescent children are similar to those of adults. Prior to puberty notable differences from adult IIH are (1) an equal incidence in males and females, (2) higher rates of spontaneous resolution, and (3) less of an association with obesity.[16]

IIH can be caused by elevated levels of unbound vitamin A in the cerebrospinal fluid, which appears to reduce outflow at the level of the arachnoid granulations. Vitamin A (Danzole) and thyroxine ingestion, corticosteroid withdrawal, and recovery from malnutrition cause IIH. Other agents implicated include tetracycline and naladixic acid.

Children rarely require surgical intervention for IIH due to their high rate of spontaneous resolution (especially following lumbar puncture) and good response to medical treatment. Children should be treated with furosemide and/or high-dose acetazolamide. Surgical treatment for nonresponsive patients includes optic nerve sheath fenestration or lumboperitoneal shunting.[17–19]

Hydrocephalus

Papilledema is relatively rare (12%) in infants with congenital hydrocephalus. Open cranial sutures are believed to function as a release valve for gradual elevations in intracranial pressure. Following shunt placement the cranial sutures fuse. These children are particularly at risk for papilledema and optic atrophy with subsequent shunt failure. Children with hydrocephalus present with specific eye findings, which should be familiar to any ophthalmologist or pediatrician. In infants, hydrocephalus can present with the setting sun sign, which is

characterized by eyelid retraction, conjugate downward deviation, and upgaze palsy. Older children can present with the dorsal midbrain syndrome, characterized by light-near pupil disassociation, dilated pupils, upgaze palsy, and upbeat nystagmus. Increased intracranial pressure can cause paresis of cranial nerves III, IV, and VI and often comitant horizontal strabismus. The presence of an A-pattern esotropia should alert the observer to increased cranial pressure. Parents of children who had a ventriculoperitoneal shunt placed should be advised that the appearance of strabismus may indicate shunt failure and should necessitate prompt evaluation by the neurosurgeon or ophthalmologist.

Craniosynostosis

Craniosynostosis is a condition associated with the premature closure of the cranial sutures. Papilledema is common in Crouzon's (31%), oxycephaly (23%), and Apert's (9%). A significant number of infants with craniosynostosis and papilledema will develop optic atrophy.

Intracranial Tumors

Intracranial tumors can increase intracranial pressure by mass effect or obstructive hydrocephalus. Suprasellar tumors, such as chiasmal gliomas, are often associated with papilledema by compressing the third ventricle.

Spinal Cord Tumors

Like ependymomas, spinal cord tumors are frequently associated with papilledema and back pain. Blockage of cerebrospinal fluid flow into the spinal cord causes increased intracranial pressure by reducing the pressure accommodating capacity of the spinal cord.

Child Abuse

Papilledema in an infant with shaken baby syndrome is an ominous sign. This usually indicates severe brain edema with intracranial hemorrhage.

Meningitis and Subarachnoid Hemorrhage

Meningitis and subarachnoid hemorrhage may cause increased intracranial hypertension by the cellular and inflammatory mediated obstruction of the arachnoid granulations.

Compressive Optic Nerve Head Swelling

Optic nerve gliomas are the most common retrobulbar process causing optic nerve head swelling in the pediatric population. They are associated with neurofibromatosis. Optic nerve sheath meningiomas are rare in children but may be associated with neurofibromatosis 2.

Metabolic Optic Nerve Head Swelling

Diabetic Papillopathy

Diabetes-related optic neuropathy is thought to be a mild form of anterior ischemic optic neuropathy. The papillopathy is typically bilateral and presents in young type I diabetics without significant visual complaints. The condition resolves spontaneously in approximately 6 months without sequellae.

Malignant Hypertension

Malignant hypertension in children is rare. It is usually seen in various autoimmune disorders that affect the renal system. Optic nerve head swelling is a sign of advanced disease and is associated with ischemic retinopathy and choroidopathy. Blood pressure must be reduced gradually to avoid brain and optic nerve infarctions.

Infiltrative/Inflammatory Optic Neuropathy

Leukemia

Leukemia can cause optic nerve head swelling by three mechanisms: (1) direct infiltration of the optic nerve head by leukemic cells, (2) ischemia secondary to hypervisocity of the hematological system, and (3) papilledema secondary to central nervous system involvement. Leukemic optic nerve infiltration is indicative of central nervous system involvement and is one of the few neuroophthalmic emergencies requiring prompt radiation therapy to prevent severe visual loss.[20]

Optic Neuritis

Optic neuritis in children is usually preceded by either a viral infection or vaccination with live or attenuated viruses. Children typically present with bilateral prelaminar swelling and profound visual loss. Although the traditional belief is that pediatric optic neuritis is distinct from the adult form, recent evidence suggests that more than 50% of children with optic neuritis will eventually develop multiple sclerosis.

Complete visual recovery usually occurs by 6 months but may take as long as 1 year. Work-up is focused on ruling out other forms of optic nerve head swelling and should include (1) neuroimaging studies to exclude hydrocephalus, tumors, or demyelinating plaques; (2) lumbar puncture to exclude inflammatory cells and intracranial hypertension; (3) chest X-ray to exclude sarcoidosis and tuberculosis, and, most importantly; (4) a good history and physical examination. Treatment is primarily supportive. Children with acute encephalomyelitis should be treated with high-dose corticosteroids, but high-dose systemic steroids have been advocated by some authors.

Bilateral optic neuritis accompanied by neurological findings suggests the diagnosis of (1) acute disseminated encephalomyelitis (central nervous system demyelination), (2) multiple sclerosis (central nervous system demyelination), or (3) Devic's disease (ascending spinal cord dysfunction).

Leber's Idiopathic Stellate Neuroretinitis

Leber's idiopathic stellate neuroretinitis is characterized by unilateral optic nerve head swelling accompanied by a macular star. Visual acuity is usually reduced to the 20/100 to 20/200 range. The disc swelling resolves spontaneously in a period of 3 months with near full recovery of vision. The two most common causative agents are *Bartinelae henselae* (cat scratch disease) and *Borrelia burgdorferi* (Lyme disease). Work-up should include a careful history for cat associations, recent febrile illnesses, and rashes. Laboratory testing for cat scratch disease, lyme disease, toxoplasmosis, toxocara, mononucleosis, tuberculosis, and syphilis should be performed.[21,22]

Posterior Visual Pathway

Except for the rubric known as DVM, central nervous system pathology restricted to the visual system is rare. The majority of infants with lesions of the posterior visual pathway causing visual impairment will have multiple neurological handicaps and will be referred to the ophthalmologist by the neurologist or pediatrician. Infants or children who present directly to the ophthalmologist with "posterior visual impairment" (normal ocular examination and absence of nystagmus) should have neuroimaging studies and neurological examination performed. Recall that nystagmus in the congenitally blind infant occurs at approximately 2 months of age and does not occur in acquired vision loss after 2 years of age.

Posterior Visual Pathway Pathology

Congenital CNS Disorders

Neuronal migration and proliferation disorders (lissencephaly, macrogyria, microgyria, and microcephaly)

Developmental (cleavage) defects (holoprosencephaly, schizencephaly, and porencephaly)

Congenital infections (TORCHES)

Congenital vascular abnormalities

Acquired CNS Disorders

Perinatal hypoxia/asphyxia

Ischemia (periventricular leukomalacia of prematurity)

Trauma (intracranial hemorrhage)

Infection (meningitis)

Hydrocephalus

Neurometabolic disease

Cortical Visual Impairment

CVI is a term used to describe patients with poor vision, a normal ocular examination (including pupillary responses), and absence of nystagmus. However, in contrast to adults with CVI, some children may present with abnormal pupillary responses, optic atrophy (secondary to transsynaptic degeneration), roving eye movements, bursts of nystagmus, and strabismus.

Most cases of CVI are diagnosed by neuroimaging studies (MRI). Etiologies include (1) ischemia/hypoxia; (2) periventricular and intraventricular hemorrhages; (3) hydrocephalus; (4) cerebral malformations; (5) head trauma; (6) meningitis, encephalitis and sepsis; and (7) neurodegenerative, toxic, and metabolic conditions.[23] Management of CVI is generally supportive (unless treatable etiology is encountered). It must be emphasized that, due to the tremendous cortical plasticity of the young brain, infants and young children typically recover more visual function than could be predicted based on the degree of cortical injury.

Delayed Visual Maturation

DVM is a diagnosis that is usually made following the profound visual recovery of an infant who was thought to have CVI. Features of DVM are (1) poor visual behavior for age, (2) normal ocular examination, (3) normal pupillary responses, (4) normal electrophysiological testing (ERG), (5) absence of nystagmus, and (6) normal neuroimaging studies. As the name implies, DVM is believed to be caused by either a delay in the normal maturation of the visual system (i.e., myelination or extrastriate processing) or a mild form of CVI involving, perhaps, the subcortical geniculostriate system. Infants with DVM will ultimately develop normal or near normal visual function. However, many children with a history of DVM will later suffer from mild to moderate developmental or neurological defects.[23]

■ Disorders of the Efferent Visual Pathway

Ocular Motor Disorders

Ocular motor disorders are a group of conjugate gaze abnormalities that affect the efferent system of the oculomotor (3rd cranial nerve), trochlear (4th cranial nerve), and abducens (6th cranial nerve) pathways. These lesions affect the "final common pathway" and thus are not overcome by ocular–cephalic and Bell's reflexes, thus distinguishing them from the supranuclear disorders to be described. Children with acquired deficits generally develop incomitant strabismus resulting in diplopia and abnormal head positions. Congenital forms may be incomitant or comitant and are often associated with amblyopia and more-generalized neurological deficits. An important exception to this is an acquired comitant esotropia that has been associated with posterior fossa tumors and the Arnold Chiari malformation. Any eye movement disorder represents a neurological sign that may be focal or generalized in nature.

Third Cranial Nerve Palsy

Approximately 75% of isolated oculomotor palsies are congenital, posttraumatic, or related to meningitis. The remaining quarter may be associated with tumors, aneurysms, or migraines.[24,25] The 3rd cranial nerve exits the midbrain and traverses the skull in the subarachnoid space where it is susceptible to (1) aneurysms of the posterior communicating or internal carotid arteries, (2) basilar skull fractures, and (3) arachnoiditis. It enters the cavernous sinus and exits anteriorly as a superior branch innervating the levator and superior rectus muscles and an inferior branch innervating the medial rectus, inferior rectus, and inferior oblique muscles. The inferior branch also innervates the ciliary ganglion affecting the pupil and accommodation. In the absence of orbital disease, isolated muscle paresis is extremely rare. If an isolated inferior rectus palsy is suspected, rule out myasthenia gravis; if an isolated inferior oblique dysfunction is apparent, consider Brown's syndrome.

Almost half of the pediatric oculomotor deficits are congenital in nature, and many probably represent trauma during delivery. Those not associated with a difficult delivery may be nuclear in origin and come about as the result of prenatal brainstem infarction. Due to the tremendous central nervous system plasticity in the pediatric age group, marked reorganization (rewiring) resulting in cyclic spasm (alternate cycles of spasm and paresis that occur every 2 minutes) or synkinesis may occur.[26] Strabismic amblyopia is common and must be treated appropriately.[27]

Traumatic 3rd nerve injury can occur anywhere in its pathway. Surgical correction should be delayed a minimum of 6 months following injury. Affected children should be monitored and treated for strabismic amblyopia in the interim. Purulent meningitis usually affects multiple cranial nerves. Etiology is determined by history. In the acute setting, intracranial hypertension should be excluded.

Ophthalmic migraine may be associated with transient or permanent oculomotor paresis. Most occur in the first decade of life and may occur in the absence of headache. Diagnosis is made by recurrence in the setting of normal neuroimaging studies.

Fourth Cranial Nerve Palsy

Clinical features of a 4th nerve palsy are (1) hypertropia on the side of lesion that increases in adduction, (2) head tilt opposite to lesion (75%), (3) mild excyclotorsion (5 degrees or less) that is within fusional range, and (4) absence of amblyopia. Secondary contractures of vertical recti are common in long-standing 4th nerve palsies in children with fixation preferences. Spread of comitance (large hypertropia is seen in both adduction and abduction) is caused by ipsilateral superior rectus contracture and occurs when the patient routinely fixes with the nonparetic eye.[28]

One of 10 4th nerve palsies is bilateral. Bilateral cases should be recognized prior to surgical correction. Bilateral 4th nerve palsies (1) have more cyclotorsion (10 degrees in primary and 20 in down gaze), (2) "flip-flop" on the second step of the three-step test, and (3) are esotropic in down gaze (V pattern secondary to bilateral inferior oblique overaction).[29]

The two most common etiologies for trochlear nerve palsies are trauma and congenital disorders (likely birthing trauma). Congenital palsies are recognized by (1) facial asymmetry (face is shorter on opposite side of palsy), (2) high vertical fusional amplitudes (up to 16 diopters compared with 2 in normals), and (3) absence of cyclotorsional complaints. Other causes of 4th nerve palsy include synostotic plagiocephaly and hydrocephalus.

Sixth Cranial Nerve Palsy

Abducens palsy is characterized by (1) incomitant esotropia (35 diopters in primary), (2) large face turn, and (3) divergence paralysis (esotropia greater at distance than at near). The abduction deficit usually results in contracture of the ipsilateral medial rectus, which may worsen the esotropia or cause the esotropia to persist following the resolution of the abducens palsy. The most common etiologies are (1) benign recurrent, (2) trauma, (3) meningitis, (4) hydrocephalus, and (5) pontine glioma.[30] Although some authors have advocated watchful waiting for children with 6th nerve palsies, a computed tomography (CT) or magnetic resonance image (MRI) should be obtained immediately if there are any neurological signs or if there is no sign of improvement in 4 weeks.

Congenital 6th nerve palsies are rare, present at birth (congenital esotropias do not usually appear until 6 weeks of age), and are probably caused by birthing trauma. The incidence is approximately 1 in 150 neonates, and the majority of such palsies resolve spontaneously. Other rare causes of acquired 6th nerve palsy include migraine, following lumbar puncture, internal carotid aneurysm (within cavernous sinus), and other posterior fossa tumors (medulloblastoma, ependymoma, and cerebellar astrocytoma).[31]

Benign recurrent abducens palsies are acute in onset and usually resolve in 2 to 3 months. Amblyopia and residual esotropia may occur. The precise mechanism is unknown, although an infectious cause has been postulated.[32]

Duane's syndrome may be considered an "embryonic" 6th nerve palsy with aberrant innervation of the lateral rectus by the superior branch of the oculomotor nerve. Clinical features include (1) retraction of the globe on adduction (co-contraction of the medial and lateral rectus), (2) V pattern (contraction of the lateral rectus on upgaze), (3) up or down shoot on adduction, and (4) rare amblyopia (rare, usually orthotropic within 15 degrees of primary). A face turn may be employed to compensate for a small angle strabismus in primary gaze.

Duane's is usually a sporadic condition, although family history is positive in 10% of cases. Hearing deficits have been reported in 10% of children with Duane's. Surgical correction should be considered for (1) large face turn, (2) significant enophthalmos (retraction), or (3) severe up- or downshoots.[33]

Supranuclear Disorders of Eye Control

Supranuclear eye movements are mediated by the saccadic (frontal lobe), pursuit (occipitoparietotemporal area), fixation (brainstem), and vestibular systems. Any abnormality in the initiation of eye movements is supranuclear. Saccadic eye movements are initiated by the frontal eye fields. Vertical saccades are mediated by the rostral interstitial nucleus of the medial longitudinal fasciculus (riMLF), which in turn projects to the oculomotor and trochlear nuclei. Horizontal eye movements are mediated by the paramedian pontine reticular formation (PPRF), which project to the abducens nucleus and the oculomotor nucleus by way of the medial longitudinal fasciculus (MLF).

Vertical Supranuclear Palsies

Skew Deviation

Skew deviation is a horizontally and vertically comitant vertical strabismus caused by a lesion in the brainstem or cerebellum (relative vertical deviation the same in all fields of gaze). The lesion is thought to affect the tonic vertical control of the eye, which is regulated by the vestibular system. A high pontine lesion (pontomesencephalic) results in loss of downward eye tone (the ipsilateral eye is hypertropic), whereas a lower pontine lesion (pontomedullary) results in a hypotropic ipsilateral eye.

Alternating Skew

Alternating skew is a horizontally incomitant vertical deviation that appears similar to bilateral superior oblique overaction (hypotropia in adducting eye). Alternating skew is associated with posterior fossa lesions and may be related to the A-pattern strabismus seen in neurological children.[34]

Double Elevator Palsy

Double elevator palsy is a congenital deficit of *monocular* elevation. Supranuclear (contralateral pretectum, ipsilateral riMLF fibers), nuclear (ipsilateral superior rectus subnucleus), and infranuclear lesions (inferior rectus restriction) have been reported. Other considerations include (1) Brown's syndrome, (2) 4th nerve palsy, (3) congenital absence of the superior rectus (Crouzon's), (4) myasthenia gravis, (5) 3rd nerve palsy, and (6) congenital fibrosis syndrome. Congenital fibrosis syndrome (congenital fibrosis of the inferior rectus) is the most common cause of double elevator palsy and can be excluded by normal vestibular reflexes and normal forced ductions.[35]

Vertical Gaze Palsies

Unlike skew deviation, vertical gaze palsies are conjugate (binocular) disorders in vertical eye movements caused by defects in the saccadic pathway.

Downgaze palsies are very rare and are caused by bilateral midbrain lesions affecting the riMLF. Tonic upgaze is a rare transient episodic downgaze palsy that is often associated with downbeat nystagmus. The condition resolves spontaneously by 4 months.[36] Eccentric fixation ("overlooking" of macular disease–neuronal ceroid lipfuscinosis) should be excluded.

Upgaze palsies are commonly seen as part of the dorsal midbrain syndrome, which commonly involve pineal region and third ventricle tumors, encephalitis, and hydrocephalus.

Ocular Findings Associated with Hydrocephalus

Upgaze palsy (tonic downgaze)

Eyelid retraction
  (coinnervation of functional levator)

Convergence–retraction
  (simulation of the medial rectus on attempted upgaze)

Light-near dissociation of pupils

Setting sun sign
  (combination of upgaze palsy and eyelid retraction)

A pattern esotropia

Tonic downgaze is a transient upgaze palsy seen in normal infants that may be associated with upbeat nystagmus. It is thought to be caused by excessive vertical tone of the maturing vestibular system, which is absent in sleep. The condition resolves spontaneously by 6 months of age.[37]

Horizontal Supranuclear Palsies

Horizontal gaze palsies can be caused by lesions in the (1) frontal eye field (contralateral to gaze palsy), (2) PPRF (ipsilateral), or (3) abducens nucleus (ipsilateral). The vestibular system (doll's/caloric testing) requires an intact PPRF and abducens nucleus for horizontal eye movements.[38]

Mobius syndrome is a rare congenital disorder characterized by poor horizontal eye movements and mask facies. It is a sporadic genetic anomaly that results in various limb, face, cardiac, and brainstem developmental anomalies.

Congenital ocular motor apraxia is characterized by the inability to initiate volitional horizontal saccades in the context of normal vertical eye movements. In contrast to the acquired form (which is actually a saccadic or true gaze palsy), congenital ocular motor apraxia spares horizontal OKN and vestibular saccades. Infants develop "compensatory" head thrusts to achieve fixation beginning at 6 months of age. Blinking is often used to disrupt normal fixation reflexes. The head thrusts improve spontaneously in the first decade of life. Due to associations with (1) various central nervous system malformations (posterior fossa tumors/hypoplasia and hypoplastic corpus callosum), (2) Joubert's syndrome (cerebellar vermis hypoplasia), (3) ataxia telangectasia, and (4) Gaucher's disease, neuroimaging and neurological work-up are recommended, especially if vertical movements are involved.[39,40]

Ophthalmoplegia

Ophthalmoplegia is a disorder affecting conjugate gaze. "Supranuclear" ophthalmoplegias are discussed. Other causes include (1) myasthenia gravis, (2) botulism toxicity, (3) multiple sclerosis, and (4) orbital processes.

Internuclear ophthalmoplegia is characterized as a unilateral or bilateral adduction deficit in lateral gaze. The ipsilateral eye may adduct slowly while the abducting eye exhibits horizontal nystagmus. Convergence is typically preserved. The clinical findings indicate damage to the ipsilateral MLF (midbrain and pons), which can be caused by (1) demyelinating disease, (2) stroke, (3) brainstem tumors (pontine glioma), (4) vasculitis, (5) postinfectious encephalitis, (6) structural malformations (Arnold Chiari), (7) drug intoxication, and (8) trauma. Most cases improve spontaneously.

Fisher's syndrome, or one-and-a-half syndrome, is a variant of the Guillain-Barre syndrome and is characterized by an ipsilateral horizontal gaze palsy (lesion in the PPRF or abducens nucleus), a contralateral adduction deficit on lateral gaze (lesion also affects the MLF), and intact convergence. Males are affected twice as often as females, and the majority of patients report a viral prodrome 1 to 3 weeks prior to the onset of diplopia and ataxia. Most cases resolve spontaneously within 1 to 3 months.[41]

Chronic progressive external ophthalmoplegia (CPEO) is a nonspecific diagnosis that indicates a mitochondrial neurodegenerative disorder that causes a slowly progressive bilateral ptosis and inability to move the eyes. The pupils are usually spared. Mitochondrial disorders are often diagnosed by muscle biopsy, which reveals "ragged red fibers."

Kearns-Sayre syndrome is a CPEO associated with a pigmentary retinopathy that manifests prior to age 20 years. Additionally, the patient must have one of the following: (1) heart block, (2) elevated cerebral spinal fluid protein levels (>100 mg/dL), or (3) cerebellar dysfunction.

Nystagmus and Eye Movement Disorders

Nystagmus is a rhythmic oscillation of the eyes that is defined by the (1) direction, (2) amplitude, (3) frequency, and (4) velocity of phases. Jerk nystagmus consists of an initial slow phase followed by a fast "corrective" phase. Pendular nystagmus has two phases that are equal in velocity. Physiological nystagmus includes (1) endpoint nystagmus and (2) OKN. In contrast to adult nystagmus, the majority of pediatric nystagmus is "congenital" (onset <6 months) and usually represents pathology in the afferent sensory visual pathway. Acquired pediatric (onset >6 months) nystagmus, like adult nystagmus, may be neurological in nature (particularly if the child is older than 2 years of age) and represent a lesion in the efferent motor pathway. It must be noted, however, that nystagmus is conspicuously absent in children with cortical visual loss.

Congenital Nystagmus

Congenital nystagmus (sensory or motor) is a horizontal pendular or jerk nystagmus that has several distinct clinical features that distinguish it from the more ominous acquired forms: (1) fast phase changes direction in right and left gaze (fast phase always in direction of abducting eye), (2) fixation enhances nystagmus intensity, (3) convergence (adduction) dampens nystagmus intensity, (4) oscillopsia is absent, (5) a null zone is present (gaze position related reduction of nystagmus intensity) that is often associated with a face turn, and (6) onset, typically between 8 and 12 weeks of age.[42]

Congenital sensory nystagmus becomes evident between 8 and 12 weeks of age and is usually caused by pathology in the anterior visual pathway resulting in bilateral loss of vision beyond the 20/70 level. Typical causes include (1) anterior segment pathology (corneal opacities, cataract, and aniridia), (2) optic nerve anomalies (colobomas, hypoplasia, and atrophy), and (3) retinal pathology (Leber's congenital amaurosis, albinism, achromatopsia, blue cone monochromism, and congenital stationary night blindness).[43]

Albinism is a heterogeneous disorder of pigmentation that has two main forms: ocular (neuroectoderm defect), which is inherited in an X-linked and autosomal recessive manner, and oculocutaneous (defect in neuroectoderm and neural crest derivatives), which is inherited in an autosomal dominant or recessive manner. The oculocutaneous form can further be divided into tyrosinase-positive and -negative subtypes. Tyrosinase negative albinos have very poor vision, white hair, and pink eyes. Tyrosinase positive albinos may have associated potentially lethal systemic diseases: (1) Chediak-Higashi syndrome (immune disorder, bleeding diatheses, or neuropathy) and (2) Hermansky-Pudlak syndrome (pulmonary fibrosis or bleeding diatheses).

Features of albinism include (1) reduced visual acuity with associated nystagmus and myopia, (2) strabismus (usually esotropia) with associated amblyopia, (3) iris and ocular translucency with associated photophobia, and (4) typical funduscopic findings, which include (a) signs of foveal hypoplasia (reduced foveal reflex, macula lutea pigment and foveal retinal pigment epithelium pigmentation, and retinal vessels coursing over the fovea), (b) clear view of choroid in the mid-periphery (reduced retinal pigment epithelium pigmentation), and (c) optic nerve anomalies (small cupless disk that may have a gray cast, oblique cup with situs inversus). Albinism is a clinical diagnosis that may be confirmed by an abnormal hemispheric visual evoked response caused by excessive chiasmal ducussation of temporal ganglion axons.[44]

Congenital motor nystagmus represents 10% of cases of congenital nystagmus. As the name implies, the pathology is thought to involve the efferent (motor) system. Many cases may actually represent a mild form of ocular albinism with only modest (20/40 to 20/70) reductions of visual acuity.[45] The diagnosis is made by reasonable vision in the context of a normal neurological and funduscopic examination. The nystagmus generally manifests by 3 months and improves with age.[43]

Strabismic Nystagmus

Nystagmus associated with congenital and infantile esotropia is common. The nystagmus is usually latent, becoming manifest when one eye is occluded. This is important to remember when testing visual acuities in children with infantile esotropia. Latent nystagmus is a sign of lost binocular vision during a critical period in the developing visual system. It is associated with persistence of nasotemporal disparity on optokinetic testing that normally resolves by 22 weeks of age. Like congenital nystagmus, the slow phase is in (adduction) and fast corrective phase is out (abduction).

Manifest latent nystagmus is a term that has been used to describe a latent nystagmus that has become "manifest" through amblyopia or strabismus (suppression).

Ciancia's syndrome, or nystagmus blockage syndrome, is congenital nystagmus associated with a variable esotropia. The esotropia is believed to be an adaptive mechanism used to dampen the nystagmus (congenital nystagmus dampens with adduction). Interestingly, if a convergence pathway is responsible, it is dissociated from accommodation (absence of miosis and myopia).

Monocular Nystagmus

Monocular (or highly asymmetric) nystagmus usually indicates spasmus nutans (90%), although it may be caused by severe unilateral visual loss or chiasmal gliomas.

Spasmus nutans is characterized by (1) nystagmus (fine/rapid, horizontal, or asymmetrical), (2) head nodding (low frequency and resolves at sleep), and (3) torticollis (head turn or tilt) beginning at 6 to 12 months of age. The nystagmus generally resolves spontaneously by 1 to 2 years of age without sequellae. If optic atrophy or subnormal vision is encountered, suprasellar pathology (chiasmal glioma) should be excluded with neuroimaging.

Neurological Nystagmus

Positional nystagmus is akin to benign positional nystagmus seen in adults and is elicited by head movements. In children, the most common etiology is labyrinthitis or trauma (injuring the peripheral vestibular system).

Upbeat nystagmus usually indicates anterior visual pathway disease (optic nerve hypoplasia, cataract, or retinal pathology) in children.[46] If ERG and neuroimaging studies are normal, tonic downgaze or benign hereditary etiologies may be considered. In adults, cerebellar or brainstem pathology is common.

Downbeat nystagmus in early childhood indicates craniocervical junction abnormalities including (1) Arnold-Chiari malformation, (2) syringobulbia, (3) Klippel-Feil anomaly, and (4) glioma. Improvement usually occurs following surgical decompression of the herniated cerebellum. Other causes are (1) intracranial hypertension, (2) cerebellar degeneration, and (3) medications (lithium and anticonvulsants). Like upbeat nystagmus, a benign congenital motor form has been reported.[47]

Periodic alternating nystagmus (PAN) is an underdiagnosed form of nystagmus that alternates between right beating and left beating every few minutes. Between fast phase reversal, there may be a vertical component. The congenital form may have underlying neurological pathology but more commonly is associated with albinism. PAN is differentiated from other forms of congenital nystagmus because the nystagmus dampens with fixation. The acquired form is associated with (1) spinocerebellar degeneration, (2) posterior fossa tumors/malformations, and (3) encephalitis. Baclofen (inhibitor of glutamate release) may help diminish acquired PAN, suggesting that the pathology may lie in the vestibular system.[48]

See-saw nystagmus is characterized by one eye that elevates and intorts while the other depresses and extorts. Sea-saw nystagmus is associated with large suprasellar tumors (craniopharyngioma and chiasmal gliomas) that affect the optic chiasm. It is associated with bitemporal hemianopsia, suggesting a sensory etiology. Clonazepam and baclofen may help eliminate nystagmus.[49]

Other Oscillatory Eye Movements

Ocular flutter is bursts of back-to-back horizontal saccades without intrasaccadic interval. These "saccadic intrusions" are seen in association with postviral encephalopathy.

Opsoclonus is characterized as chaotic multidirectional bursts without intrasaccadic intervals. It is a profound form of ocular flutter that suggests cerebellar dysfunction. Infantile opsoclonus is usually transient and benign. Opsoclonus in childhood may be caused by (1) benign encephalitis (of Kinsbourne's), also known as "dancing eyes and dancing feet" (associated lower extremity myoclonus), which resolves spontaneously in weeks to months, (2) toxins, (3) encephalitis/meningitis, and (4) hydrocephalus. Either flutter or opsoclonus may be a paraneoplastic effect of neuroblastoma.[50]

■ Conclusion

This chapter has outlined the examination techniques required to diagnose common pediatric neuro-ophthalmic disorders. The practitioner is commonly confronted with the decision of when a patient should be referred to pediatric neurology and which patients require neuroimaging. Although there are certainly no specific criteria, the following findings should initiate a consultation and/or imaging:

1. Afferent pupil defect.
2. New onset squint in a patient complaining of diplopia.
3. Swollen or atrophic optic nerve.
4. Multiple cranial nerve palsies.
5. Any child losing developmental milestones.
6. New onset nystagmus.
7. Amblyopia not responding to compliant occlusion therapy.
8. Congenital exotropia.

REFERENCES

1. Brodsky M. Congenital optic disk anomalies. *Surv Ophthalmol.* 1994;39(2):89–112.
2. Hoyt C, Good W. Do we really understand the difference between optic nerve hypoplasia and atrophy? *Eye.* 1992;6:201–204.
3. Skarf B, Hoyt C. Optic nerve hypoplasia in children: association with anomalies of the endocrine and CNS. *Arch Ophthalmol.*1984;102:62–67.
4. Brodsky M, Conte F, Taylor D, Hoyt C, Mrak R. Sudden death in septo-optic dysplasia. *Arch Ophthalmol.*1997;115:66–70.
5. Caprioli J, Lesser R. Basal encephalocoele and morning glory syndrome. *Br J Ophthalmol.*1983;67:349–351.

6. Hoyt C, Billson F, Ouvrier R, Wise G. Ocular features of Aicardi's syndrome. *Arch Ophthalmol.* 1978;96:291–295.

7. Repka M, Miller N. Optic atrophy in children. *Am J Ophthalmol.* 988;96:195–199.

8. Eliott D, Traboulsi E, Maumenee I. Visual prognosis in autosomal dominant optic atrophy (Kjer type). *Am J Ophthalmol.*1993;115:360–367.

9. Hoyt C. Autosomal dominant optic atrophy: a spectrum of disability. *Ophthalmology.* 1980;80:245–259.

10. Marzan K, Barron T. MRI abnormalities in Berh syndrome. *Pediatr Neurol.* 1994;10:247–248.

11. Hagemoser K, Weinstein J, Bresnick G. Optic atrophy, hearing loss, and peripheral neuropathy. *Am J Med Genet.* 1989;33:61–65.

12. Weiner H, Wisoff J, Rosenberg M. Craniopharyngiomas: a clinicopathological analysis of factors predictive of recurrence and functional outcome. *Neurosurgery.* 1998;6:1001–1011.

13. Dutton J. Gliomas of the anterior visual pathway. *Surv Ophthalmol.* 1994;38:427–452.

14. King K, Cronin C. Ocular findings in premature infants with grade IV intraventricular hemorrhage. *J Pediatr Ophthalmol Strabismus.* 1993;30:84–87.

15. Folz S, Trobe J. The peroxisome and the eye. *Surv Ophthalmol.* 1991;35:353–368.

16. Babikian P, Corbett J, Bell W. Idiopathic intracranial hypertension in children. *J Child Neurol.* 1994; 9:144–149.

17. Schoeman J. Childhood pseudotumor cerebri: clinical and intracranial pressure response to acetazolamide and furosemide treatment in a case series. *J Child Neurol.* 1994;9:1301–1334.

18. Baker R, Baumann R, Bruncic J. Idiopathic intracranial hypertension (pseudotumor cerebri) in pediatric patients. *Pediatr Neurol.* 1989;5:5–11.

19. Lessel S. Pediatric pseudotumor cerebri (idiopathic intracranial hypertension). *Surv Ophthalmol.* 1992; 37:155–166.

20. Rennie I. Ophthalmic manfestations of childhood leukaemia. *Br J Ophthalmol.* 1992;76:641–645.

21. Bar S, Segal M, Shapira R, Savir H. Neuroretinitis associated with cat scratch disease. *Am J Ophthalmol.* 1990;1990:702–705.

22. Weiss A, Beck R. Neuroretinitis in childhood. *Pediatr Ophthalmol Strabismus.* 1989;26:198–203.

23. Hamed L. Visual impairment in infants: localizing the lesion on a clinical basis. *Semin Ophthalmol.* 1997; 12(2):96–108.

24. Keith C. Oculomotor palsy in children. *Aust NZ J Ophthalmol.* 1987;15:181–184.

25. Miller N. Solitary oculomotor nerve palsy in childhood. *Am J Ophthalmol.* 1977;83:106–111.

26. Hamed L. Associated neurologic and ophthalmologic findings in congenital oculomotor nerve palsy. *Ophthalmology.* 1991;98:708–714.

27. Ing E, Sullivan T, Clarke M, Buncic J. Oculomotor nerve palsies in children. *J Pediatr Ophthalmol Strabismus.* 1992;29:331–336.

28. Von Noorden G, Murray E, Wong S. Superior oblique paralysis. A review of 270 cases. *Arch Ophthalmol.* 1986;104:1771–1776.

29. Keane JR. Fourth nerve palsy: historical review and study of 215 patients. *Neurology.* 1993;43:2439–2443.

30. Robertson D, Hines J, Rucke C. Acquired sixth nerve paresis in children. *Arch Ophthalmol.* 1970;83:574–579.

31. Archer S, Sondhi N, Helveston E. Strabismus in infancy. *Ophthalmology.* 1989;96:133–137.

32. Afifi A, Bell W, Bale J, Thompson H. Recurrent lateral rectus palsy in childhood. *Pediatr Neurol.* 1990; 6:315–318.

33. Shauly Y, Weissman A, Meyer E. Ocular and systemic characteristics of Duane syndrome. *J Pediatr Ophthalmol Strabismus.* 1993;30:178–183.

34. Hamed L, Maria B, Quisling R, Mickle J. Alternating skew on lateral gaze: neuroanatomic pathway and relationship to superior oblique overaction. *Ophthalmology.* 1993;100:281–286.

35. Metz H. Double elevator palsy. *J Pediatr Ophthalmol Strabismus.* 1981;18:31–35.

36. Ahn J, Hoyt W, Hoyt C. Tonic upgaze in infancy. *Arch Ophthalmol.* 1989;107:57–58.

37. Hoyt C, Mousel D, Weber A. Transient supranuclear disturbances of gaze in healthy neonates. *Am J Ophthalmol.* 1980b;89:708–713.

38. Yee R, Duffin R, Baloh R. Familial congenital paralysis of horizontal gaze. *Arch Ophthalmol.* 1982;1449–1452.

39. Zee R, Yee R, Singer H. Congenital ocular motor apraxia. *Brain.* 1977;100: 581–599.

40. Steinlin M, Martin E, Largo E. Congenital ocular motor apraxia: a neurodevelopmental and neuroradiological study. *Neuro-Ophthalmology.* 1990;10:27–32.

41. Berlit P, Rakicky J. The Miller Fisher syndrome: review of the literature. *J Clin Neuro-Ophthalmol.* 1992;12:57–63.

42. Leigh R, Zee D. *The Neurology of Eye Movements.* Philadelphia, PA: FA Davis;1991.

43. Gelbart S, Hoyt C. Congenital nystagmus: a clinical perspective in infancy. *Graefeis Arch Clin Exp Ophthalmol.* 1988;226:178–180.

44. Kinnear P, Jay B, Witkop C. Albinism. *Surv Ophthalmol.* 1985;30:75–101.

45. Simon J, Kandel G, Krohel C, Nelsen C. Albinotic characteristics in congenital nystagmus. *Am J Ophthalmol.* 1984;97:320–327.

46. Good W, Brodsky M, Hoyt C, Ahn J. Upbeating nystagmus in infants: a sign of anterior visual pathway disease. *Binoc Vis Q.* 1990;5:13–18.

47. Schmidt D. Downbeat nystagmus: a clinical review. *Neuro-Ophthalmology.* 1991;11:247–262.

48. Gradstein L, Reinecke R, Wizov S, Goldstein H. Congenital periodic alternating nystagmus. *Ophthalmology.* 1997;104:918–929.

49. Zelt R, Biglan A. Congenital seesaw nystagmus. *J Pediatr Ophthalmol Strabismus.* 1985;22:13–16.

50. Shawkat F, Harris C, Wilson J, Taylor D. Eye movements in children with opsoclonus. *Neuropediatrics.* 1993; 24:218–223.

51. Sharpe J, Johnston J. Ocular motor paresis versus apraxia. *Ann Neurol.* 1989;25:209–210.

Pediatric Ophthalmology
Edited by P. F. Gallin
Thieme Medical Publishers, Inc.
New York © 2000

11

Motor and Sensory Tests

SALLY A. MOORE

To understand strabismus in patients of any age, it is necessary to thoroughly evaluate motor and sensory status. With this evaluation, the examiner makes a diagnosis, plans therapy, and predicts the prognosis.

To accurately perform the various tests, it is necessary that the patient maintains fixation on the object of regard (target). To assure this, a constant flow of conversation by the examiner is helpful. In the verbal patient, this conversation is usually in the form of questions. Most children want to answer correctly and enjoy this rapport with the examiner. Ask the child about clothes, activities, siblings, birthdays, and nursery school. Also, attentive fixation assures better control of the accommodation.

■ Motor Evaluation

Heterophoria vs. Heterotropia

The first step in evaluating motor status is to determine whether the eye alignment is a latent (hiding), intermittent, or constant deviation. If stabismus is present, it is essential to be aware of any variability in the angle of deviation.

Cover–Uncover Test

Currently, one of the most accurate methods of evaluating the motor picture is the cover–uncover test. Each eye in turn is covered and uncovered, allowing binocularity to exist in the interval between the covering maneuver. The occlusion can be with a plastic occluder, the hand, or the fingers. Fixation is controlled by an accommodative target (at distance or near) throughout the testing procedure.

Two observations are made (Table 11–1). (1) The uncovered eye is observed when the other eye is covered. No movement of either eye when one eye is covered indicates no strabismus. Movement of the uncovered eye indicates strabismus. Care is taken that alternate fixation does not occur during the binocular situation. An esotropia is present if the uncovered eye moves out to fixate the target, an exotropia is present if the uncovered eye moves in to fixate, and a hypertropia or hypotropia is present if the uncovered eye moves up or down to fixate, respectively. (2) A tropia is present when the uncovered eye moves. A phoria is present when the covered eye moves. The covered eye is observed as the cover is removed. In the presence of heterophoria, the eye under the cover assumes a fusion-free position. When the cover is removed, the eye performs a fusional movement to resume bifoveal fixation. After determining the status of the deviation (i.e., heterophoria vs. heterotropia) with the cover–uncover test, the next step is to measure the amount of the deviation.

TABLE 11–1. Cover–Uncover Test

Cover–Uncover Alternate Cover	Prism Direction	Diagnosis
No movement	No movement	No strabismus (orthophoria)
Uncovered eye moves out	Prism base out	Esotropia
Uncovered eye moves in	Prism base in	Exotropia
Covered eye moves out	Prism base out	Esophoria
Covered eye moves in	Prism base in	Exophoria

Alternate Cover and Prism Test

Clinically, the most accurate test to measure the full amount of the deviation in patients with central fixation is the alternate cover and prism test. The patient fixates a target, controlling accommodation by having the child identify different optotypes or features of a picture or toy. The cover is alternated from one eye to the other eye. If there is no movement of the eyes after prolonged alternate cover, orthophoria is suspected. However, to prove that orthophoria exists, a 2-prism diopter (pd) is introduced base in, base out, base up, and base down. If reverse movement is noted in all four directions, then orthophoria exists. If there is movement of the eyes with alternate cover, a deviation is present. The cover is alternated from one eye to the other as appropriately held prisms are increased until the end point is reached (i.e., no movement of the eyes).

> Prism base-out for esodeviation
> Prism base-in for exodeviation
> Prism base-down or -up for hyperdeviation

The point of the prism is in the direction of the deviation, for example, eye moves *in* in esotropia so base *out*/point in. However, to ensure the maximum end point, the prisms are increased until reversal of movement is noted. To uncover the full amount of the deviation, prolonged dissociation of the eyes with the cover along with slowly increasing the prism strength is helpful. The patient should never be allowed to see binocularly until the measurements are determined. At times, more deviation can be elicited by asking the patient to relax and give up eye control. This is particularly true for patients with heterophoria or intermittent deviations, yielding a range of prism measurements. Correcting both horizontal and vertical deviations to the end point with the appropriate prisms is advised. Correcting one meridian may

influence the amount of deviation in the other meridian. The secondary component of a deviation may become more prominent postoperatively, and this could be disturbing if not previously detected and measured. These measurements are done and recorded at distance fixation in primary position. (They are also done at distance fixation in right and left gaze to rule out lateral gaze incomitance and in up and down gaze to rule out A and V patterns. If a vertical deviation is measured in any of the previosly mentioned directions, then the measurements are done at distance with the head tilted to either side approximately 30 degrees. The results of this head tilt test will help incriminate the offending vertical muscle. The prism is held parallel to the lower lid fissure.[1]) Alternate cover–prism measurements are repeated at near fixation, with and without +3.00 in primary position. (Measurements are done at near fixation in four diagnostic positions of gaze: right, up and down, and gaze left, up and down.) The results of these measurements are recorded as follows:

Latent Deviation		Manifest Deviation	
Esophoria	= S or E	Esotropia	= ST or ET
Exophoria	= X	Exotropia	= XT
Right hyperphoria	= RH	Right hypertropia	= RHT
Left hyperphoria	= LH	Left hypertropia	= LHT

The amount of the deviation is expressed in pd. A prime (′) after the initial indicates the measurements were done at near fixation, i.e., ST 30 distance esotropia and ST′ 40 near esotropia.

For example,

SC	CC
ST = 10	ST = 5
ST′ = 20	ST′ = 10
	bifocal = 0
	[+3 or +3.50
	(state amount)]

Note: SC (without optical correction)
        CC (with spectacles)
        bifocal

Corneal Reflection Tests

These tests are used for infants and patients with marked amblyopia.

Hirschberg Method

The patient fixates on a light while the examiner compares the relative location of the corneal reflection of each eye. Strabismus is usually present if the corneal reflections are not symmetric. The angle of strabismus can be grossly estimated by the amount of horizontal displacement of the corneal reflections. (This can be done vertically but is classically applied horizontally.) Each millimeter of displacement is roughly equivalent to 14 pd of deviation. For example, in general

Center = 0
Midpupil
    (half way from center to iris margin) = 15
Iris margin = 30
Mid-iris = 45
Limbus = 60

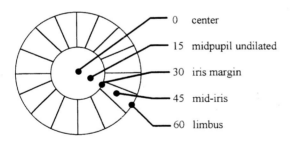

- 0   center
- 15   midpupil undilated
- 30   iris margin
- 45   mid-iris
- 60   limbus

Krimsky Method

In this method the corneal reflexes are centered by the use of prisms. The amount and type of deviation should be determined with the fixating eye remaining in primary position at near fixation. Therefore, it is suggested that the prisms be placed over the deviating eye until the corneal reflexes are centered. At distance fixation it is difficult to accurately evaluate the corneal reflections. In this case the prism is placed over the fixating eye until the usually deviating eye appears straight in the orbit.

Simultaneous Prism and Cover Test

Strabismus frequently exhibits a certain variability in amount of deviation for various reasons, i.e., physical or emotional state, the accommodative and proximal convergence, poorly developed reflexes, amblyopia, etc. The examiner should be aware of any variability in the angle of deviation under different testing as well as under nontesting conditions (casual observation of the patient) and the parents' history of variations of the deviation. Therefore, every effort is made to determine the minimum as well as the maximum angle of deviation. Both these angles of deviation may have functional as well as cosmetic importance. The prolonged alternate cover and prism test is used to elicit the full amount of the deviation, whereas the simultaneous prism and cover test is used to measure the ordinary binocular condition deviation. While the patient fixates a target, the fixating eye is covered with an occluder at the same time that a prism is placed over the deviated eye. The prism is held base out if an esotropia is present and base in with an exotropia. Covering the fixating eye forces the deviating eye to fixate. If the appropriate prism is used, there is no movement of the newly fixating eye, as the prism has deflected the image onto the fovea. However, if there is movement, the prism is used inappropriately, and the test is repeated with a deterrent prism starting again from a binocular situation.

4Δ Base-Out Test

Another test that is useful in determining whether bifixation (central fusion) or monofixation (absence of central fusion) exists is the 4Δ base-out test. While the patient fixates on a letter at distance, a 4Δ prism base out is introduced before each eye separately. There are three basic responses to this test.

1. A convergence movement indicating a heterophoria with bifoveal fusion
2. No movement indicating a heterotropia, and the prism has been placed before the suppressed nonfixating eye
3. Parallel movement of the eyes toward the apex of the prism indicating a heterotropia, and the prism has been placed before the fixating eye

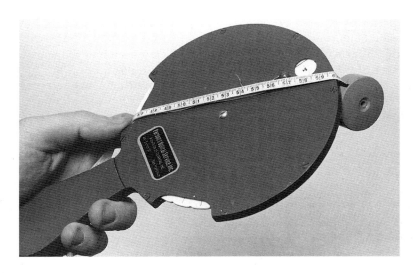

FIGURE 11–1. The accommodometer: side facing patient.

Near Point of Convergence

The distance inside which convergence (disjunctive inward movement of the eyes) can no longer occur is termed the near point of convergence (NPC). An accommodative target is held in line with the bridge of the nose and slowly moved closer until the patient reports diplopia or the examiner observes cessation of convergence (i.e., a deviation of one eye). At this point, a millimeter ruler is placed near the inner canthus of one eye, and the NPC is recorded. The normal NPC for an adult is 50 to 70 mm. Children normally have an NPC limited only by their nose.

Near Point of Accommodation

The distance inside which the eyes can no longer effectively accommodate is termed the near point of accommodation (NPA). This is routinely measured in patients with strabismus, patients with symptomatic heterophoria, and patients successfully treated for amblyopia as the last step before treatment is discontinued. It is done monocularly, and it is preferable to start from a nonseeing position (inside the NPA) and slowly move the target away until proper identification is made and recorded. The NPA is normal if equal and within the normal range.[2] The Costenbader accommodometer[3] (Fig. 11–1) and the RAF rule (Fig. 11–2) are two instruments that can be used to determine the NPA.

Rotations are composed of versions and ductions. Versions are parallel movements of the eyes. To study versions, the patient is requested to follow a fixation target into the diagnostic positions of gaze. Drawing an imaginary line from the two upper limbi in eyes down (or lower limbi in eyes up), the limbus of each eye should touch the imaginary line. If one eye is too high or low in relation to the other eye, then it is recorded as overaction or underaction. It is suggested that versions be done with either eye fixating. When a dissociated vertical deviation (DVD) is present, the adducted eye will appear relatively higher than the fixating

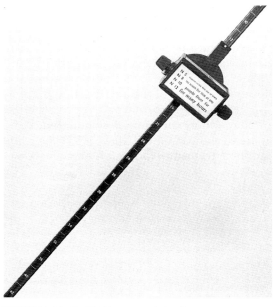

FIGURE 11–2. RAF near point rule.

abducting eye in all lateral gaze positions. (This could give the erroneous impression of an overacting inferior oblique and an underacting superior oblique muscle.) However, if versions are repeated with the adducting eye fixating, a more reliable diagnostic picture can be made. If the nonfixating eye is always higher than the fixating eye, a DVD is most likely present. However, if the right eye, for example, is always higher, regardless of which eye is fixating, a relative over- or underaction of a muscle is present. Combined types exist. It is not uncommon to find versions that do not correspond to prism measurements in the cardinal position of gaze. The reason for this is that versions are done in extreme of gaze, whereas cardinal fields are limited to the binocular field.

Ductions are monocular movements of one eye into the farthest possible diagnostic position of gaze. The limbus test of motility of Kestenbaum[4] provides a measurement of the amount of ductions in each eye. The test is performed by holding a transparent millimeter ruler horizontally in front of the cornea. When measuring adduction, the location of the temporal limbus is noted on the ruler in primary position and in maximum adduction. The amount of adduction can be recorded in millimeters. Abduction is measured using the same method by noting the nasal limbus point on the ruler in primary position and in maximum abduction. To measure elevation and depression, the ruler is held vertically. The normal values of motility as stated by Kestenbaum[4] are 9 to 10 mm for adduction and abduction, and 5 to 7 mm for depression and elevation. However, the relative values are as important as the normal values, i.e., the left eye may abduct the normal 10 mm, but, if the right eye abducts 14 mm, there is a relative limitation of abduction of the left eye.

Vergences

Horizontal and vertical vergences are disjunctive compensatory reflex movements of the eyes to establish fusion. These movements are the motor arc of the fusion reflex and are referred to as fusional amplitudes. They are measured directly by prisms and can also be measured indirectly by plus and minus lenses. The patient with heterophoria bifoveally fixates an appropriate target and is requested to report when the target becomes doubled or blurred. Using a prism bar (Fig. 11–3), the prism strength is increased slowly until the limit of vergence is exceeded, which is termed the break point. It is detected by the patient by constant diplopia and by the examiner by cessation of disjunctive eye movements. The prism strength is then decreased until fusion is regained, which is termed the recovery point. Probably the most important patient observation in detecting horizontal vergence is the point at which blurred visual acuity occurs. This represents the dissociation point of harmony between accommodation and horizontal vergences.

Base out for convergence
Base in for divergence
Base down over OD for positive vergences
Base up over OD for negative vergences

The indirect method of determining horizontal fusional amplitudes utilizes plus and minus lenses for testing patients with heterophoria. Because accommodation is varied by using different lenses, the vergences are evaluated. The patient reads print at near fixation as minus lenses are introduced. Accommodation is exerted, and convergence is elicited by reflex action. To avoid heterotropia, fusional divergence is needed. The minus lenses are increased until the limit of divergence is reached and

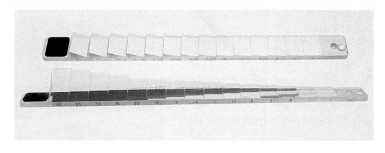

FIGURE 11–3. Prism bar: vertical and horizontal.

bifoveal fixation is no longer present. The angle of deviation is measured with the prism and alternate cover test using the highest strength of minus lenses that the patient can overcome and still remain heterophoric. This test is repeated using plus lenses that will relax accommodation and convergence. Fusional convergence is now needed to keep the exodeviation latent. Normally, a child shows a fusional range sufficient to remain a heterophoric reading through −3.00 and +3.00 diopter lenses.

■ Sensory Evaluation

After analyzing the motor anomaly, the next step is to evaluate the sensory status, that is, (1) fusion, which is a cortical phenomenon wherein the two retinal images are perceived as one; (2) suppression, which is an adaptive mechanism that protects the strabismus patient from diplopia and visual confusion; and (3) diplopia, which is double vision in the absence of peripheral suppression.

All sensory testing requires a subjective response. Therefore, only certain pediatric patients will be able to be tested. The objective of sensory testing is to establish if the patient is fusing or has a potential to fuse. Fusion is usually classified as peripheral or foveal. There are numerous sensory tests described in other texts. The examiner soon learns to depend on a few reliable tests to understand the sensory status. Only the tests we use will be described in this chapter.

The most common clinical method of testing fusion is evaluating stereopsis in patients with heterophoria and intermittent or small angle strabismus. The eyes are dissociated with Polaroid spectacles. The target plate is constructed to stimulate fusion of disparate elements. The least disparity seen in depth is recorded in seconds of arc (60″ or better indicates foveal fusion). For near fixation the following tests may be used: Titmus Stereoacuity (Fig. 11–4), Random Dot E, TNO, and WIRT. For distance fixation, the stereopsis portion of the American Optical Vectographic Projectoslide may be used (Fig. 11–5). This slide is used in conjunction with a nonpolarizing illuminated screen for Polaroid glasses. There are four lines of five circles with one circle in each line with stereoscopic qualities (Fig. 11–5).

$$1\text{st line} = 240''$$
$$2\text{nd line} = 180''$$
$$3\text{rd line} = 120''$$
$$4\text{th line} = 60''$$

Another portion of this slide also is used to test for foveal suppression (Fig. 11–6). Each of the three lines of letters is presented so that the first letter is seen by both eyes, the second letter is seen only by the left eye, and the third letter is seen only by the right eye. Then the sequence is repeated. Exposing the first three or four letters of each line will suffice. This test is used primarily for patients who appear to be bifoveally fixating. The patient with bifoveal fixation and no suppression

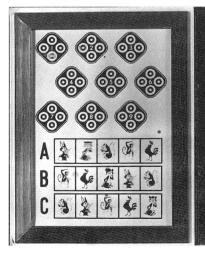
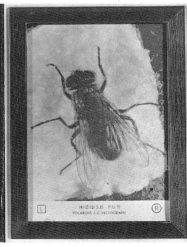

FIGURE 11–4. Titmus Stereo-acuity test.

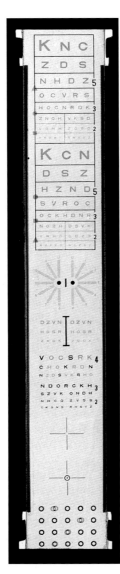

FIGURE 11–5. American Optical Vectographic Projectoslide.

reads or counts all the letters. The patient with central suppression will not see all the letters. For the patients with a larger deviation of strabismus, the *prism adaptation test*[5,6] is helpful to determine potential fusional ability. Also, the results of this test aid in deciding the surgical approach in correcting the strabismus. The full amount of the distance deviation is corrected with the appropriate Fresnel prism. The patient's adjustment to the prism is evaluated after 1 month. If with the cover–uncover test the eyes appear straight or a small-angle deviation is observed with the prism in place, fusion testing is done. Because the plastic prism usually creates some blurred visual acuity, more peripheral fusion tests are used, i.e., Worth four-dot test. The *Worth four-dot test* consists of four lighted dots, one red, two green, and one white, arranged in a diamond shape. The patient wears colored filters, one red and the other green. The colors of the filters and the lights are complementary so that through the red filter only two lights are seen, the red one and the white one, which appears red. Through the green filter, three lights are seen, two green ones and the white one, which appears green. If the two eyes are being used together, the patient fuses the white light, which is the only one common to both eyes and sees four lights. Anything less than four lights is suppression; anything more is diplopia. Diplopia is an infrequent symptom of the pediatric strabismus patient. However, it is an annoyance in the adult patient with a recently acquired strabismus. The Fresnel prisms[5,6] (Fig. 11–7) are of considerable help for these patients.

General Principles for Fresnel Prisms for Patients with Diplopia

The least amount of prism is applied that will allow comfortable fusion. In most cases, the amount usually is less than the strabismus measurements with alternate cover and prism. After the full amount of the deviation is determined

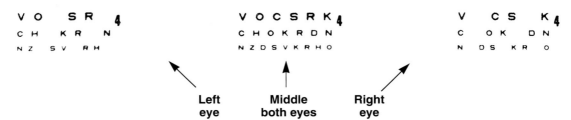

FIGURE 11–6. Testing for foveal suppression. Left: left eye. Middle: both eyes. Right: right eye.

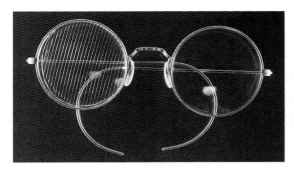

FIGURE 11–7. Fresnel press-on prism.

with alternate cover and prism, different prisms are introduced with the patient in a binocular condition. The patient selects the prism that is most comfortably fused. The prism is used over only one eye. It can be used over the entire lens or over one segment, or a different prism can be used on upper and lower segments. The prism is placed over the nondominant eye or over the eye with the poorer visual acuity. It is placed over the eye with the paretic muscle if primary and secondary deviation is demonstrated, or it is placed over the eye with greatest restriction of movement.

The prism is cut on the outside of the lens $\frac{1}{2}$ mm inside the frame. If the prism touches the frame, air bubbles will form. The prism and glasses are submerged into a bowl of warm water or held under gently flowing tap water. The prism is applied to the inside (face side) of the lens and is allowed to self-dry or is patted dry with a soft cloth, forcing out all the bubbles.

Patient discomfort from the prism may be blurred visual acuity. The higher the prism power the more the blur. Patients may complain of the prism lines or the glare. The prism needs to be changed every 6 to 9 months. The plastic absorbs pollutants in the environment, which turns the plastic yellow.

At times oblique prismation is needed to correct a compound vertical and horizontal muscle imbalance.[7] The determination of what power prism at what angle is a general trigonometric problem involving a right-angle triangle. We use our computer charts. Two types of charts are necessary, that is, the patient is able to fuse with a base-out 28 and base-down 10. The first chart determines the power of the prism to be used (Fig. 11–8). Tracing horizontally across to 28 and then vertically down to 10

gives the power of the prism to be used (#30). The second chart gives the angle at which the prism is to be placed (Fig 11–9). Again across to 28 and down to 10 shows that the axis is to be 20 degrees from the vertical meridian. Placing the base above or below the midline will be determined by whether a right or left hypertropia is present. With a protractor the 30 prism base out is rotated 20 degrees to correct both the horizontal and the vertical deviation.

If the primary vertical deviation is associated with an exotropia, seldom does the exotropia need to be corrected. Just the vertical needs to be corrected. However, if the primary vertical deviation is associated with an esotropia, frequently both the horizontal and the vertical components need to be corrected.

Types of Cases

The following are the types of conditions associated with prism therapy.

Neural

Due to the gross incomitance, patients with a *third nerve paresis* do not respond well with the prism. Bangerter film (Fig. 11–10) or scotch tape is used for occlusion. As recovery is occurring, a prism may be helpful.

Patients with a unilateral *fourth nerve paresis* respond well with prism therapy. At times, the patient may need two prisms, one for distance fixation and a different power prism for near reading. Patients with bilateral fourth nerve paresis do not respond well to prisms. Usually the involvement is asymmetric. A prism may be helpful at distance fixation, but, due to the torsion in reading position, the prism is not helpful at near fixation. Tape over the lower segment will be necessary, or reading glasses are prescribed so that the patient is not forced to look down through the bifocals.

Patients with *sixth nerve paresis* are most grateful for the prism help. They adjust extremely well to the prism. The prism is usually placed over the involved eye, especially if primary and secondary deviations are present. If the patient is fusing well in primary position with the prism but still is bothered by diplopia when looking to the involved side, the prism power is increased, which will help the annoying diplopia to the involved side. This creates an exodeviation that is easily fused in primary position and in the uninvolved side.

	1	2	3	4	5	6	7	8	9	10	11	12	13	14	15	16	17	18	19	20	21	22	23	24	25	26	27	28	29	30
1	1	2	3	4	5	6	7	8	9	10	11	12	13	14	15	16	17	18	19	20	21	22	23	24	25	26	27	28	29	30
2	2	3	4	4	5	6	7	8	9	10	11	12	13	14	15	16	17	18	19	20	21	22	23	24	25	26	27	28	29	30
3	3	4	4	5	6	7	8	9	9	10	11	12	13	14	15	16	17	18	19	20	21	22	23	24	25	26	27	28	29	30
4	4	4	5	6	6	7	8	9	10	11	12	13	14	15	16	16	17	18	19	20	21	22	23	24	25	26	27	28	29	30
5	5	5	6	6	7	8	9	9	10	11	12	13	14	15	16	17	18	19	20	21	22	23	24	25	25	26	27	28	29	30
6	6	6	7	7	8	8	9	10	11	12	13	13	14	15	16	17	18	19	20	21	22	23	24	25	26	27	28	29	30	31
7	7	7	8	8	9	9	10	11	11	12	13	14	15	16	17	17	18	19	20	21	22	23	24	25	26	27	28	29	30	31
8	8	8	9	9	9	10	11	11	12	13	14	14	15	16	17	18	19	20	21	22	22	23	24	25	26	27	28	29	30	31
9	9	9	9	10	10	11	11	12	13	13	14	15	16	17	17	18	19	20	21	22	23	24	25	26	27	28	28	29	30	31
10	10	10	10	11	11	12	12	13	13	14	15	16	16	17	18	19	20	21	21	22	23	24	25	26	27	28	29	30	31	32
11	11	11	11	12	12	13	13	14	14	15	16	16	17	18	19	19	20	21	22	23	24	25	25	26	27	28	29	30	31	32
12	12	12	12	13	13	13	14	14	15	16	16	17	18	18	19	20	21	22	22	23	24	25	26	27	28	29	30	30	31	32
13	13	13	13	14	14	14	15	15	16	16	17	18	18	19	20	21	21	22	23	24	25	26	26	27	28	29	30	31	32	33
14	14	14	14	15	15	15	16	16	17	17	18	18	19	20	21	21	22	23	24	24	25	26	27	28	29	30	30	31	32	33
15	15	15	15	16	16	16	17	17	17	18	19	19	20	21	21	22	23	23	24	25	26	27	27	28	29	30	31	32	33	34
16	16	16	16	16	17	17	17	18	18	19	19	20	21	21	22	23	23	24	25	26	26	27	28	29	30	31	31	32	33	34
17	17	17	17	17	18	18	18	19	19	20	20	21	21	22	23	23	24	25	25	26	27	28	29	29	30	31	32	33	34	34
18	18	18	18	18	19	19	19	20	20	21	21	22	22	23	23	24	25	25	26	27	28	28	29	30	31	32	32	33	34	35
19	19	19	19	19	20	20	20	21	21	21	22	22	23	24	24	25	25	26	27	28	28	29	30	31	31	32	33	34	35	36
20	20	20	20	20	21	21	21	22	22	22	23	23	24	24	25	26	26	27	28	28	29	30	30	31	32	33	34	34	35	36
21	21	21	21	21	22	22	22	22	23	23	24	24	25	25	26	26	27	28	28	29	30	30	31	32	33	33	34	35	36	37
22	22	22	22	22	23	23	23	23	24	24	25	25	26	26	27	27	28	28	29	30	30	31	32	33	33	34	35	36	36	37
23	23	23	23	23	24	24	24	24	25	25	25	26	26	27	27	28	29	29	30	30	31	32	33	33	34	35	35	36	37	38
24	24	24	24	24	25	25	25	25	26	26	26	27	27	28	28	29	29	30	31	31	32	33	33	34	35	35	36	37	38	38
25	25	25	25	25	25	26	26	26	27	27	27	28	28	29	29	30	30	31	31	32	33	33	34	35	35	36	37	38	38	39
26	26	26	26	26	26	27	27	27	28	28	28	29	29	30	30	31	31	32	32	33	33	34	35	35	36	37	37	38	39	40
27	27	27	27	27	27	28	28	28	28	29	29	30	30	30	31	31	32	32	33	34	34	35	35	36	37	37	38	39	40	40
28	28	28	28	28	28	29	29	29	29	30	30	30	31	31	32	32	33	33	34	34	35	36	36	37	38	38	39	40	40	41
29	29	29	29	29	29	30	30	30	30	31	31	31	32	32	33	33	34	34	35	35	36	36	37	38	38	39	40	40	41	42
30	30	30	30	30	30	31	31	31	31	32	32	32	33	33	34	34	34	35	36	36	37	37	38	38	39	40	40	41	42	42

FIGURE 11–8. Prism chart: the power of the prism.

	1	2	3	4	5	6	7	8	9	10	11	12	13	14	15	16	17	18	19	20	21	22	23	24	25	26	27	28	29	30
1	45	27	18	14	11	9	8	7	6	6	5	5	4	4	4	4	3	3	3	3	3	3	2	2	2	2	2	2	2	2
2	63	45	34	27	22	18	16	14	13	11	10	9	9	8	8	7	7	6	6	6	5	5	5	5	5	4	4	4	4	4
3	72	56	45	37	31	27	23	21	18	17	15	14	13	12	11	11	10	9	9	9	8	8	7	7	7	7	6	6	6	6
4	76	63	53	45	39	34	30	27	24	22	20	18	17	16	15	14	13	13	12	11	11	10	10	9	9	9	8	8	8	8
5	79	68	59	51	45	40	36	32	29	27	24	23	21	20	18	17	16	16	15	14	13	13	12	12	11	11	10	10	10	9
6	81	72	63	56	50	45	41	37	34	31	29	27	25	23	22	21	19	18	18	17	16	15	15	14	13	13	13	12	12	11
7	82	74	67	60	54	49	45	41	38	35	32	30	28	27	25	24	22	21	20	19	18	18	17	16	16	15	15	14	14	13
8	83	76	69	63	58	53	49	45	42	39	36	34	32	30	28	27	25	24	23	22	21	20	19	18	18	17	17	16	15	15
9	84	77	72	66	61	56	52	48	45	42	39	37	35	33	31	29	28	27	25	24	23	22	21	21	20	19	18	18	17	17
10	84	79	73	68	63	59	55	51	48	45	42	40	38	36	34	32	31	29	28	27	25	24	24	23	22	21	20	20	19	18
11	85	80	75	70	66	61	58	54	51	48	45	43	40	38	36	35	33	31	30	29	28	27	26	25	24	23	22	21	21	20
12	85	81	76	72	67	63	60	56	53	50	47	45	43	41	39	37	35	34	32	31	30	29	28	27	26	25	24	23	22	22
13	86	81	77	73	69	65	62	58	55	52	50	47	45	43	41	39	37	36	34	33	32	31	29	29	27	27	26	25	24	23
14	86	82	78	73	70	67	64	60	57	54	52	49	47	45	43	41	39	38	36	35	34	32	31	30	29	28	27	27	26	25
15	86	82	79	74	72	68	65	62	58	56	54	51	49	47	45	43	41	40	38	37	36	34	33	32	31	30	29	28	27	27
16	86	83	79	76	73	69	66	63	59	58	55	53	51	49	47	45	43	42	40	39	37	36	35	34	33	32	31	30	29	28
17	87	83	80	76	74	71	68	65	61	60	57	55	53	51	49	47	45	43	42	40	39	38	36	35	34	33	32	31	30	30
18	87	84	81	77	75	72	69	66	62	61	59	56	54	52	50	48	47	45	43	42	41	39	38	37	36	35	34	33	32	31
19	87	84	81	78	76	72	70	67	63	62	60	58	56	54	52	50	48	47	45	44	42	41	40	38	37	36	35	34	33	32
20	87	84	81	79	77	73	71	68	65	63	61	59	57	55	53	51	50	48	46	45	44	42	41	40	39	38	37	36	34	34
21	87	85	82	79	77	74	72	69	66	64	63	60	58	56	54	53	51	49	48	46	45	44	42	41	40	39	38	37	35	35
22	87	85	82	80	78	75	73	70	67	65	64	61	59	58	56	54	52	51	49	48	46	45	44	43	41	40	39	38	36	36
23	88	85	83	80	78	75	74	71	68	66	65	62	61	59	57	55	54	52	50	49	48	46	45	44	43	41	40	39	38	37
24	88	85	83	81	79	76	74	72	69	67	66	63	62	60	58	56	55	53	52	50	49	47	46	45	44	43	42	41	39	39
25	88	85	83	81	79	77	75	72	69	67	67	64	63	61	59	57	56	54	53	51	50	49	47	46	45	44	43	42	41	40
26	88	86	83	81	80	77	75	73	70	68	68	65	63	62	60	58	57	55	53	52	51	50	49	47	46	45	44	43	42	41
27	88	86	83	82	80	77	75	74	71	69	68	66	64	63	61	59	58	56	55	53	52	51	50	48	47	46	45	44	43	42
28	88	86	84	82	80	78	76	74	72	70	69	67	65	63	62	60	59	57	56	54	53	52	51	49	48	47	46	45	44	43
29	88	86	84	82	81	78	76	75	73	71	69	68	66	64	63	61	60	58	57	55	54	53	52	50	49	48	47	46	45	44
30	88	86	84	82	81	79	77	75	73	72	70	68	67	65	63	62	60	59	58	56	55	54	53	51	50	49	48	47	46	45

FIGURE 11–9. Prism chart: the angle of the prism.

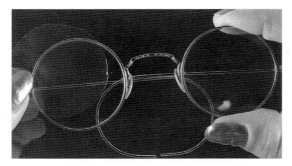

FIGURE 11–10. Bangerter film.

Internuclear

In the patient with unilateral or bilateral internuclear ophthalmoplegia, prisms are not used. Fusion is usually present in primary position.

Supranuclear

A skew deviation is a vertical deviation that is either concomitant or incomitant. It is an acquired vertical deviation caused by a supranuclear dysfunction. There may be one type of vertical deviation to one side with an opposite vertical deviation to the other side. It is associated with lesions of the brainstem or cerebellum or damage to the pontine or the tonic otolith–ocular pathways. The vertical deviation is not large usually, and the more concomitant the deviation the more likely the prism will be helpful.

Neuromuscular Conduction Defect

Ocular myasthenia is usually characterized by a variable deviation. However, there are cases in which the deviation remains sufficiently stable for prisms to eliminate diplopia for a long period of time. From a recent study of 41 patients with ocular myasthenia, 26 were pleased with the prism help.[8] The deviations were still variable but not on short cycles of hour-to-hour or even week-to-week periods. The deviation would remain fairly constant for months at a time then subsequently change to a remission or change in the amount or type of deviation. Most patients soon learned when to remove the prism or when a different one was necessary.

Muscular: Restrictive/Nonrestrictive

Prior to muscle surgery, prisms are used to keep the patient comfortable while waiting for a stable deviation. Our goal is single vision in the primary and the reading positions. If this in not accomplished with surgery, prisms are used again postoperatively. Usually more than one muscle is involved in *Graves' disease* causing a compound strabismus; therefore, most of the time oblique prismation is necessary.

Basically there are three types of conditions involving patients with pseudophakia. A sensory exotropia may develop as the *cataract* dims the visual acuity of the eye. After cataract surgery and the restoration of visual acuity, the exotropia may remain with annoying diplopia. Prisms help stimulate fusion, and frequently with time the exodeviation lessens and is well controlled without the prism.

The second condition is convergence insufficiency at near fixation, which is helped with the prisms. Most often, the prisms need to be continued and are eventually built into the glass correction.

The third condition is a vertical deviation, at times of large amounts. This also is helped with a prism. Usually the vertical deviation remains.

With newer techniques for *retinal* surgery and fewer cases where the muscles need to be detached or large buckles used, fewer patients are seen with diplopia after retinal surgery. In the few patients where prisms are used, they usually allow fusion, but most cases will eventually need muscle surgery.

Adults with diplopia with *childhood-onset strabismus* are helped with prisms either to aid in fusing of the two images or to place the second image onto a suppression area that was developed in childhood. Patients with marked amblyopia with newly experienced diplopia are helped with prisms. Symptomatic adults with early-onset intermittent exotropia at times present a problem. The smaller the amount of the exodeviation, the more likely the prism will help. The patients with larger angles will need a surgical correction to relieve the symptoms.

Symptomatic Phorias

1. Patients with small latent vertical deviations are helped with the prism. All or nearly all of the amount of deviation needs to be corrected.
2. Patients with convergence insufficiency, if convergence training has been unsuccessful, will benefit with prism help. Usually only half or less of the amount of deviation needs to be corrected.

3. Patients with accommodative effort syndrome will not be helped with a prism. This is an accommodative problem that will be helped with plus-reading correction.

Degenerative Diseases

Patients with multiple sclerosis can present with a variety of ocular-motor problems. Bilateral internuclear ophthalmoplegia, cerebellar eye signs, sixth nerve paresis, and pendular nystagmus are most common. At times, the deviation is variable. Only certain conditions can be helped with prisms.

Others

1. Retinal wrinkling. Patients with retinal wrinkling do not respond to prism therapy. They have vague symptoms that may include diplopia or ghostlike images. Therefore, they are referred for prisms. However, when they complain of dips or curves in the images, they cannot be helped with prisms.
2. Homonymous hemianopsia. Smith[9] reported that a prism helped patients with homonymous hemianopsia visual field defects. For example, a patient with a left homonymous hemianopsia can have a 30-diopter base-left (base-out) prism placed on the temporal half of the left lens. A small 1- to 1.5-mm portion can be cut out of the center to prevent diplopia.
3. Divergence insufficiency.[10] One of the groups of patients that are most grateful for prism help present with what is categorized as divergence insufficiency type of esodeviation. Usually it is found in the older age group that complains of off–on diplopia at distance, during mainly at the theater or night driving, both conditions in dim light with loss of peripheral clues. Gradually, the condition becomes worse with more annoying constant diplopia at distance only. There is a relatively small esotropia at distance, usually concomitant. However, some patients may show mild (2 to 3 pd) incomitance to either or both lateral sides. Lateral ductions are normal. The condition remains the same. The base-out prism is needed only for distance fixation. If the patient complains of the line of the prism cut at the bifocal

level, the base-out prism is placed over the entire lens. This will increase the exodeviation at near fixation, but most patients will overcome the exodeviation with fusion.

The patients are seen monthly to monitor the muscle problem and to adjust the prism appropriately. After a reasonable length of time, if the prism needs to be continued or the prism blur is annoying and the deviation is 15 pd or less, the patient is given the option of prism incorporated into the glass correction. Surprisingly, many patients prefer to continue Fresnel prism. However, if they opt to have built-in prisms, the prism is then divided equally between the two lenses if the deviation is concomitant. If the deviation is incomitant, the prisms are divided unequally, and more prism is given toward the field of the greater restriction.

If the deviation is larger, surgery is offered. If this is refused, as much prism is built into the glass correction as is practical, and the rest is made up with the Fresnel prisms.

REFERENCES

1. Parks MM. Isolated cyclovertical muscle palsy. *Arch Ophthalmol.* 1958;60:1027.
2. Duane A. Studies in monocular and binocular accommodation with their clinical applications. *Am J Ophthalmol.* 1922;5:865.
3. Costenbader F. The accommodometer, *Trans Am Acad of Ophthalmol.* 1949;3:362.
4. Kestenbaum A. *Clinical Methods of Neuro-ophthalmologic Examination.* 2nd ed. New York: Grune & Stratton;1961:237.
5. Jampolsky A. A simplified approach in strabismus diagnosis. In *Symposium on Strabismus: Transactions of the New Orleans Academy of Ophthalmology.* St. Louis, MO: Mosby;1971:66.
6. Jampolsky A, Flom M, Thorson JC. Membrane Fresnel prisms: a new therapeutic device. In *The First Congress of the International Strabismological Association*, Fells P, ed. St. Louis, MO: Mosby;1971:183.
7. Moore S, Stockbridge L. Fresnel prisms in the management of combined horizontal and vertical strabismus. *Am Orthoptic J.* 1972;22:14–21.
8. Moore S, Welter P. Ophthalmic diagnosis and evaluation of prism therapy for ocular myasthenia. *Am Orthoptic J.* 1993;43:97–101.
9. Smith JL et al. Hemianopic Fresnel prisms. *J Clin Neuro-Ophthalmol.* 1982;2:19–22.
10. Moore S, Harbison J, Stockbridge L. Divergence insufficiency. *Am Orthoptic J.* 1971;21–59.

Pediatric Ophthalmology
Edited by P. F. Gallin
Thieme Medical Publishers, Inc.
New York © 2000

12

Horizontal Strabismus

CAROLINE J. SHEA AND J. BRONWYN BATEMAN

Horizontal strabismus forms the basis of strabismus in pediatric ophthalmology. The nuances of the condition are so subtle that the reader may need to read this chapter numerous times to understand it fully. The term *strabismus* has its origin in the Greek word *strabismos*, which means a squinting. Strabismus is defined as a misalignment of the visual axes and has a prevalence ranging from 1.3[1] to 7%.[2] Strabismus may be subclassified in several ways with the most basic reflecting the direction of deviation: horizontal, vertical, or torsional. Horizontal strabismus may be divided into convergent (eso-) or divergent (exo-), with esodeviations being more common than exodeviations.[3] The suffix *phoria* refers to a latent deviation whereby the deviation is controlled by fusion; under binocular viewing conditions, the eyes are aligned and only when fusion is disrupted is the deviation demonstrable. In contrast, the suffix *tropia* refers to a "manifest" deviation that is evident under binocular conditions and, presumably, beyond the control of fusion; the deviation is intermittent when it is controlled some of the time. All deviations occur on a spectrum related to fusional mechanisms and defined by control under binocular conditions and frequency, ranging from phoria to intermittent tropia to manifest deviation (tropia). Strabismus may also be classified as concomitant or incomitant. The term *concomitant* implies that the angle of deviation is the same in all fields of gaze; incomitant strabismus varies by the field of gaze and is usually associated with paralytic, restrictive, or special syndromes (i.e., Duane's and Mobius' syndromes).

■ Esodeviations

Esodeviations represent the most common type of strabismus and account for over 50% of ocular misalignment in childhood.[4] Most esodeviations are manifest tropias. Esodeviations are broadly classified as infantile (congenital) or acquired (Table 12–1).

Pseudoesotropia

Often families are told that a "turn" will disappear or will be outgrown. This is incorrect. **All children suspected of having a deviation must be examined**. Many children aged less than 1 year have the optical illusion of crossing.

Pseudoesotropia refers to the appearance of esotropia when, in fact, the eyes are straight by cover test (see Chapter 11). These infants usually have prominent epicanthal folds and a broad flat nasal bridge; the epicanthal folds mask more of the sclera nasally and the appearance of crossing may be more evident in side gaze. Often the parents have an intermittent appearance of cross-

TABLE 12–1. Classification of Esodeviations

I. Infantile (congenital)
   A. Classic type
   B. Early onset with accommodative/refractive
      component
   C. Duane's syndrome
   D. Abducens palsy
   E. Nystagmus blockage syndrome
   F. Mobius' syndrome
   G. Ciancia syndrome

II. Acquired
   A. Accommodative
      1. Refractive
      2. Nonrefractive
      3. Combined
   B. Nonaccommodative
      1. Cyclic
      2. Idiopathic
      3. Decompensated accommodative
   C. Sensory
   D. Divergence insufficiency
   E. Divergence paralysis
   F. Spasm of the near synkinetic reflex
   G. Medial rectus restriction
   H. Lateral rectus weakness

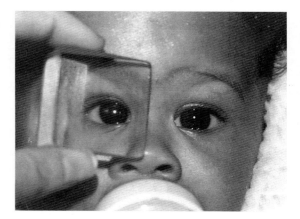

FIGURE 12–1. Baby with infantile esotropia. Angle of deviation is neutralized by prism.

ing. When there is a history of crossing from the parents, it is important to ask if they think the child's eyes are crossed at the time of the examination. Often the illusion created by the epicanthal folds "fools" the parents and primary care physicians. The ultimate determination of straight or crossed eyes is to use the Hirschberg (corneal light reflex test) or Krimsky (Hirschberg with prism) tests in conjunction with cover and alternate cover testing (see Chapter 11). Some children with pseudoesotropia may have an intermittent deviation or develop esotropia later; they should be monitored.

Infantile (Congenital) Esotropia

The onset of infantile esotropia (Fig. 12–1) is by the age of 6 months and the incidence is probably less than 1%.[1,2] Infantile esotropia is synonymous with congenital esotropia; the term *congenital* is inappropriate as the deviation is not present since birth. Large population studies have shown that the vast majority of neonates are either straight or exotropic and usually become aligned by 2 months of age.[5,6] Although esotropia typically occurs in an otherwise healthy child, it is frequently associated with a positive family history. Developmental and motor delays such as cerebral palsy, Down syndrome (Fig. 12–2), and hydrocephalus often have an associated strabismus during infancy. There is no single gene inheritance pattern, but strabismus often clusters in families.[7,8]

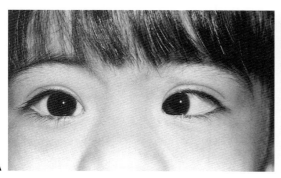
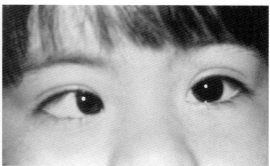

FIGURE 12–2. (A) Child with Down syndrome and esotropia: OD is fixating. **(B)** OS is fixating.

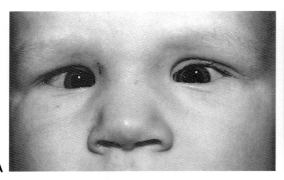
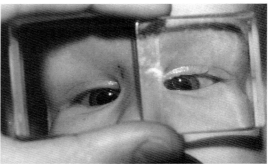

FIGURE 12–3. (A) Infantile esotrope exhibiting large angle of deviation. **(B)** Same child with prisms neutralizing angle of deviation.

Characteristic Features

The angle of deviation is usually very large, greater than 30 prism diopters (pd), and is approximately the same at distance and at near (Fig. 12–3). If the infant cross-fixates, he views targets by looking across his nose with the adducted eye toward the opposite field (Fig. 12–4).

Amblyopia

The equality of vision is of paramount importance and must be established before further treatment. However, the assessment of fixation preference in preverbal children is quite subjective, is difficult to establish, and requires judgment (see Chapter 2).

If there is a fixation preference, amblyopia treatment must be instituted. Generally, however, cross-fixators have equal vision because they use each eye half of the time. Patching is not usually necessary.

Deficient Abduction

As a result of cross-fixation, abduction may be difficult to demonstrate, and clinically the infant may appear to have bilateral sixth nerve palsies. Occlusion of one eye in the office for as little as 1 hour may demonstrate abduction. Other useful maneuvers include stimulating the vestibulocular reflex or performing a doll's head maneuver. If these do not prove fruitful, patching at home for 1 to 2 days before the next visit will usually demonstrate abduction. A radiological scan should be obtained if abduction cannot be proven. Over time, abduction gradually improves so that by the age of 2 years the cross-fixator becomes a spontaneous alternator maintaining one eye straight at a time.

Refraction

Cycloplegic refraction usually reveals mild hyperopia of less than 2 diopters. Significant refractive

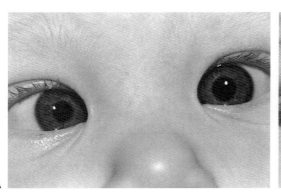
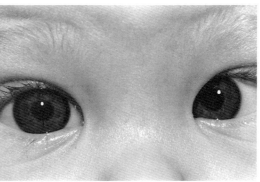

FIGURE 12–4. (A) Infantile exotrope who is cross-fixating. Note that the right eye is esotropic. **(B)** Left eye is now esotropic.

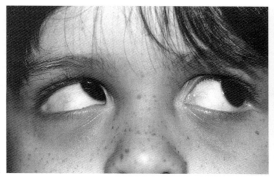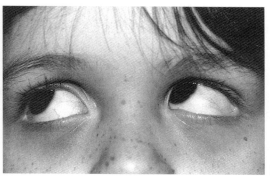

FIGURE 12–5. (A) Child with inferior oblique overaction OS 1+. **(B)** Inferior oblique overaction OS 2+.

errors should be optically corrected before surgery. Although preoperative glasses are usually not indicated, more than 50% of patients will need correction at some point after surgery.[9] Although rare, accommodative esotropia may be evident as early as 4 months of age.[10,11]

Inferior Oblique Overaction

Over time, vertical deviations develop. Inferior oblique overaction (Fig. 12–5) is best identified by elevation in adduction; a vertical deviation in primary position is uncommon. The amount of overaction has been graded by the differences in elevation between the two eyes in upgaze and to the side; the scale ranges from 1 to 4+, with 4+ being the greatest. Inferior oblique overaction results in a "V pattern" esotropia, whereby the deviation decreases in upgaze secondary to the abducting effects of the inferior obliques. Significant inferior oblique overaction may be associated with superior oblique underaction.

Inferior oblique overaction often develops after the horizontal strabismus. Overall incidence ranges from 36[13] to 78%,[9] and the onset is usually after 1 year of age and most frequently between the ages of 2 and 4 years. Neither early surgical correction nor binocularity seems to change the rate of development of inferior oblique overaction.[9,13,14] Inferior oblique overaction is most commonly associated with infantile esotropia but also can be seen with accommodative esotropes and intermittent exotropes.

Dissociated Vertical Deviation

Dissociated vertical deviation (DVD) is characterized by elevation, abduction, and excy-

clotorsion of the nonfixing eye without corresponding hypotropia of the contralateral eye; thus, DVD does not obey Hering's law. On alternate cover test, the occluded eye will spontaneously "float up" and outward, and, when fixation recurs, there is no redress movement of the other eye. DVD is usually bilateral but asymmetrical; it is most noticeable in the nondominant eye during periods of visual inattentiveness. DVD usually is apparent by 18 months of age, although it may be seen as early as 8 months[15]; the prevalence seems to be unrelated to surgical alignment. It occurs most frequently with infantile esotropia.[16,17] Stereopsis is generally poor, and the deviation is concomitant.[17,18] The cause is not known but is believed to be central.[19]

DVD and inferior oblique overaction may occur simultaneously; differentiating between the two is clinically important and may be difficult. The deviation is greatest in adduction for overaction of the inferior oblique and concomitant for DVD. Another important distinguishing feature is the hypotropia of the nonfixing eye when the adducting eye of the overacting inferior oblique fixates; there is no corresponding hypotropia in DVD. Key differentiating features are summarized in Table 12–2.

Treatment

The goal in the management of infantile esotropia is ocular alignment with binocularity. However, affected children rarely achieve 40 seconds of stereoacuity regardless of the age of surgical alignment.[20] Thus, the best outcome of

TABLE 12–2. Key Differentiating Features between Inferior Oblique Overaction and Dissociated Vertical Deviation

Features	Inferior Oblique Overaction	Dissociated Vertical Deviation
Elevation in adduction	X	X
Elevation in abduction and primary		X
Concomitant deviation		X
Associated V pattern	X	
Associated torsional movement		X
Corresponding hypotropia of abducted eye	X	
Variable hyperdeviation		X

treatment is the creation of a monofixation syndrome with alignment within 8 to 10 prism diopters of orthotropia.[4,21,22] It is generally agreed that ocular alignment is rarely obtained without surgery. Prior to surgery, hyperopia greater than 2 diopters should be corrected; with higher amounts of hyperopia, some of the esotropia may be controlled with glasses. Amblyopia should be treated before surgery to optimize postoperative alignment and binocularity. The end point of patching should be spontaneous alternation or no fixation preference. Surgery should be performed for the residual esotropia.

Although the optimal timing of surgery remains controversial, **evidence supports "early" surgery (before the age of 2 years)**.[4,13,22–27] Historically, some surgeons prefer to wait until the age of 2 years so that they can better identify associated vertical deviations, diagnose and treat amblyopia, and obtain accurate distance measurements.[20,28] The first choice of surgical methodology is usually bilateral medial rectus recession. If there is unilateral visual loss (more than two lines), surgery may be restricted to the nonfixing eye with a recession of the medial rectus and a resection of the lateral rectus.

Surgical correction is not a cosmetic procedure. The purpose is binocularity. In children with delayed motor development due to a central neurological process (e.g., prematurity, cerebral palsy, or nonspecific delayed maturation), postoperative alignment may aid their motor development.[73]

Final surgical alignment is assessed 6 weeks after surgery. A residual esotropia or exotropia of more than 15 diopters 6 weeks postoperatively warrants surgical reintervention. In the case of persistent esotropia, hyperopia (generally greater than 1.5 diopters) should be cor-rected. If the esotropia persists, repeat surgery should be undertaken. The same principles apply for persistent exotropia of more than 15 diopters; any myopia should be corrected. Surgical reintervention is warranted if the deviation persists.

As hyperopia increases during the first several years of life, cycloplegic refractions should be monitored.[29,30] Recurrent esotropia usually responds well to correction of low levels of hyperopia. Hiles and colleagues[9] reported that 65% of infantile esotropes that underwent surgery required hyperopic spectacles at some time postoperatively to control the deviation.

Accommodative Esotropia

The onset of accommodative esotropia is typically between the ages of 2 and 3 years; it has been described as occurring as early as 6 months and as late as 7 years of age.[31] Affected children are presumed to have ocular alignment and some level of binocularity prior to the onset of the deviation. Amblyopia is more common in accommodative esotropia than in infantile esotropia. Accommodative esotropia is considered an "acquired" deviation. Acquired esotropia is a "daytime emergency" in visually immature children as suppression may develop rapidly; the onset is usually coincident with the child becoming more aware of the environment. The subset of children with an onset prior to 1 year of age is sometimes classified separately as early-onset accommodative esotropia; the infants tend to exhibit features of both the infantile and the accommodative forms.

Accommodative esotropia is caused by accommodative dysfunction and may be completely or partially controlled with spectacles. Accom-

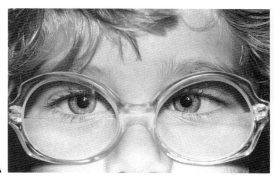 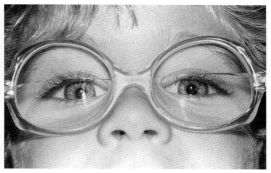

FIGURE 12–6. (A) Accommodative esotrope who is crossing at near. **(B)** Same child is straight with bifocals.

modative esotropia is caused by significant hyperopia and/or a high accommodative convergence to accommodation ratio (AC/A ratio). Patients with a high AC/A ratio have a deviation that measures more at near than at distance, usually defined by 10 prism diopters or more. The AC/A ratio is defined as the amount of convergence in prism diopters per diopter change in accommodation; a normal ratio is 3. When the esotropia measures more at near than at distance by at least 10 prism diopters, this is a "clinical" (qualitative) AC/A ratio.

Accommodative Esotropia (Normal AC/A Ratio)
In accommodative esotropia with a normal AC/A ratio, the deviation is usually between 20 and 45 diopters, which is smaller than in infantile esotropia. Hyperopia, usually greater than + 3.00 diopters, is characteristic; Parks[31] found

an average of + 4.75 diopters. Individuals with refractive errors above + 7.00 diopters are less likely to develop accommodative esotropia, presumably because the effort is too much to maintain.[31]

Accommodative Esotropia (High AC/A Ratio)
Patients with a greater deviation at near than at distance have a high clinical AC/A ratio; bifocals may control the near deviation (Figs. 12–6, 12–7). Patients with a high AC/A ratio possess an abnormal synkinesis between accommodation and convergence such that a given accommodative effort elicits excessive convergence. This type of accommodative esotropia occurs not just in hyperopes but also in myopes and emmetropes. The majority of affected patients have a refractive error around + 2.25 diopters.[31]

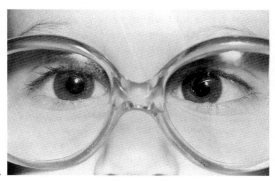 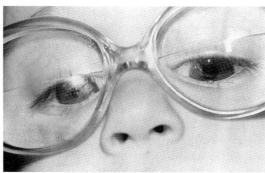

FIGURE 12–7. (A) Accommodative esotrope who is crossing at near. **(B)** Same child is straight with bifocals.

Treatment

The goal of treatment is to treat amblyopia and reestablish and maintain ocular alignment and fusion. In children less than 3 years of age, the interval between the onset of the esotropia and treatment is the key factor in determining the prognosis.[32] The mainstay of treatment for accommodative esotropia is prescribing the hyperopic correction. In children less than 4 years of age, the full cycloplegic refraction should be prescribed; children older than 4 years may not tolerate the full hyperopic correction especially if they have not previously worn glasses and compliance is improved by reducing their correction by 1 to 1.5 diopters. Atropine refractions may be particularly important in uncovering the full hyperopia. Some children may require a period of cycloplegia to relax accommodation and foster compliance with the glasses. Patching should be instituted if amblyopia is evident. Once the glasses have been prescribed, the effect may be evident within days. Surgery should be performed for any residual deviation greater than 15 diopters. As in infantile esotropia, a bimedial rectus recession is the procedure of choice.

A child who is orthotropic or has only a small esophoria after wearing the glasses should be monitored for the amblyopia and recurrence of deviation. Cycloplegia should be done every 6 months. If the deviation recurs, a cycloplegic refraction should be repeated to identify any uncorrected hyperopia. Generally, hyperopia continues to increase until the age of 7 years.[29,33] Some affected individuals previously controlled will decompensate and exhibit a nonaccommodative component requiring surgical intervention. Once the child reaches 5 or 6 years of age and demonstrates fusion, the hyperopic correction may be gradually reduced at each visit to maintain either orthotropia or a small esophoria.

Bifocals

The use of a +2.50 or +3.00 bifocal will minimize the near deviation and may promote fusion in the child with a high AC/A ratio; the method is useful for children with acceptable ocular alignment at distance and a deviation at near that precludes fusion (see Figs. 12–6, 12–7).

When fitting bifocals, the line of the bifocal segment should bisect the pupil, and the flat top or executive type works best. When properly positioned, a chin-up position at near is evidence that the child is using the bifocal. Cycloplegic agents can be used to encourage compliance.

The strength of the bifocals may be decreased gradually when binocularity is established, usually around the age of 8 years. Successful weaning may require several years and is coincident with the natural decrease in the high AC/A ratio with age.[31,34]

Miotics can be used in the treatment of high AC/A ratio. The first line of therapy is heatedly debated among pediatric ophthalmologists. Miotics are useful for children who swim for extended periods.

Miotics

Glasses are the treatment of choice for accommodative esotropia if the child needs a distance hyperopic correction. If the child has only a near deviation, miotics may be considered. Mitotics reduce the AC/A ratio by minimizing accommodation. Miotics such as echothiopate iodide [Phospholine iodide (PI), Wyeth-Ayerst, Philadelphia] and isofluorophate [Floropryl (DFP), Merck & Co., Inc., West Point, PA] may be diagnostically useful and, less commonly, are an adjunctive therapy in accommodative esotropia. Both are long-acting anti-cholinesterases and indirectly inhibit the breakdown of acetylcholine, potentiating its action on the ciliary muscle and iris sphincter. DFP is a wonderful medication that is no longer produced.

Topically applied echothiopate iodide reaches significant blood levels within a few weeks, irreversibly depressing both plasma and erythrocyte cholinesterase activity; **its use should be avoided in patients using cholinesterase inhibitors because of possible respiratory and cardiovascular collapse.**[12] Cholinesterase inhibitors should be discontinued at least 6 weeks prior to undergoing general anesthesia with succinylcholine. Other important side effects are associated with marked vagotonia. These drugs should be used with caution in patients with bronchial asthma, bradycardia, spastic gastrointestinal disease, epilepsy, and peptic ulcer disease. Iris cysts at the pupillary border are seen in 20 to 50% of cases and may regress slowly after discontinuing the drug.[35,36] The concomitant use of phenylephrine has been reported to reduce iris cysts by decreasing miosis.[35] Initially, phenylephrine 2.5% is given twice weekly at bedtime. This can be downwardly titrated as the dose of echothiophate iodide is decreased.

The initial dose of echothiophate iodide is a low percentage (.125%) at bedtime. Patients should be re-evaluated in 1 months' time. The dose can be downwordly titrated depending on the residual near deviation. As the frequency decreases, the examination intervals decrease. Generally, a patient with a good result is on this medication for a few months to a year. During that time the amplitudes of divergence build up.

Special Forms of Esotropia

Monofixation Syndrome

The "monofixation syndrome," originally described by Marshall Parks in his 1969 American Ophthalmological Society thesis, is a sensory adaptation associated with a small deviation or straight eyes. Key features include (1) deviation of 8 to 10 prism diopters or less, (2) peripheral fusion with central scotoma, (3) horizontal fusional vergences, (4) amblyopia, (5) reduced stereoacuity, and (6) latent component. All features need not be present to make the diagnosis.

Although the monofixation syndrome is most commonly a consequence of strabismus, it frequently occurs secondary to anisometropia or, less commonly, unilateral macular lesion; it may exist as a primary condition. In patients with strabismus who develop the monofixation syndrome following surgery, nearly 90% are esotropes.[22] Amblyopia varies from mild to profound. Postoperative esotropes must be watched carefully for a secondary amblyopia from this entry.

Over one third of patients with the monofixation syndrome do not manifest a detectable deviation on cover–uncover testing; the majority were anisometropes.[22] If a deviation exists, it typically measures less than 8 to 10 prism diopters on cover–uncover testing. When binocular vision is disrupted on alternate cover testing there is an apparent increase in the size of the deviation as peripheral fusion is disrupted, revealing the phoric component; the deviation under binocular conditions is measured by the simultaneous prism-cover test; 40% of monofixating patients will exhibit this feature.[22]

Duane's Retraction Syndrome

The ocular abnormality that bears Alexander Duane's name[37] consists of retraction of the globe with narrowing of the palpebral fissure on attempted *addu*ction, *abdu*ction deficiency, and variable adduction deficiency and up- or downshoot of the involved eye on adduction. The incidence is 1 to 4% of all strabismus patients with a preponderance in females and the left eye[38,39]; the prevalence of bilaterality is 15 to 20%.[38,40,41] Amblyopia can occur, but the reported incidence varies widely.[38,42]

Although numerous theories concerning the pathogenesis have been proposed, aplasia of the sixth nerve nucleus was first demonstrated in 1980 by autopsy[43]; Miller[44] reported the next case. Paradoxical innervation of the lateral rectus with cocontraction of the medial and lateral recti as demonstrated by electromyogram best describes the characteristic features.[45]

Duane's syndrome has been associated with other ocular and nonocular abnormalities including Goldenhar's syndrome. Nystagmus, anisocoria, ptosis, epibulbar dermoids, and crocodile tears have been reported.[46] There is a 50% incidence of associated anomalies, which include bony and vertebral anomalies, sensorineural deafness, and external ear defects.[46] Autosomal dominant inheritance has been reported.[40,46]

In 1974, Huber[47] devised the following classification scheme based on electromyography. All types exhibit narrowing of the palpebral fissure in attempted adduction (globe retraction) and widening of the palpebral fissure on abduction. The simultaneous cocontraction of the medial and lateral recti produces the globe retraction.

Type I: marked limitation or absent abduction with normal or slightly decreased adduction (esotropic in primary position)

Type II: marked limitation or absent adduction with normal or slightly decreased abduction (exotropic in primary position)

Type III: limitation or absence of both abduction and adduction (orthotropic in primary position)

Type I is the most common type, accounting for approximately three quarters of all cases.[38,40] Type II is the least common of the three types and represents approximately 1 to 7%; type III accounts for the remaining cases.[38,40]

Most patients with Duane's syndrome have strabismus in primary gaze with esotropia being the most common.[40,41,48] A face turn is often present to maintain fusion. Orthotropia is the second most common primary position alignment.[40,41,48] Exotropia occurs more frequently in type II.[48] The frequency of deviation in bilateral Duane's is 15 to 18%.[38,39,41]

Vertical deviation of the adducted eye can be seen in Duane's syndrome. Upshoots occur more frequently than downshoots.[40,41,49] The proposed mechanisms include cocontraction of the horizontal recti causing the "tight" muscles to "slide" over the globe,[49] simultaneous innervation of both the medial rectus and superior rectus on adduction, and overaction of the inferior obliques.[45,50]

Sixth Nerve Palsy

Acquired sixth nerve palsy causes an incomitant deviation with a deviation that increases toward the field of gaze of the paretic lateral rectus muscle. In other words, with a left sixth nerve palsy, there is an esotropia greatest on left gaze as the left eye cannot abduct. The child may develop a head turn to avoid diplopia; turning the head to the left allows the left medial and right lateral recti to maintain orthotropia in right gaze. With a straight head the field of alignment is shifted to the right. Occlusion may be employed to minimize symptoms. Because of its long intracranial course the sixth nerve is susceptible to various forms of trauma such as meningeal inflammation, increased intracranial pressure, contrecoups head injury (head injury where head hits head rest), as well as postinfectious processes and vascular occlusion. One third of sixth nerve palsies in children are due to intracranial tumors.[51] Neurological evaluation should be considered in a child with an acquired sixth nerve palsy. Patching the nonparetic eye and Botulinum toxin injection into the antagonist medial rectus can be performed to minimize contractures and improve alignment while the patient is observed for resolution. If after 6 to 12 months the paresis is stable and does not resolve, surgery is indicated.

Sensory Esotropia

Unilateral organic visual loss such as congenital cataract, optic atrophy corneal opacity, or retinoblastoma may cause an eso- or an exotropia. A near equal incidence of esotropia and exotropia has been demonstrated when the onset of visual impairment occurred between birth and 5 years of age, whereas exotropia was more common when visual loss occurred after the age of 5 years.[52]

■ Exodeviations

Childhood exodeviations consist of exophoria, intermittent exotropia (Fig. 12–8), and constant exotropia. Sensory exotropia and consecutive exotropia are more common in the adult population. The natural history of intermittent exotropia has not been as extensively studied. Although it is commonly believed that most intermittent exotropes progress over time to become constant exotropes,[53] Hiles and colleagues[54] found no significant rate of deterioration in the frequency or deviation over 22 years of observation.

Exodeviations are less common than esodeviations. Generally, exodeviations have a later onset, begin as an intermittent deviation, and may increase in frequency or magnitude over time. The prevalence of amblyopia is usually less than in esodeviations, presumably because they are intermittent and good binocularity may be demonstrated in the phoric phase.

Exodeviations may be classified according to fusional mechanisms and distance/near relationships (see Table 12–3). The most common classification based upon distance/near relationships derives from Duane.[55] (see Table 12–4) Basic type exotropia describes a patient whose

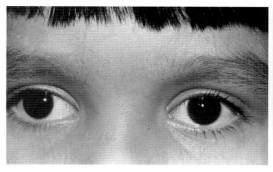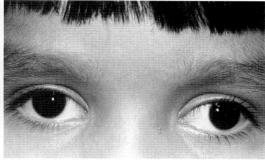

A   B

FIGURE 12–8. (A) Child with exotropia manifest in her right eye. **(B)** Child alternates spontaneously and is now exotropic in her left eye.

TABLE 12–3. Classification of Exodeviations

1. *Basic exodeviation.*
   The distance deviation is approximately equal to the near deviation
2. *Divergence excess.*
   The exodeviation is at least 10 to 15 pd more at distance than at near
3. *Simulated divergence excess.*
   The exodeviation appears to be greater at distance than at near but, after fusion is disrupted and the measurements are repeated, the near deviation amount approaches the distance deviation.
4. *Convergence insufficency.*
   The near deviation is larger than the distance deviation by 10–15 pd
5. *Consecutive exodeviations.*
   The exodeviation follows an esodeviation most commonly after surgery.
6. *Secondary exodeviation or sensory exodeviation.*

near deviation measurement approximately equals the distance deviation. The divergence excess type refers to the patient whose distance deviation exceeds the near deviation measurement by more than 10 pd. A subset of the divergence excess type patients have simulated or pseudodivergence excess where the near deviation increases to within 10 pd after suspending fusion with 30 to 45 minutes of monocular occlusion ("patch test"). Others have reported that utilizing a +3.00 lens also differentiates divergence and pseudodivergence excess[30]; Helveston[56] has argued that a +3.00 lens suspends accommodative convergence and does not affect fusion and should not be substituted for the patch test.[56]

Exotropic patients may exhibit a high or low AC/A ratio; this should be evaluated after performing the patch test in divergence excess patients [see Accommodative Esotropia (High AC/A ratio)]. Knowing if the exotropic patient has a high AC/A ratio is helpful in surgical planning. Exotropic patients also may exhibit a low AC/A ratio. These patients are typically referred to as having convergence insufficient type exotropia where the near deviation is greater than the distance deviation measurement.

Treatment

The goals of treatment in exotropia include establishing or preserving binocularity and ocular alignment. Generally, any significant refractive error should be corrected and the patient's deviation should be reassessed. The use of minus lenses has been advocated[57] as a treatment for intermittent exotropia (2.00 to 4.00 diopters of minus lenses over the cycloplegic refraction). This is not uniformly accepted and is discouraged by many pediatric ophthalmologists as ineffective because of the optical blur that may result.

Part-time occlusion of the dominant or preferred eye can be employed, even if amblyopia is not evident, to improve control of the deviation.[58] If amblyopia is evident, patching is warranted but usually does not substitute for surgical correction of the alignment.

The timing of surgery has been debated. Some advocate "early" surgery[59,60]; others believe delaying surgery past the age of 4 years is advisable.[53,61,62] Others found no significant difference between early and late surgery.[63] By consensus, surgery should be seriously considered when the intermittent exotropia increases in frequency (usually manifesting more than

TABLE 12–4. Duane's Classification of Exodeviations

Exodeviation	Distance	Near
Basic exotropia	A	A
Divergence	A + 10 (at least)	A
Simulated or pseudodeviation excess after fusion disrupted		
Patch test	A + 10+	A
+ 3.00 at near	A + 10+ ≅	A = (10±)
Convergence insufficiency	A	A = (10–15)

A = measurement in prism diopters.

50% of the waking hours) and measures over 15+ prism diopters at distance and near.

Although there has been considerable debate as to which type of procedure results in the best alignment, most advocate symmetric surgery (bilateral lateral rectus recession). Unilateral recession-resection surgery may create a lateral incomitance. When significant amblyopia is present, surgery restricted to the amblyopic eye is preferred, so there is no risk to the only seeing eye.[64]

An initial overcorrection of up to 20 pd is the desirable surgical result as the alignment tends to diverge during the healing period.[60,61,65–67] This is usually accompanied by diplopia that usually resolves over the first 2 to 3 weeks as ocular alignment occurs. Patching may be instituted to prevent suppression and amblyopia. If after 3 to 4 weeks the esotropia persists, prisms or hyperopic correction may be prescribed to minimize diplopia and preserve binocularity.[60] Because children less than 4 years of age can easily develop suppression and loss of fusion, they should be monitored closely and treated accordingly.[59,60,63,67–69] Some advocate waiting up to 6 months and utilizing prisms before considering a second surgery.[60,67]

There is much disagreement among pediatric ophthalmologists regarding treatment of intermittent exotropia.

Special Forms of Exotropia

Congenital Exotropia

Congenital exotropia (Fig. 12–9) and early onset exotropia (before the age of 2 years) are uncommon and usually associated with neurological deficits.[70] These patients often have poor fusional convergence and a large angle of deviation and require more than one surgery.[63,70]

Any patient with an early-onset exotropia is presumed to have a structural lesion (retinoblastoma, cataract, intracerebral tumor) **unless explicitly proven otherwise.** This is a diagnosis of exclusion.

Pseudoexotropia

Pseudoexotropia refers to the appearance of exotropia without a shift on cover testing (Fig. 12–10). Causes of pseudoexotropia include a wide interpupillary distance, a positive angle kappa, or a temporally dragged macula as in retinopathy of prematurity. Pseudoexotropia is

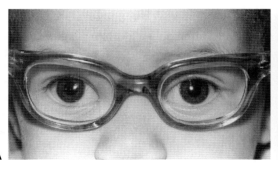
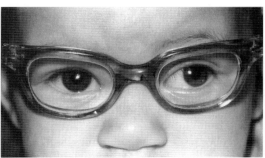

A   B

FIGURE 12–9. (A) Baby with congenital exotropia. The right eye is deviating. **(B)** The left eye is now exotropic.

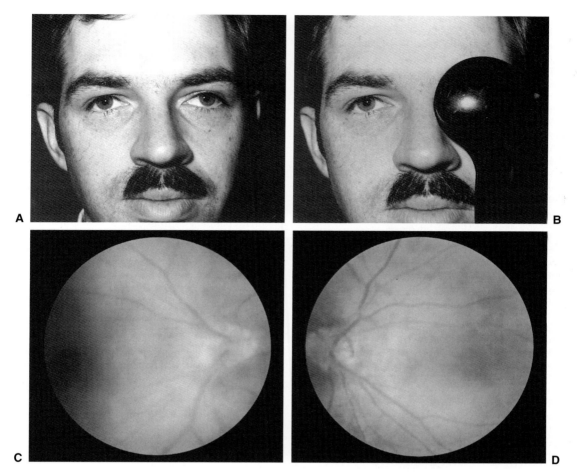

FIGURE 12–10. **(A)** This patient appears exotropic. **(B)** Covering the left eye shows no redress of the right eye, and on alternate cover test there is no shift. This patient has pseudoexotropia. **(C)** Fundus photograph of the right eye shows a dragged macula. **(D)** Fundus photograph of the left eye also shows a dragged macula as the cause of this patient's pseudoexotropia.

far less common than pseudoexotropia (negative angle of kappa).

The optical line from the macula through the lens extends nasally (pseudoexotropia) or temporally (pseudoesotropia) through the cornea, thus giving a Hirschberg-like appearance of a horizontal deviation.

Third Nerve Palsy

A third nerve palsy results in ptosis, hypotropia, and exotropia of the involved eye. Causes of third nerve palsies can be congenital (most common), traumatic, inflammatory, and postviral.[71,72] Congenital third nerve palsy is usually incomplete and unilateral.[71,72] Surgical correction is necessary but should be delayed for up to

1 year to allow for any spontaneous improvement. Correction of the ptosis should be delayed until the eye is straightened as a large inferior rectus recession may change the vertical lid fissure. Aberrant regeneration can occur in traumatic third nerve palsies resulting in anomolous horizontal and vertical eye movements as well as lid and pupil changes; surgical management can be complicated.

REFERENCES

1. Friedman Z, Neuman E, Hyams SW, Peleg B. Ophthalmic screening of 38,000 children, age 1 to 2½ years, in child welfare clinics. *J Pediatr Ophthalmol Strab.* 1980; 17:261–267.
2. Graham PA. Epidemiology of strabismus. *Br J Ophthalmol.* 1974; 58:224–231.

3. Fletcher ML. Natural history of idiopathic strabismus. In: Burian HM, ed. *Symposium on Strabismus: Transactions of the New Orleans Academy of Ophthalmology.* St. Louis, MO: Mosby; 1971:15.

4. Ing MR. Early surgical alignment for congenital esotropia. *Trans Am Ophthalmol Soc.* 1981; 79:625–663.

5. Nixon RB, Helveston EM, Miller K, Archer SM, Ellis FD. Incidence of strabismus in neonates. *Am J Ophthalmol.* 1985; 100:798–801.

6. Archer SM, Sondhi N, Helveston EM. Strabismus in infancy. *Ophthalmology.* 1989; 96:133–137.

7. Podgor MJ, Remaley NA, Chew E. Associations between siblings for esotropia and exotropia. *Arch Ophthalmol.* 1996; 114:739–144.

8. Maumenee IH, Alston A, Mets MB, Flynn JT, Mitchell TN. Inheritance of congenital esotropia. *Trans Am Ophthalmol Soc.* 1986; 84:85–93.

9. Hiles DA, Watson A, Biglan AW. Characteristics of infantile esotropia following early bimedial rectus recession. *Arch Ophthalmol.* 1980; 98:697–703.

10. Pollard Z. Accommodative esotropia during the first year of life. *Arch Ophthalmol.* 1976; 94:1912–1913.

11. Baker JD, Parks MM. Early onset accommodative esotropia. *Am J Ophthalmol.* 1980; 90:11–18.

12. Ellis PP, Esterdahl M. Echothiophate iodide therapy in children. *Arch Ophthalmol.* 1967; 77:598–601.

13. Ing MR, Costenbader FD, Parks MM, Albert DG. Early surgery for congenital esotropia. *Am J Ophthalmol.* 1966; 61:1419–1427.

14. Wilson ME, Parks MM. Primary inferior oblique overaction in congenital esotropia, accommodative esotropia, and intermittent exotropia. *Ophthalmology.* 1989; 96: 950–957.

15. Anderson JR. Latent nystagmus and alternating hyperphoria. *Br J Ophthalmol.* 1954;38:217–231.

16. Parks MM. The overacting inferior oblique muscle. *Am J Ophthalmol.* 1974;77:787–797.

17. MacDonald AL, Pratt-Johnson JA. The suppression patterns and sensory adaptations to dissociated vertical divergent strabismus. *Can J Ophthalmol.* 1974; 9:113–119.

18. Noel LP, Parks MM. Dissociated vertical deviation: associated findings and results of surgical treatment. *Can J Ophthalmol.* 1982;17:10–13.

19. Harcourt B, Mein J, Johnson F. Natural history and association of dissociated vertical divergence. *Trans Ophthal Soc UK.* 1980; 100:495–497.

20. Nelson LB, Wagner RS, Simon JW, Harley RD. Congenital esotropia. *Surv Ophthalmol.* 1987; 31:363–383.

21. Zak TA, Morin JD. Early surgery for infantile esotropia: results and influence of age upon results. *Can J Ophthalmol.* 1982; 17:213–218.

22. Parks MM. The monofixation syndrome. *Trans Am Ophthalmol Soc.* 1969; 57:609–615.

23. Costenbader FD. Infantile esotropia. *Trans Am Ophthalmol Soc.* 1961; 59:397–429.

24. Taylor DM. How early is early surgery in the management of strabismus? *Arch Ophthalmol.* 1963; 70:752–756.

25. Taylor DM. Congenital strabismus: the common sense approach. *Arch Ophthalmol.* 1967; 77:478–484.

26. Taylor DM. Is congenital esotropia functionally curable? *Trans Am Ophthalmol Soc.* 1972;70:529–576.

27. Bateman JB, Parks MM, Wheeler N. Discriminant analysis of congenital esotropia surgery. *Ophthalmology.* 1983; 90:1146–1153.

28. Lang J. The optimum time for surgical alignment in congenital esotropia. *J Pediatr Ophthalmol Strab.* 1984; 21:74–75.

29. Slataper FJ. Age norms of refraction and vision. *Arch Ophthalmol.* 1950;43:466–481.

30. Brown HW. Aids in the diagnosis of strabismus. In: Haik GM, ed. *Strabismus: Symposium of the New Orleans Academy of Ophthalmology.* St. Louis, MO: Mosby; 1962:238.

31. Parks MM. Abnormal accommodative convergence in squint. *Arch Ophthalmol.* 1958; 59:364–380.

32. Pratt-Johnson JA, Barlow JM. Binocular function and acquired esotropia. *Am Orthop J.* 1973; 23:52–59.

33. Brown EVL. Net average yearly changes in refraction of atropinized eyes from birth to beyond middle life. *Arch Ophthalmol.* 1938; 19:719–734.

34. Pratt-Johnson JA, Tillson G. Sensory outcome with nonsurgical management of esotropia with convergence excess (a high accomodative convergence/accommodation ratio). *Can J Ophthalmol.* 1984; 19:220–223.

35. Chin NB, Gold AA, Breinin GM. Iris cysts and miotics. *Arch Ophthalmol.* 1964; 71:611–616.

36. Abraham SV. Intra-epithelial cysts of the iris. *Am J Ophthalmol.* 1954; 37:327–331.

37. Duane A. Congenital deficiency of abduction associated with impairment of adduction, retraction movements, contraction of the palpebral fissure and oblique movements of the eye. *Arch Ophthalmol.* 1905; 34:133–159.

38. deRespinis PA, Caputo A, Wagner RS, Guo S. Duane's retraction syndrome. *Surv Ophthalmol.* 1993; 38:257–288.

39. Yang M, Yee RD, Bateman JB. Electrooculography and discriminant analysis in Duane syndrome and sixth cranial nerve palsy. *Graef Arch Ophthalmol.* 1991; 229:52–56.

40. Raab EL. Clinical features of Duane's syndrome. *J Pediatr Ophthalmol Strab.* 1986; 23:64–68.

41. Isenberg S, Urist MJ. Clinical observations in 101 consecutive patients with Duane's retraction syndrome. *Am J Ophthalmol.* 1977; 84:419–425.

42. Tredici TD, von Noorden GK. Are anisometropia and amblyopia common in Duane's syndrome? *J Pediatr Ophthalmol Strab.* 1985; 22:23–25.

43. Hotchkiss MG, Miller NR, Clark AW, Green WR. Bilateral Duane's retraction syndrome. *Arch Ophthalmol.* 1980; 98:870–874.

44. Miller NR, Kiel SM, Green WR, et al. Unilateral Duane's retraction syndrome (type I). *Arch Ophthalmol.* 1982; 100:1468–1472.

45. Breinin, GM. Electromyography—a tool in ocular and neurologic diagnosis. II. Muscle palsies. *Arch Ophthalmol.* 1957; 57:165–167.

46. Pfaffenbach PD, Cross HE, Kearns TP. Congenital anomalies in Duane's retraction syndrome. *Arch Ophthalmol.* 1972; 88:635–639.

47. Huber A. Electrophysiology of the retraction syndromes. *Br J Ophthalmol.* 1974; 58:293–300.

48. O'Malley ER, Helveston EM, Ellis FD. Duane's retraction syndrome—plus. *J Pediatr Ophthalmol Strab.* 1982; 19:161–165.

49. von Noorden GK, Murray E. Up- and downshoot in Duane's retraction syndrome. *J Pediatr Ophthalmol Strab.* 1986; 23:212–215.

50. Scott AB, Wong GY. Duane's syndrome. *Arch Ophthalmol.* 1972; 87:140–147.

51. Robertson DM, Hines D, Rucker CW. Acquired sixth nerve paresis in children. *Arch Ophthalmol.* 1970; 83:574–579.

52. Sidikaro Y, von Noorden GK. Observations in sensory heterotropia. *J Pediatr Ophthalmol Strab.* 1982; 19:12–19.

53. Jampotsky A. Management of exodeviations. In: Haik GM, ed. *Strabismus: Symposium of the New Orleans Academy of Ophthalmology.* St. Louis, MO: Mosby; 1962:140–156.

54. Hiles DA, Davies GT, Costenbader FD. Long-term observations on unoperated intermittent exotropia. *Arch Ophthalmol.* 1968; 80:436–442.

55. Duane A. A new classification of the motor anomalies of the exotropias based upon physiological principles. *Ann Ophthalmol.* 1897; 6:84–122.

56. Helveston EM. The use and abuse of +3.00 D lenses. *J Pediatr Ophthalmol Strab.* 1974;11:175–176.

57. Caltrider N, Jampotsky A. Overcorrecting minus lens therapy for treatment of intermittent exotropia. *Ophthalmol.* 1983; 90:1160–1165.

58. Iacobucci I, Henderson JW. Occlusion in the preoperative treatment of exodeviations. *Am Orthop J.* 1965; 15:42–47.

59. Pratt-Johnson JA, Barlow JA, Tilson G. Early surgery in intermittent exotropia. *Am J Ophthalmol.* 1977; 84:689–694.

60. Hardesty HH. Management of intermittent exotropia (major review). *Binocular Vis.* 1990; 5:145–152.

61. Jampotsky A. Surgical management of exotropia. *Am J Ophthalmol.* 1958; 46:646–648.

62. von Noorden GK. Simulated divergence excess diagnosis and surgical management. *Doc Ophthalmol.* 1969; 26:719–728.

63. Richards JM, Parks MM. Intermittent exotropia: surgical results in different age groups. *Ophthalmology.* 1983; 90:1172–1177.

64. Kushner BJ. Exotropia deviations: a functional classification and approach to treatment. *Am Orthoptic J.* 1988; 38:81–93.

65. Burian HM, Spivey BE. The surgical management of exodeviations. *Trans Am Ophthalmol Soc.* 1964; 62:276–306.

66. Raab EL, Parks M. Recession of the lateral recti. *Arch Ophihalmol.* 1969; 82:203–208.

67. Hardesty HH, Boynton JR, Keenan JP. Treatment of intermittent exotropia. *Arch Ophthalmol.* 1978; 96:268–274.

68. Hardesty HH. Treatment of overcorrected intermittent exotropia. *Am J Ophthalmol.* 1968; 66:80–86.

69. Pratt-Johnson J, Wee HS. Suppression associated with exotropia. *Can J Ophthalmol.* 1969; 4:136–143.

70. Reynolds JD, Wackerhagen M. Early onset exodeviations. *Am Orthop J.* 1988; 38:94–100.

71. Harley RD. Paralytic strabismus in children: etiologic incidence and management of the 3rd, 4th and 6th N, palsies. *Ophthalmology.* 1980; 87:24–43.

72. Miller NR. Solitary oculomotor nerve palsy in childhood. *Am J Ophthalmol.* 1977; 83:106–111.

73. Hiles DA, Wallar PH, McFarlane F. Currrent concepts in the management of strabismus in children with cerebral palsy. *Ann Ophthalmol.* 1975; 7:789–798.

Pediatric Ophthalmology
Edited by P. F. Gallin
Thieme Medical Publishers, Inc.
New York © 2000

13

∎∎∎

Vertical Deviations

EMILY J. CEISLER AND RENEE RICHARDS

Vertical deviations pose special challenges to the beginning ophthalmology resident as well as to the experienced strabismus surgeon. The muscles involved in vertical deviations are ones that have multiple functions that vary in different fields of gaze. This results in incomitance (variable deviation in different fields of gaze) and adds layers of complexity to the understanding, diagnosis, and management of vertical strabismus. Other complicating factors include the issue of torsion (not a factor when dealing only with horizontal deviations) and the small margin of error from both a cosmetic and a functional viewpoint when treating conditions of vertical misalignment. This is true functionally because normal vertical fusional amplitudes are much smaller than horizontal fusional amplitudes; therefore, a procedure to improve vertical misalignment must be much more precise so that little is left to the fusional vergence mechanisms. Cosmetically, a vertical misalignment is much more noticeable than a horizontal misalignment of similar magnitude because of the changes in the eyelids and palpebral fissures that accompany any vertical strabismus.

Vertical strabismus remains a difficult topic to organize, and we have chosen to separate it into congenital and acquired disorders, further categorizing it by the major division of paralytic versus mechanical. As this is a text of pediatric ophthalmology, we have not discussed disorders that are seen purely or primarily in adults.

∎ Congenital Vertical Strabismus

Paralytic Vertical Strabismus

Superior Oblique Muscle Palsy
Paresis of the fourth cranial nerve (to the superior oblique muscle) is the most common cause of a paretic vertical deviation in childhood. Many strabismologists find that superior oblique paresis is the most common cause of a vertical strabismus at all ages. Although unilateral paresis is more common than bilateral, a bilateral palsy may be masked by asymmetry and only become manifest when treatment is instituted for one side.

A patient with a congenital superior oblique palsy presents either with a head tilt and/or face turn (to the opposite side) to compensate for the vertical misalignment or, if the patient does not have binocular fusion, without a compensatory head posture but with a manifest hypertropia of the affected side. Soon after onset (i.e., early in childhood for a congenital etiology), the hyperdeviation is frequently greatest in the field of action of the involved superior oblique muscle (i.e., down and to the left for a paretic right superior oblique). As time passes, the ipsilateral inferior oblique muscle, the direct antagonist of the paretic superior oblique, begins to overact, and the hyperdeviation may be greatest in its field of action (i.e., up and to the left for a paretic right superior oblique) (Fig. 13–1C). Later, spread of comitance may be seen as the hyperdeviation spreads to other fields of gaze, and precise diagnosis of the original palsy becomes difficult.

The wide range of possible patterns that can be observed in a patient with a superior oblique paresis led Knapp to propose a classification scheme for superior oblique muscle paresis depending on which fields of gaze manifested the greatest vertical deviation. Knapp's classification is still in use today and is helpful in assessment of motility and in planning for surgery. This classification should not be memorized but rather understood as an approach to management by directing surgery to the muscles, that act in the fields of greatest deviation (Fig. 13–2).[1,2]

There are four consequences of a palsy of an extraocular muscle.[3] For the case of the superior oblique, these include (1) underaction of the paretic muscle (superior oblique), (2) overaction of the antagonist to the paretic muscle (ipsilateral inferior oblique), (3) secondary overaction of the yoke muscle of the other eye when the paretic eye is fixating (contralateral inferior rectus), and (4) inhibitional palsy of the contralateral antagonist (contralateral superior rectus).

Despite the spread of comitance, it is usually possible to diagnose a superior oblique paresis by the three-step test that utilizes this information as well as the Bielschowsky head tilt phenomenon.[4–6]

Three-Step Test
The three-step test is an attempt to find a single cyclovertical muscle palsy. It is not useful if the problem is a restrictive one or if more than one muscle is weak.

Step 1: Determine which eye is hypertropic in the primary position (done by cover testing) (Fig. 13–3). As an example, we will say that the right (R) eye is hypertropic. This being the case, the paretic muscle is therefore either a depressor of

the hypertropic eye (R superior oblique or R inferior rectus) or an elevator of the hypotropic (contralateral) eye (L inferior oblique or L superior rectus). At this point, the involved muscle has been narrowed from eight possibilities to four.

Step 2: Determine whether the deviation is greater in gaze R or L (Fig. 13–4). In our example, we will say that the deviation is greater in left gaze. The paretic muscle is the muscle whose field of action corresponds to the side in which the deviation is greater (R superior oblique or L superior rectus). At this point, the involved muscle has been narrowed from four possibilities to two.

Step 3: Determine whether deviation is greater in head tilt to the R or L (Fig. 13–5). Let us say that the deviation in our example is greater in right head tilt. When the head is tilted to one side (e.g., to the right), the ipsilateral eye must intort (right) and the contralateral eye must extort (left). The two superior muscles (superior oblique and superior rectus) are the intorters. If the ipsilateral superior oblique is paretic, the superior rectus of that side performs all or most of the intorsion. The superior rectus, however, also elevates the eye, and this elevation is unopposed by the paretic superior oblique whose function is to depress the eye. Therefore, if the deviation increases with head tilt to the same side, then the ipsilateral superior oblique is paretic (R superior oblique); if the deviation is greater with head tilt to the opposite side, the contralateral superior rectus is paretic. At this point, the involved muscle has been identified by a process of elimination (Fig. 13–6).[7]

The presence and degree of torsion can be helpful in the diagnosis and management of superior oblique paresis. Subjective extorsion can be measured most readily by the double Maddox rod test. The Bagolini striated glasses and the synoptophore and/or the Lancaster red–green projection test (done with bars of light rather than circles) are other options.

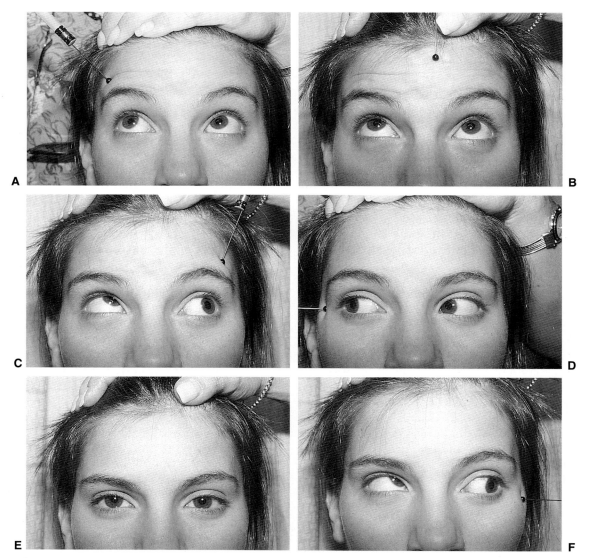

FIGURE 13–1. (A–I) Fifteen-year-old girl with a right superior oblique palsy. She has a small left face turn (not demonstrated). A small right hypertropia is seen in forced primary gaze. The right hypertropia is markedly worse in left gaze and right head tilt. Poor depression of the right eye is seen, most marked in adduction, which represents paresis of the superior oblique muscle. There is marked overaction of the right inferior oblique muscle (the direct antagonist of the paretic superior oblique) best seen in gaze to the left and gaze up and to the left. **(J,K)** The right hypertropia is seen to be markedly worse in right head tilt and essentially absent in left head tilt.

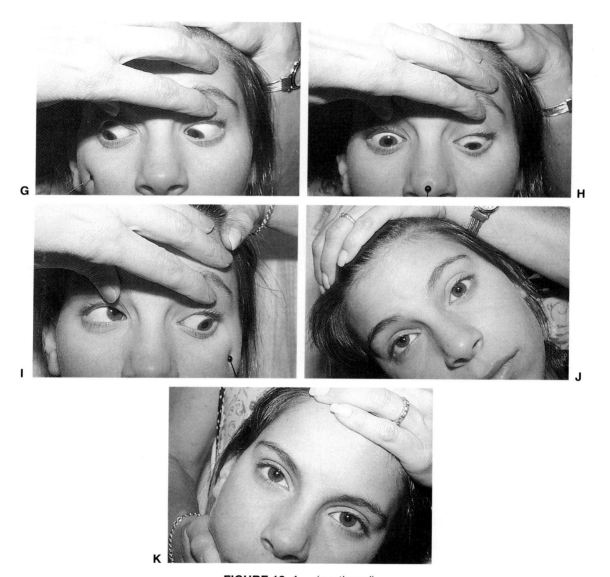

FIGURE 13–1.   *(continued)*

KNAPP'S TREATMENT SCHEME FOR SUPERIOR OBLIQUE MUSCLE PARESIS

Class	Measurements Obtained as Shown Above	Diagnosis	Surgery
I	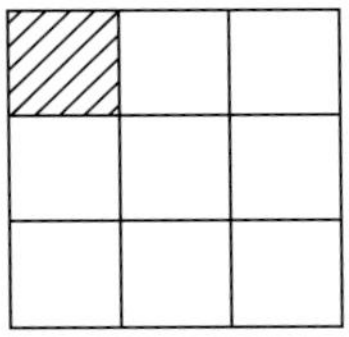	LSO paresis Class I	LIO weakening
II	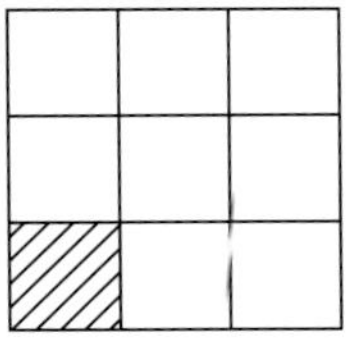	LSO paresis Class II	LSO strengthening (tuck)
III	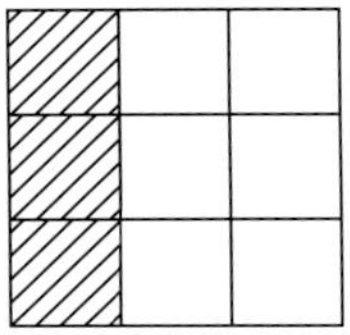	LSO paresis Class III	Tuck LSO if LH < 25Δ. if >25Δ tuck LSO and weaken LIO.
IV	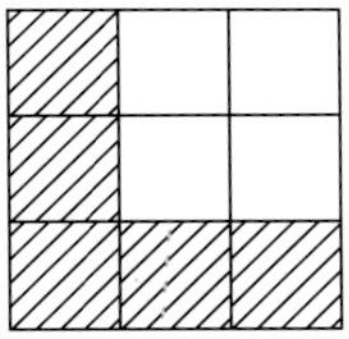	LSO paresis Class IV	1st surgery: Tuck LSO, weaken LIO < 25Δ 2nd surgery: Strengthen LIR
V	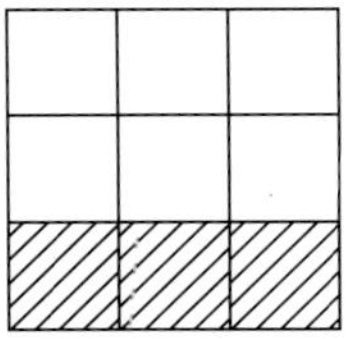	LSO paresis Class V	Tuck LSO or recess RIR
VI	1. Underaction SO, OU 2. Overaction IO, OU 3. V pattern 4. Bilaterally positive Bielschowsky test	Bilateral SO SO paresis	Bilateral SO tuck
VII			"Canine tooth syndrome." Underaction inferior oblique (acquired Brow's), underaction superior oblique. Usually due to trauma in the area of the trochlea.

*Shaded area represents field of greatest vertical deviation.

FIGURE 13–2. Knapp's classification and treatment scheme for superior oblique muscle paresis.

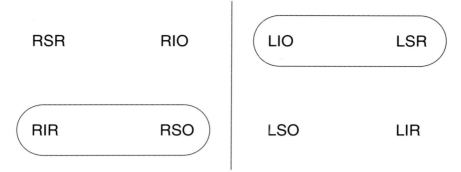

FIGURE 13–3. Three-step test. *Step 1:* Decide which eye is higher in primary gaze (in this example, the right eye). Circle the muscles that could cause a hypertropia on that side (i.e., depressors of right eye [RIR or RSO] or elevators of left eye [LIO or LSR]).

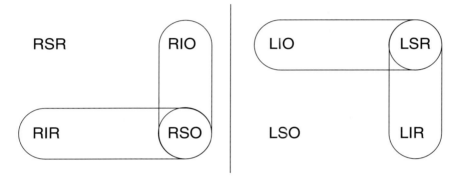

FIGURE 13–4. Three-step test. *Step 2:* Decide whether the deviation is greater in gaze R or L (in this example, deviation is greater in left gaze). Circle the muscles whose field of action corresponds to the side in which the deviation is greater (i.e., RSO, RIO or LSR, LIR). At this point, the involved muscle has been narrowed from four possibilities to two (because only two muscles are circled twice).

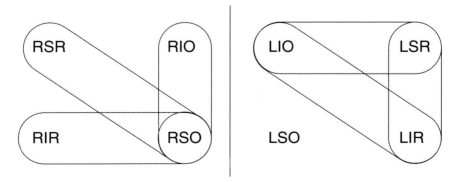

FIGURE 13–5. Three-step test. *Step 3:* Decide whether the deviation is greater in head tilt to the R or L (in this example, deviation is greater in right head tilt). Circle the muscles whose field of action corresponds to the side in which the deviation is greater (i.e., RSR, RSO or LIO, LIR). (See text for more detail on why these are the muscles involved.) At this point, the involved muscle has been identified by a process of elimination (the RSO, this is the only muscle circled three times).

BIELSCHOWSKY HEAD-TILT TEST

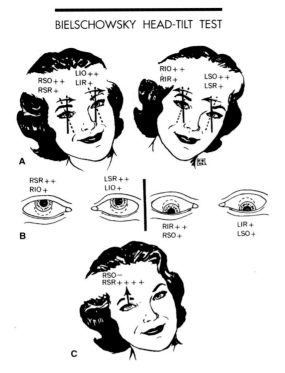

FIGURE 13–6. Bielschowsky head tilt test.[7] Physiologic principles: **(A)** When the head is moved around an anteroposterior axis, compensatory eye movements occur around an anteroposterior axis of the globe because of reflex innervation originating in the otolith apparatus. Thus, when the head is tilted to the right, the right superior oblique and rectus muscles contract to provide incycloduction of the right eye. In the left eye the left inferior oblique and rectus muscles contract to effect excycloduction of that eye. Analogously, cycloductions occur in the opposite direction when the head is tilted to the left. The compensation of the head inclination by wheel rotations of the eyes is incomplete and does not fully offset the angle of inclination. **(B)** Muscles that act synergistically during cycloductions become antagonists when elevating and depressing the globes. Under normal conditions, however, the vertical action of the rectus muscles exceeds that of the oblique muscles; conversely, the effect of the oblique muscles on cycloductions is greater than that of the vertical rectus muscles. **(C)** When the head is tilted toward the involved side in a case of right superior oblique paralysis, the vertical and adducting action of the RSR is unopposed. Contraction of this muscle in an attempt to incycloduct the eye results in an upward movement of the right eye (positive Bielschowsky head tilt test), thus increasing the vertical deviation. (From von Noorden,[52] with permission.)

Objective extorsion can be assessed by examination of the fundus by indirect ophthalmoscopy. The presence of extorsion is further evidence for a superior oblique paresis (although its absence does not rule out the diagnosis) and must be taken into consideration when deciding on a surgical plan.[4]

As discussed previously, a superior oblique paresis is most often congenital. In many cases the patient will deny a previous problem and presents as an adult with diplopia secondary to a decompensated congenital paresis. Evaluation for a compensatory head posture (which the patient may not recognize) and review of old photographs (which may show a head tilt) are good evidence for a congenital etiology (Fig. 13–7). Facial asymmetry from longstanding ocular torticollis may be present and, some studies suggest, may be at least partly reversible if early surgical intervention is undertaken to correct the compensatory head posture. Large vertical fusional amplitudes also speak to a congenital etiology.

When not congenital, the second most common etiology for a superior oblique paresis is traumatic. A history of head trauma should be elicited if possible, but may not have been severe enough to cause this problem. The fourth cranial nerves decussate at the roof of the midbrain and are particularly susceptible to traumatic injury (hemorrhage) in this area, which may lead to bilateral superior oblique weakness.[8] In adult patients, when not congenital or traumatic, a microvascular etiology may be the cause. If none of these etiologies can be identified as the cause, neurological evaluation with neuroimaging is indicated to rule out the possibility of neoplasm or other acquired disease of the brainstem or orbit.

The Fixing Eye

If the patient maintains fusion through a compensatory head posture, there may not be a "fixing eye." However, if there is a manifest deviation, there will be a fixing eye. If the fixing eye is the nonparetic eye, the surgery should be undertaken on the paretic eye (often addressing a contracture of the inferior oblique from longstanding unopposed overaction). If the fixing eye is the paretic eye, surgery can be undertaken on either eye as determined by other factors.

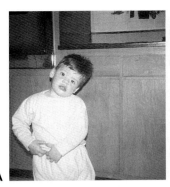
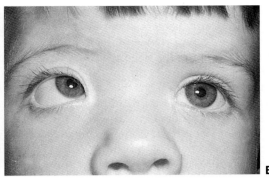

FIGURE 13–7. (A) Young boy demonstrates a large left head tilt due to a congenital right superior oblique palsy. **(B)** Same child demonstrates a large right hypertropia in left gaze.

Treatment

Prisms. Prisms may be used occasionally in the treatment of superior oblique paresis, particularly during the observation period for an acquired deviation while the diagnosis is being solidified and the stability of the deviation is observed. Incomitance, the presence of torsion, and the magnitude of the deviation are often factors that prevent the utility of prisms on a long-term basis; however, in unusual cases, prisms can be the sole means of therapy.

Surgery. Surgery is indicated in children (or adults) to relieve an anomalous head posture or diplopia. There is debate in the literature regarding whether early surgery for congenital superior oblique paresis can prevent or ameliorate the development of facial asymmetry. In long-standing deviations, it is wise to aim for a small undercorrection because the patient has built up large fusional vergence amplitudes to control the hypertropic eye and will easily compensate for a small residual deviation but has no mechanism to deal with a hypertropia of the opposite eye as would occur with an overcorrection.

Depending on the clinical picture (and evaluating which fields of gaze have the greatest deviation—as outlined by Knapp[2]), the surgery indicated may be a strengthening of the ipsilateral superior oblique, a weakening of the ipsilateral inferior oblique, or a weakening of the contralateral inferior rectus. Less commonly, a weakening of the ipsilateral superior rectus or strengthening of the ipsilateral inferior rectus

may be needed. A combination of these procedures may be performed in one patient either simultaneously or sometimes sequentially in a staged fashion.

In young children who present with a superior oblique paresis, a floppy, redundant, or missing tendon may be found.[9] Helveston classifies the anatomic abnormalities found in superior oblique paresis and underlines the importance of assessing the tendon at the time of surgery to perform the most appropriate surgical procedure.[10] Plager recommends exaggerated traction testing as a means to identify a floppy or missing tendon.[11] Many authors recommend a superior oblique tuck for children who demonstrate a floppy tendon.[12] Parks advocates a superior oblique tuck for children with anomalous head tilt.

More typically, a floppy tendon is not found, and the most important surgical principle is to operate on the muscles acting in the fields of greatest deviation.[2] Commonly, a large overaction of the ipsilateral inferior oblique may be present with a large deviation up and to the opposite side. In such cases, a weakening procedure of the inferior oblique is indicated.

If there is a large deviation down and to the opposite side, this can be addressed with either a strengthening procedure of the ipsilateral superior oblique or a weakening of the contralateral inferior rectus (the yoke muscle of the paretic superior oblique). Deciding between these two options should take into account the presence and magnitude of a torsional component (more torsion favors the superior oblique procedure) and the magnitude of the deviation in down gaze (if there is little or no downgaze deviation, an inferior rectus recession can cause overcorrection). The importance of the field of downgaze also underlines the need to avoid the addition of poor depression in the fellow eye to an eye that already suffers from this problem. The use of a Faden, or posterior fixation, suture of the inferior rectus can be useful in cases where the primary deviation is small but the downgaze deviation is more significant.

These procedures can be combined if the deviation is largest in all fields of gaze opposite to the affected eye. More often the ipsilateral inferior oblique and contralateral inferior rectus procedures are combined because operating on the inferior and superior obliques of the same eye may result in an iatrogenic "Brown's" syndrome (decreased elevation in adduction). Weakening of the ipsilateral inferior oblique muscle will correct up to approximately 15 prism diopters (pd) of hypertropia. Inferior rectus weakening contributes an additional ~3pd per mm of recession and in older, cooperative patients is often performed on an adjustable suture. If more correction is needed, attention is turned to additional muscles on an individualized basis applying the same principles as outlined previously.

If the deviation also is present in gaze up and to the same side, the ipsilateral superior rectus can be weakened. If present in gaze down and to the same side, the ipsilateral inferior rectus can be resected. These procedures can be added as necessary to the previously detailed options.

If there is no significant hyperdeviation in primary position, but there is torsional diplopia and the presence of significant extorsion as measured with double Maddox rod testing, a Harada-Ito procedure is indicated.[13] This procedure is an anteriorization and temporal advancement of the anterior fibers of the superior oblique tendon. This is indicated because the anterior fibers are responsible for intorsion and the posterior fibers for depression.

Bilateral Superior Oblique Paresis

Although these may be traumatic, bilateral superior oblique pareses can also be congenital. Sometimes surgery to correct a seeming uni-

lateral problem "unmasks" a paresis of the opposite side due to significant asymmetry. A classic bilateral case manifests a left hyperdeviation on right gaze and a right hyperdeviation on left gaze. Signs that should raise suspicion of bilaterality include measurable extorsion of greater than 15 degrees, objective evidence of bilateral torsion on fundus exam, reversal of the deviation in any gaze or tilt position (particularly in gaze toward the side of the paretic eye), and V-pattern esotropia.[14]

Bilateral surgery may be indicated for bilateral superior oblique paresis and often consists of bilateral inferior oblique weakening or superior oblique strengthening procedures. Asymmetry can be addressed by titrating the amount of surgery done to each side and/or by the addition of a single inferior rectus recession when indicated.

Double Elevator Palsy

As Wilson points out,[9] "double elevator palsy" is a misnomer; he suggests replacing the term with monocular elevation deficiency (MED). Double elevator palsy implies a paresis of both the inferior oblique and the superior rectus muscles of one eye, but, in fact, these patients may have deficient elevation due to inferior rectus restriction or to paresis of just one of the elevator muscles. We agree with this appropriate change in terminology. It is unlikely that one muscle innervated from the superior division and one muscle innervated from the inferior division of the third cranial nerve would be selectively paretic in so many cases.

Incidence

Although the incidence of this disorder is unknown, it is documented less frequently among series of general pediatric ophthalmology patients and appears to be present more often in studies of congenital ptosis populations.[9,15–17] It may be even more frequent in patients with the Marcus-Gunn jaw-winking phenomenon.[18]

Findings

The patient presents with a monocular deficiency of elevation of the involved eye. The elevation deficit is often worse in abduction, helping to distinguish this disorder from Brown's syndrome in which there is deficient elevation in adduction. There may be a hypotropia in primary gaze that increases in upgaze. When fixating with the uninvolved eye, the affected eye will be hypotropic and often ptotic (this may be true ptosis, pseudoptosis, or a combination of both) (Fig. 13–8). When fixating with the affected eye, a large hypertropia will be seen in the uninvolved eye. A chin-up head position may be adopted to maintain fusion. Horizontal strabismus and amblyopia are not uncommon and should be evaluated. Bell's phenomenon is absent in restrictive and infranuclear paretic cases but may be preserved in supranuclear cases.

Etiologic Subtypes

The first type of MED is due to elevator muscle paresis. Forced ductions are normal with no evidence of restriction. Force generation and saccadic velocity testing are consistent with a paretic etiology. True ptosis is often present. Bell's phenomenon may be preserved if the paresis has a supranuclear etiology or missing if the cause is infranuclear (such as superior division third nerve palsy or absent muscle).[9] Many authors feel that the true etiology of this subtype of MED may be a solitary superior rectus palsy, which over time has exhibited spread of comitance through all superior fields of gaze. This would be consistent with the view that the superior rectus is the principle elevator not only in abduction and primary gaze but also in adduction.[19] Additionally, at least one case has been documented to have normal electromyography of the inferior oblique muscle.

The second type of MED is due to inferior rectus restriction. Forced ductions are positive. Saccadic velocity testing is normal. Active force in the superior rectus may be felt when the eye is held in depression with forceps. This type of MED is more common than the paretic type and may not have a primary gaze hypotropia.[20]

The third type of MED is a combination of both types. Long-standing elevator paresis leads to contracture of the inferior rectus muscle. Forced ductions are mildly positive. Saccadic velocity to upgaze is slowed, and ptosis may be present or absent.[9]

Treatment

Surgery is indicated for MED if there is a primary gaze deviation that requires a compensatory chin-up head position. The most important initial step in surgical evaluation is forced duction testing. This cannot be overemphasized because the results of forced duction testing absolutely dictate surgical management. If forced ductions are positive, an ipsilateral inferior rectus recession is indicated. If forced ductions are negative, implicating a paretic etiology, the surgical decision rests on which is the fixating eye. If the sound eye fixates, surgery should be performed on the paretic eye and usually consists of the Knapp procedure, in which both horizontal recti are transposed to the insertion of the superior rectus muscle.[21] If the paretic eye is the fixating eye, the procedure of choice is either to elevate both horizontal recti of the paretic eye or to weaken the elevator muscles in the secondarily deviating sound eye. This may be done in two stages if necessary.

Timing and Considerations. It is generally better to defer ptosis repair until after correction of the strabismus so that (1) any component of the ptosis that is actually pseudoptosis (secondary to the hypotropia) is not erroneously addressed in the surgical planning and (2) the position of the upper limbus after vertical muscle surgery is established, which is an important guide for the desired height of the upper eyelid ptosis procedure. It is also very important to take into account the presence or absence of Bell's phenomenon when deciding how much elevation of the lid is appropriate. However, although strabismus surgery is usually first, the degree of ptosis may dictate the timing of all surgical intervention because a severe ptosis without a compensatory head posture may lead to severe amblyopia. If amblyopia is untreatable without ptosis repair, this procedure may necessitate earlier intervention than would otherwise be performed.

Frontalis fixation is usually the procedure of choice for ptosis surgery because levator function is commonly absent. This is generally indicated by the absence of a lid crease and the lack of eyelid elevation when the brow is held still by the examiner's hand.

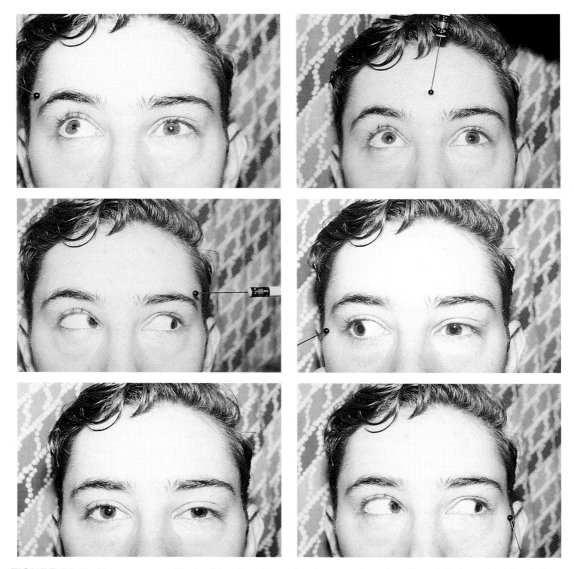

FIGURE 13–8. Young man with double elevator palsy (monocular elevation deficiency) of the left eye. He demonstrates a pseudoptosis of the left eye in primary gaze due to the relative hypotropia OS when he is fixating with the OD. He demonstrates poor elevation in adduction, primary, and abduction.

Inferior Oblique Paresis

Isolated inferior oblique paresis is extremely rare but it can be seen on occasion. It can be congenital or acquired but is almost always congenital. A primary position hypotropia of the involved side is usually seen, and the greatest deviation is measured on elevated adduction of the affected eye. An anomalous head posture is often seen, as is a head tilt to the side of the affected inferior oblique; the three-step test including the Bielschowsky head tilt maneuver will identify the affected muscle.[4–6] A paresis of the right inferior oblique will demonstrate a left hypertropia (right hypotropia) worse on left gaze and with left head tilt. Incyclotorsion can be demonstrated with double-Maddox rod testing.

Inferior oblique palsy, usually of mild degree, may be bilateral. It is frequently seen in A-pattern horizontal strabismus (e.g., Down syn-

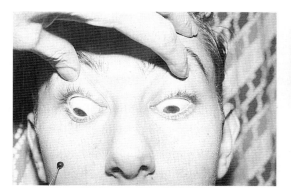
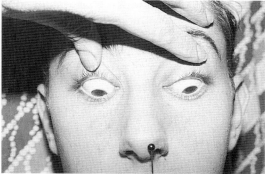
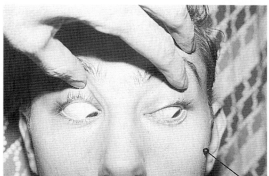

FIGURE 13–8.   *(continued).*

drome) but can sometimes suggest neurological disease.

Differential from Brown's Syndrome

Evaluation of an inferior oblique paresis requires differentiating this entity from a Brown's superior oblique tendon sheath syndrome (decreased elevation in adduction). One of the most important distinguishing features between these two entities is that inferior oblique paresis will be accompanied by an overaction of the ipsilateral superior oblique (the direct antagonist to the inferior oblique). In Brown's syndrome, there is usually no or only slight overaction of the ipsilateral superior oblique muscle. The only definitive way to differentiate between the two diagnoses is by forced duction testing in which Brown's syndrome (see subsequent discussion) demonstrates positive forced ductions, and inferior oblique paresis has negative forced ductions in elevation in the adducted position.

Treatment

Surgery for inferior oblique paresis generally consists of a weakening procedure of the ipsilat-

eral overacting superior oblique muscle because efforts at strengthening the paretic inferior oblique muscle are notoriously ineffective. Tenotomy, tenectomy, and graded superior oblique lengthening procedures (with nonabsorbable suture or a silicone band) can be considered. If the deviation is too large to be managed simply by superior oblique weakening, a contralateral superior rectus recession may be necessary in addition. Much care must be taken in embarking on superior oblique weakening in a patient with high-grade stereopsis, as torsional diplopia can result and be extremely disabling. In such cases a reversible procedure (i.e., one of the graded lengthening procedures) is a better choice than free tenotomy.

Structural Vertical Strabismus

Brown's Syndrome

Brown's syndrome, previously referred to as "superior oblique tendon sheath syndrome," because Brown postulated a taut tendon sheath as an etiology, is well recognized in both congenital and acquired forms. It is now understood that the tendon sheath is not the cause of the restriction.[22] Current thinking postulates congenital Brown's syndrome to be secondary to a taut, inelastic tendon or to limitation of movement of the tendon through the trochlea due to adhesions in the region of a narrowed trochlea.[23]

Clinical Findings and Diagnosis

The classic clinical picture consists of limitation of elevation in adduction but fairly good elevation of the eye in abduction. The eye is seen to travel as if it is on a guidewire as it moves from a normally elevated position in abduction to the opposite side into adduction. A slight widening of the lid fissure on adduction is also seen, and occasionally a downshoot of the adducting eye is also present (Fig. 13–9). Definitive diagnosis is made at the time of surgery by demonstrating positive forced duction testing for restricted passive elevation of the eye in adduction.

Important to the diagnosis is the absence of overaction of the ipsilateral superior oblique muscle, which would overact in the case in an inferior oblique palsy (the most important other consideration in the differential diagnosis). However, in some cases a slight overaction can be seen. An inferior oblique palsy would also have negative forced duction testing. Double elevator palsy should demonstrate a limitation of elevation in both abduction *and* adduction as well as negative forced duction testing.

More difficult to differentiate are diseases of inferior rectus restriction such as the fibrosis syndrome, thyroid disease, or traumatic floor fracture. In these cases forced ductions are positive for restricted elevation in abduction as well as adduction, unlike Brown's syndrome in which the restriction is most pronounced for elevation in adduction. Another differentiating factor is

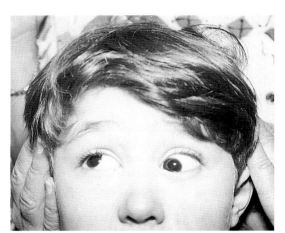

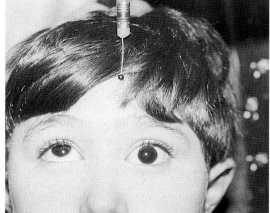

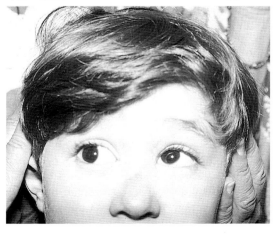

FIGURE 13–9. Young boy with Brown's syndrome OS. He demonstrates poor elevation in adduction but reasonable elevation in abduction.

that, in Brown's syndrome, the forced ductions show more evidence of restriction when the eye is retropulsed, putting the superior oblique on stretch. If forced ductions show that more resistance is noted when the eye is proptosed, the muscles causing the restriction are more likely to be the rectus muscles, which are placed on stretch by this proptosing maneuver.

Patients with Brown's syndrome may show an exotropia in upgaze. Various compensatory head postures are seen; most common is a chin-up head position, face turn away from the affected side, head tilt toward the affected side, or combinations of all three to maintain binocularity and fusion. Some patients with Brown's syndrome do not demonstrate compensatory head postures because no deviation is present in primary gaze.

Treatment

In many cases of congenital Brown's syndrome, no treatment is necessary. Surgical intervention is only indicated if there is an anomalous head position and a manifest deviation in primary position. Timing of surgery must be balanced between early surgery to avoid structural orthopedic changes due to head posturing and waiting to allow a good period for development of binocularity. Generally, surgical timing is dictated by the severity of the head position and primary gaze deviation.

It must again be emphasized that forced ductions must be done at surgery to definitively make the diagnosis of Brown's syndrome. Brown's initial attempts at correction by stripping the anterior tendon sheath from the superior oblique tendon proved disappointing, and this procedure is no longer used. Currently, a superior oblique weakening procedure is the procedure of choice.

Superior oblique tenotomy and/or tenectomy have been advocated as treatment for congenital Brown's syndrome.[24–26] Although these procedures demonstrate improvement in elevation in adduction, subsequent superior oblique palsy and inferior oblique overaction can occur.[26–29] Because of the connections between the superior oblique and the superior rectus muscle, if only a tenotomy is performed and the sheath left untouched, a superior oblique palsy is less likely, although undercorrection may

occur.[26] A superior oblique tenectomy, in which a small segment of tendon is actually removed, is less likely to result in undercorrection but more likely to result in paralysis and inferior oblique overaction. Ipsilateral inferior oblique recession at the time of superior oblique weakening has been suggested by some to avoid the subsequent superior oblique palsy with inferior oblique overaction.[30]

Some authors advocate a controlled lengthening procedure either with 6-0 prolene suture or a silicone band spacer.[31] The advantages of these procedures are that the amount of lengthening is quantifiable and therefore titratable and that the tendon may be recovered if reoperation is necessary to reverse an iatrogenic palsy. In point of fact, in severe cases of Brown's syndrome, undercorrection is much more common and eventual limitation may recur, requiring repeat surgical intervention for an anomalous head posture.

It is important to remember that excellent results are possible but difficult to achieve in Brown's syndrome and that surgery must be limited to those patients with anomalous head positions and/or primary gaze deviations.

General Fibrosis Syndrome

In this syndrome, the extraocular muscles, including the levator, are replaced by fibrous tissue. In some cases, the inferior recti are more selectively involved (as well as the levator), leading to the label of inferior fibrosis syndrome. In fact, the clinical appearance is quite variable and may be unilateral or bilateral, symmetric or asymmetric.[22]

The characteristic clinical findings arise from the pathophysiology in which the replacement by fibrous tissue leads to weakness of the involved muscles and restriction of the antagonists to the involved muscles. Most commonly involved is the inferior rectus, which leads to poor elevation (due to restriction) and poor depression (due to fibrous replacement of the muscle, which thereby has abnormal elasticity and contractility). Ptosis is typical due to involvement of the levator (Fig. 13–10). Frequently a chin-up head position is adopted to maintain fusion and/or because of the ptosis.

Other clinical ocular associations include Marcus-Gunn jaw winking phenomenon,

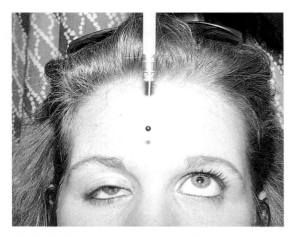

FIGURE 13–10. Young woman with fibrosis syndrome of the right eye. She manifests a significant ptosis of the right eye due to involvement of the levator and poor elevation of the right eye. Forced ductions were positive at the time of surgery.

nystagmus, optic nerve hypoplasia, and ocular colobomata. Systemic findings may include cardiac interventricular septal defects, facial palsies, and musculoskeletal abnormalities. Autosomal dominant inheritance is usually observed in these syndromes, although all modes of inheritance as well as sporadic cases have been described.[5,22,32–34]

Evaluation

As noted previously, a chin-up head position is frequently, although by no means invariably, present. Forced duction testing demonstrates a resistance to elevation (in both abduction and adduction). In some cases, the eye cannot be elevated to the primary position, even on forced duction testing.

These findings are confirmed in the operating room, where fibrosis can often be observed even in areas that do not appear abnormal clinically. Fibrosis of Tenon's fascia and extraocular muscles as well as abnormal adhesions among the extraocular structures are frequently observed. The conjunctiva may be unusually fragile and inelastic.

Differential Diagnosis

Although typically the clinical picture and family history make the diagnosis clear, other entities must be considered in the differential diagnosis. One must consider progressive external ophthalmoplegia, double elevator palsy, retraction syndrome, orbital myositis, myasthenia gravis, Mobius' syndrome, Brown's syndrome, and cranial neuropathies.

Treatment

Treatment of the strabismus associated with the fibrosis syndrome generally consists of recessions of the involved, fibrotic muscles. Typically these are the inferior recti. Ptosis surgery is often required and usually involves some type of frontalis sling procedure. Generally the strabismus surgery is performed first to establish the location of the superior limbus as a guide for the ptosis procedure.

Bilateral inferior rectus recessions are often necessary, and, if the involvement of the two eyes is asymmetric, the amount of surgery on each inferior rectus muscle must be tailored to its degree of involvement. In older patients, adjustable suture techniques can be helpful. The required recessions are generally larger than usual (6 or 7 mm may be required simply to allow the eye to elevate to a midline position).

The muscle may be densely adherent to the globe, and it may be difficult or in some cases impossible to pass a muscle hook beneath it. Persistence and careful dissection from either the medial or lateral side can usually free enough muscle to pass a hook under the insertion so that a suture can be passed. If it is impossible to pass a muscle hook, the superficial fibers of the muscle can be engaged in a double-armed suture, and the muscle can be cut from the globe, or, if necessary, a free tenotomy can be performed. In most cases the muscle can be isolated, and a suture can be placed. Any posterior adhesions to the globe behind the insertion must be carefully lysed to avoid residual restriction.

Once isolated the muscle can be recessed using a normal or hang-back technique. The latter is particularly useful for large recessions, infant eyes, and situations with difficult exposure. The taut conjunctiva is also recessed several millimeters from the limbus using the bare sclera technique.

Superior rectus resection is never indicated as a primary procedure because it does not address the underlying problem, which is one of inferior restriction, and will therefore not be useful. It can, however, be done as a secondary procedure once a large inferior rectus recession has eliminated any restriction to elevation. This may be done to elevate the eye to midline but will not allow elevation above midline.

Numerous techniques have been attempted in the past to prevent further fibrosis after surgery, such as Supramid muscle sleeves or silicone sheets. These have not proved to be useful and have been largely discarded in favor of large recessions with careful scar tissue excision. Some surgeons inject a viscoelastic around the muscle before conjunctival closure or use subconjunctival steroid injections to minimize scarring and readhesion, but there is no solid evidence to support better results with these maneuvers.

Ptosis surgery should be deferred until strabismus surgery is complete and, as mentioned previously, generally requires frontalis fixation. Care must be taken to avoid overcorrection as a poor Bell's phenomenon increases the likelihood of corneal exposure. Lagophthalmos with incomplete lid closure during sleep requires viscous artificial tears or ointment to be instilled in the eyes at bedtime.

Absence of a Vertical Muscle

There are case reports that describe congenital absence of every extraocular muscle, but this condition is exceedingly rare. The inferior rectus is the most frequently described absent muscle. Numerous associations have been reported such as craniofacial syndromes, Moebius' syndrome, and congenital ptosis.[35–42]

Clinically, these patients appear to have a complete paresis of the involved muscle, although they may compensate using other muscles to enable the eye to reach midline. As in cases of paretic muscles, the antagonist may become contracted and result in a restrictive strabismus manifest by positive forced ductions. Computed tomography (CT) and magnetic resonance imaging scans have been performed to document absent muscles and may show a muscle remnant posteriorly in some cases.

Treatments are similar to those for lost or completely paretic muscles. Large recessions of the antagonist muscle can be performed. Transpositions or modified Jensen procedures have

also been used. These procedures can be performed alone or in conjunction with each other, although anterior segment ischemia must be considered when determining the total number of muscles to be operated (taking into consideration the absent muscle).

Vertical Misalignment Secondary to Duane's Retraction Syndrome

Clinical Findings

Duane's retraction syndrome is primarily a disorder of horizontal alignment and is discussed in more detail elsewhere in this text. However, vertical misalignment can often be observed in patients with Duane's syndrome. Characteristically, these patients can demonstrate upshoot or downshoot of the involved eye in attempted adduction.

Etiology

The cause of the upshoot or downshoot is generally attributed to the lateral rectus muscle. It may be that the tight lateral rectus itself acts as a leash or tether or that the inappropriate co-contraction of the lateral rectus causes it to function as a leash or tether, such that, if the eye is just barely above or below midline, it actually shoots abruptly upward or downward.[43] Some authors argue that increased firing of the inferior or superior oblique on electromyographic tracings suggests a synkinetic, innervational etiology for the upshoot or downshoot.

Treatment

A recession of the "tight" lateral rectus muscle, which may be indicated to improve significant retraction, may also improve the up- or downshoot. If the child is orthophoric in primary gaze, this must be combined with a medial rectus recession to avoid inducing a primary gaze esotropia (this medial rectus recession will also help to decrease the retraction). This can be combined with a Y-splitting procedure, which splits the lateral rectus so that the superior half of the tendon is above and the inferior half is below the horizontal midline, thus decreasing the up- or downshoot in adduction.[44]

Another option is a posterior fixation (Faden) suture, which presumably prevents the lateral rectus from sliding above or below the midline as the eye moves into adduction. This, too, can be combined with a lateral rectus recession, if indicated, to improve significant retraction.[43]

■ Acquired Vertical Strabismus

Superior Oblique Palsy

Superior oblique palsy has been discussed at length earlier in this chapter under congenital, paralytic vertical strabismus. Possible etiologies and indications for further work-up when the palsy is not thought to be congenital are also detailed in the earlier sections.

The importance of old pictures in the evaluation of presumed acquired vertical strabismus cannot be overemphasized. Numerous "acquired" deviations are actually congenital, and convincing evidence can be found in the objective documentation of a head tilt or other anomalous head position or manifest deviation in old photographs.

Treatment is also discussed in detail previously, and the principles are similar for acquired and congenital superior oblique palsies. In cooperative older patients, the use of adjustable sutures, particularly on the contralateral inferior rectus muscle, is an important adjunct to surgical treatment for these patients.

Brown's Syndrome

Although Brown's syndrome is often congenital, it may also be acquired. When acquired, Brown's syndrome may be intermittent rather than constant, and a "click" may he heard, or sometimes felt, when the tendon is suddenly pulled through the trochlea after multiple efforts to elevate the eye in adduction.[23]

Etiology
The causes of acquired Brown's syndrome are numerous, but most are related to trauma (see later discussion on trauma) or inflammation (such as juvenile rheumatoid arthritis). Iatrogenic etiologies such as superior oblique tuck or scarring from orbital or sinus surgery are also well-described causes.[23] These situations create a narrowing of the trochlear pulley, which can lead to nodule formation around the superior oblique tendon. When the enlarged or inflamed tendon does squeeze through the trochlea, a click may be heard, and discomfort may be felt. This also explains the frequently intermittent nature of these deviations.

Treatment
Observation may be all that is required in acquired cases as spontaneous improvement can be observed over time. Massage near the trochlea, range-of-motion exercises, steroid injection near the trochlea, and oral steroids have all been reported as useful in selected patients.[23] If an underlying inflammatory disease is the presumed etiology, treatment of the underlying disease can be useful. Some patients do require surgery, and appropriate surgical therapies are discussed previously under congenital Brown's syndrome.

Other Inflammatory or Infectious Causes

Inflammatory or infectious disorders of the orbit or extraocular muscles can cause vertical misalignment. More common in children is idiopathic orbital inflammation (inflammatory pseudotumor or orbital myositis), although thyroid myopathy and orbitopathy can be seen in older children. Parasitic infiltration of the muscles is rare in this country but much more common elsewhere in the world.

Trauma

Blow-Out Fracture of the Orbital Floor
A blow-out fracture of the orbital floor is generally the result of blunt trauma to the eye and orbit, often from a fist or ball. The typical clinical findings include relative enopthalmos, diplopia with limited vertical eye movements, and hypesthesia of cranial nerve V2 (the infraorbital nerve). The diagnosis may be difficult to make, however, on initial exam as many patients will not have enophthalmos despite a floor fracture or may have diplopia and decreased motility but no fracture, both due to significant periorbital hemorrhage and swelling. Acutely, it is important to perform a complete eye exam and rule out acute ocular trauma such as a ruptured globe or intraocular hemorrhage, which takes immediate precedence over any fracture.

Imaging and Indications for Repair

Unless there is significant facial trauma or obvious signs of a large fracture necessitating immediate CT scan, we prefer to allow the acute swelling to subside for 7 to 10 days to allow for a more accurate evaluation. Many patients, even those who do have a small floor fracture, do not have symptoms or findings requiring imaging or treatment. If indicated, floor fracture repair is performed at 10 to 14 days posttrauma for large floor fractures (greater than half of the orbital floor) or for significant enophthalmos or diplopia secondary to restrictive strabismus with clinical and radiological evidence of incarceration of the inferior rectus in the fracture site.

Treatment

Once the floor fracture has been repaired, any residual restrictive strabismus can be evaluated and observed over time as strabismus repair should be deferred for at least 6 to 8 weeks. The most common abnormality of motility is a limitation of upgaze due to entrapment of inferior rectus and associated orbital tissue into the fracture area or to hemorrhage and edema in the region of the superior rectus. Poor depression is also commonly seen and may be due to injury to the inferior rectus muscle or its nerve or to a "reverse leash" effect if the inferior rectus is entrapped in a more posterior site in the orbit or to scarring of the inferior rectus to the orbital floor such that, when it contracts, it pulls against the floor and not against the globe.[45,46]

If there is hypotropia and deficient elevation with reasonable depression, a small inferior rectus recession can be performed. One should avoid large recessions so that depression is not further compromised. Adjustable sutures are particularly useful for this situation. If necessary, the contralateral superior rectus can also be recessed. If elevation is intact and the primary problem is depression, a small inferior rectus resection can be performed, sometimes accompanied by a contralateral inferior rectus recession. This does risk a primary gaze restrictive hypotropia, however, and may limit elevation. If the eyes are straight in the primary position and there is poor depression of the involved eye, a Faden operation on the contralateral inferior rectus is very useful. This will weaken the contralateral inferior rectus only in downgaze, leaving primary gaze intact but addressing the incomitant downgaze hypertropia of the involved eye.[47] It is important to remember that fusion in the primary position is the ultimate goal with minimal disturbance in downgaze if possible. It is often not realistic to achieve single binocular vision in all fields of gaze in these patients.

Following Surgery

Although far less common in children, vertical (and horizontal) strabismus can occur following sinus, orbital, and retinal detachment surgery. Although we are unable to detail the findings and treatment associated with all of these conditions within the limits of this chapter, it is important that they be recognized and addressed according to their cause. One illustrative example observed by the authors is the case of acquired Brown's syndrome caused by ethmoid sinus surgery with disruption of the superior oblique tendon–trochlea complex and subsequent scarring and limitation of rotation.

Canine Tooth Syndrome

This is a specific syndrome initially described by Knapp, which refers to trauma to the trochlear area that results in a combined superior oblique paresis and acquired Brown's syndrome.[2] This is often secondary to injury with a finger, although several of the original cases were due to dog bites (thus the name). Hemorrhage and edema near the superior oblique tendon may cause limitation of elevation in adduction (and acquired Brown's syndrome) and must be differentiated from floor fracture. Forced ductions can be helpful in differentiating these entities; if the restriction is present in both abduction and adduction, it is more likely due to inferior rectus restriction from floor fracture as opposed to acquired Brown's. Also, if the restriction is worsened by forced ductions with retropulsion of the eye, the cause is more likely Brown's syndrome; if worsened by proptosing the eye, the etiology is more likely to be inferior rectus restriction.

The treatment for acquired Brown's is conservative and consists mostly of ice to reduce edema, steroids to decrease inflammation, and time to allow hemorrhage to resolve. Any residual strabismus can be reevaluated after the acute trauma has resolved.

Primary Overaction of the Inferior Oblique Muscle

The very existence of this entity is controversial and has been debated at length by many respected strabismologists. The debate occurs primarily because of the frequent association of inferior oblique overaction (IO OA) with the congenital esotropia syndrome. Some believe that, physiologically, overaction of a muscle can occur only if there is weakness of the direct antagonist and that all cases of IO OA are in response to a weakness of the ipsilateral superior oblique muscle. These authors feel that, in cases without a superior oblique weakness (either directly demonstrable or implied by a V-pattern), the hypertropia in adduction is most likely due to dissociated vertical deviations (DVD) (which are also common in the congen-

ital esotropia syndrome) and is often misdiagnosed as IO OA.[48]

Other authors believe that the IO OA seen in congenital esotropia syndrome and, less frequently, in accommodative esotropia and exotropia patients as well is a primary muscle dysfunction not explained by an ipsilateral superior oblique (or contralateral superior rectus) weakness. These authors feel that primary IO OA is one of the great mysteries of strabismus.[49-51] Although its etiology may be a mystery, the observation of the "overelevation of the adducted eye in esotropia" was noted in the early history of strabismus, i.e., "convergens strabismus surso adductorius" (Fig. 13–11).

Although the concurrent presence of DVD in congenital esotropia may lead to misdiagnosis of IO OA in some patients, it is more difficult to explain the presence of IO OA in accommoda-

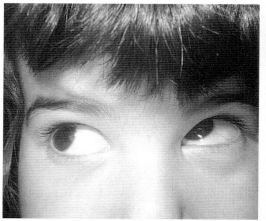

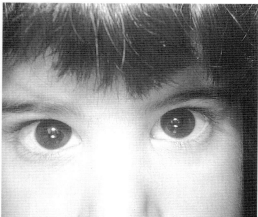

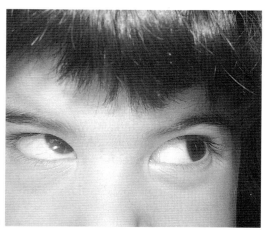

FIGURE 13–11. Young girl with a microesotropia in primary gaze **(B).** She demonstrates primary overaction of the left inferior oblique on right gaze **(A)** and primary overaction of the right inferior oblique on left gaze **(C).**

tive esotropia and exotropia patients in whom DVD is much less common. If primary IO OA does not exist, superior oblique palsy is much more common in these patients than in the normal population. This may, indeed, be true. Although neither theory is definitively proven, all authors agree that the presence of significant IO OA is very common in the congenital esotropia syndrome (~70% or more in many series[51]) and often seen in accommodative esotropia and intermittent exotropia (approximately one third of patients[51]).

IO OA sometimes occurs years after the original horizontal strabismus diagnosis and may appear despite good ocular alignment. It can be symmetrical or asymmetrical (often beginning in one eye only but involving the other within 2 to 6 months). A mild overaction may disappear after horizontal strabismus surgery (particularly in intermittent exotropes).[51] More significant overactions may result in significant V-pattern strabismus and/or large hypertropias in side gaze and may require surgery. There may be some connection between fusion and IO OA, but it is unknown whether IO OA disrupts fusion or whether patients in whom fusion is more tenuous are more apt to develop IO OA.

Treatment of this entity consists of weakening the inferior oblique muscles. Although inferior oblique myectomy can be performed, the preferred procedure is recession of the inferior oblique because it can be quantified, and the amount of surgery can be varied depending on the degree of overaction, which may be asymmetric between the two eyes.[52–54] This procedure is also preferred because it is not irreversible. In addition, it is the authors' opinion that myectomy may more often result in the adherence syndrome with limitation of upgaze than does recession.

■ Vertical Deviations Associated with Horizontal Strabismus

Dissociated Vertical Deviations

DVD is reasonably common and yet its etiology is quite obscure. DVD is the name given to situations in which the nonfixing eye elevates when fusion and/or fixation is suspended. Most of these patients have a horizontal strabismus or have been previously treated for a horizontal strabismus (usually an esotropia). Typically this is seen when a child who has a monofixational strabismus (either primary or as a consequence of treatment), which is reasonably well controlled, is in a situation in which visual inattention or the occlusion of one eye (such as by an occluder or by the child's nose in side gaze) leads to a loss of the previous tenuous control over binocular alignment. This leads to a drifting up of the nonfixing eye accompanied by an extorsion. When fixation is regained by this eye, it floats back down, but an accompanying hypotropia is not observed in the fellow eye. Rather, the fellow eye, if fixation is lost (often by moving the occluder to this side), will take its turn to float upward and extort. In a true hypertropia, one eye is up under the cover and the other eye is down under the cover. The lack of a compensatory hypotropia on alternate cover testing defines DVD as a dissociated deviation and not a true hypertropia (Fig. 13–12).

DVD is difficult to measure as it is not a true hypotropia and cannot therefore be properly neutralized with base-down prism and alternate cover testing. An attempt can be made to quantitate the DVD by placing base-down prism over the deviating eye until, when occluded, it no longer elevates beneath the occluder. Each eye must be measured separately if both demonstrate DVD with the base-down prism used in front of each eye. Because of the difficulty in reliable measurements and the variability of these measurements, DVD is often described more qualitatively on a basis of 1+ to 4+, or small/medium/large.[9]

Etiology
In spite of its frequent occurrence, the etiology of DVD is not well understood. Speculation suggests that it may be related to a tenuous control of alignment due to imperfect binocularity and sensory fusion. In fact, the better the horizontal alignment, the better the control of the DVD.

Differential Diagnosis
The principal entity that may cause confusion in differential diagnosis is IO OA. IO OA causes

ALTERNATING SURSUMDUCTION

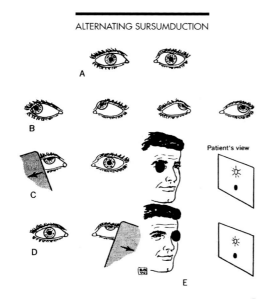

FIGURE 13–12. Dissociated vertical deviation.[7] **(A)** Patient with dissociated vertical deviation may be orthophoric when alert and maintaining fixation on a target. **(B)** Examinations of the versions may reveal overaction of the inferior oblique muscles. **(C)** Occlusion of OD may result in right hyperphoria or hypertropia. **(D)** Occlusion of OS may result in left hyperphoria or hypertropia. **(E)** With the red glass diplopia test the patient will see the red image below the white light regardless of whether he fixates with the right or with the left eye. (From von Noorden,[52] with permission.)

a true hypertropia in which the fellow eye is hypotropic on alternate cover testing; however, the hypertropia should only be observed when the eye is in adduction. In a case of bilateral IO OA, there is a true left hypertropia on right gaze and a true right hypertropia on left gaze. In primary gaze there may be no vertical deviation, or, if the IO OA is asymmetrical, there may be a true hypertropia in primary gaze on the more affected side. In contrast, in a case of DVD, the eye manifests a hyperdeviation in adduction, primary gaze, and abduction, but, as discussed previously, the deviation is not a true hypertropia because the affected eye floats down without a hypotropia being manifest in the fellow eye.

Other helpful clinical clues in differentiating DVD from IO OA include the extorsion of the elevating eye in DVD and the common association of latent occlusion nystagmus with DVD. Latent nystagmus is observed in one eye when the other eye is covered. It is a jerk nystagmus with the fast component directed toward the uncovered eye.

The Bielschowsky phenomenon is also observed in DVD. As progressively darker filters are placed over the fixating eye in a patient with DVD, the upwardly deviated eye will gradually descend, in some cases descending below the midline.[5]

In some cases, both DVD and IO OA may both be present. If an upward deviation of each eye is observed under the cover in right, primary, and left gaze, DVD is certainly present. If the upward deviation appears greater in adduction and smaller in abduction, IO OA is likely superimposed. Also, if a true hypertropia is observed, particularly in adduction on cover testing, a component IO OA must exist. The diagnostic confusion is further muddled by the fact that both the DVD and the IO OA can be asymmetric.

Associated Ocular Findings

In almost all cases, DVD accompanies a horizontal strabismus. It is extremely common in congenital esotropia patients but can accompany any type of strabismus, including monofixation syndrome.[51,55] The better the horizontal alignment and the more well established the binocularity and fusion mechanisms, the less likely it is to develop DVD. Therefore, the first strategy in treating a DVD is to improve the horizontal alignment as much as possible. If the improved horizontal alignment improves the fusional control, the DVD may be maintained the majority of the time in a latent state, and over time it often becomes less evident. If, after maximizing the alignment of the eyes horizontally the DVD is still frequently manifest, surgery can be considered for further treatment. Occasionally, if the DVD is unilateral, optical measures can be used to cause a switch in fixation to the eye that manifests the DVD. However, causing a switch in fixation may also uncover a latent DVD in the previously preferred eye, and the switching of fixation to a less preferred eye may stimulate diplopia.

Treatment

Several different procedures have gone in and out of fashion to best surgically manage DVD. The diversity of opinion on which is the best procedure perhaps reflects the frustration of surgical treatment of DVD and the fact that no procedure works perfectly for this condition. In the past, bilateral large (symmetrical or asymmetrical) inferior rectus resections had been advocated, but in recent years this procedure has fallen into disfavor with many surgeons.

Today, most surgeons prefer either large superior rectus recessions or small superior rectus recessions with a Faden (posterior fixation) suture[56] or anterior transposition of the inferior oblique muscles.[57] The authors prefer a small superior rectus recession with a Faden suture because this allows minimal disturbance of the eye in the primary position but most weakens the superior rectus in its field of action (upgaze). If there is concomitant IO OA, it is reasonable to try to address both problems through a single procedure by using anterior transposition of the inferior oblique muscles.

If the DVD is manifest only unilaterally, some surgeons perform unilateral surgery; however, this may uncover a previously latent DVD in the other eye. Therefore, bilateral surgery is preferred by many surgeons and can be performed symmetrically or asymmetrically, depending on the magnitude of the DVD in each eye.

REFERENCES

1. Knapp P. Diagnosis and surgical management of hypertropia. *Am Orthoptic J.* 1971;21:29–37.
2. Knapp P. Classification and treatment of superior oblique palsy. *Am Orthoptic J.* 1974;24:18–22.
3. Scobee RG. *The Oculorotatory Muscles.* St. Louis, MO: Mosby; 1948.
4. Parks MM. Isolated cyclovertical muscle palsy. *Arch Ophthalmol.* 1958;60:1027–1035.
5. Bielschowsky A. *Lectures on Motor Anomalies.* Hanover, NH: Dartmouth Press; 1940.
6. Bielschowsky A. Etiology, prognosis and treatment of ocular paralysis. *Am J Ophthalmol.* 1943;22:723–724.
7. von Noorden GK. *Atlas of Strabismus,* St. Louis, MO: Mosby; 1983:156–157.
8. Raskind RH. Acquired bilateral superior oblique palsy. *Doc Ophthalmol.* 1973;34:335–344.
9. Wilson ME. Vertical strabismus. In: Wright KW, ed. *Pediatric Ophthalmology and Strabismus,* pp. 211–230. St. Louis, MO: Mosby; 1995.
10. Helveston EM. Classification of superior oblique muscle palsy. *Ophthalmology.* 1992;99:1609–1615.
11. Plager DA. Traction testing in superior oblique palsy. *J Pediatr Ophthalmol Strabismus.* 1990;27:136–140.
12. Saunders RA, Tomlinson E. Quantitated superior oblique tendon tuck in the treatment of superior oblique muscle palsy. *Am Orthoptic J.* 1985;35:81–89.
13. Harada M, Ito Y. Surgical correction of cyclotropia. *Jpn J Ophthalmol.* 1964;8:88–96.
14. Kushner BJ. The diagnosis and treatment of bilateral masked superior oblique palsy. *Am J Ophthalmol.* 1988;105:186–194.
15. Scott WE, Jackson OB. Double elevator palsy: the significance of inferior rectus restriction. *Ophthalmology.* 1977;27:5–10.
16. Sevel D. Ptosis and underaction of the superior rectus muscle. *Opthalmology.* 1984;71:1080–1085.
17. Wright KW, Liu GY, Murphree AL, et al. Double elevator palsy, ptosis and jaw winking. *Am Orthoptic J.* 1989;39:143–150.
18. Pratt SG, Beyer CK, Johnson CC. The Marcus Gunn phenomenon: A review of 71 cases. *Ophthalmology.* 1984;90:27–30.
19. Boeder P. The cooperation of extraocular muscles. *Am J Ophthalmol.* 1961;51:469–481.
20. Metz HS. Double elevator palsy. *Arch Ophthalmol.* 1979;97:901–903.
21. Knapp P. The surgical treatment of double elevator paralysis. *Trans Am Ophthalmol Soc.* 1969;67:304–323.
22. Brown HW. Congenital structural muscle anomalies. In: Allen JH, ed. *Strabismus Ophthalmic Symposium,* pp. 205. St. Louis, MO: Mosby; 1950.
23. Wilson ME, Eustis HS, Parks MM. Brown's syndrome. *Surv Ophthalmol.* 1989;34:153–172.
24. Crawford JS. Surgical treatment of true Brown's syndrome. *Am J Ophthalmol.* 1976;81:289–295.
25. Parks MM. Superior oblique tendon sheath syndrome of Brown. *Am J Ophthalmol.* 1975;79:82–86.
26. Parks MM. The superior oblique tendon (33rd Doyne Memorial Lecture). *Trans Ophthalmol Soc UK.* 1977;97:288–304.
27. Crawford JS, Orton RV, Labow-Daily L. Late results of superior oblique muscle tenotomy in true Brown's syndrome. *Am J Ophthalmol.* 1980;89:824–829.
28. Eustis HS, O'Reilly C, Crawford JS. Management of superior oblique palsy after surgery for true Brown's syndrome. *J Pediatr Ophthalmol Strabismus.* 1987;24:10–17.
29. von Noorden GK, Olivier P. Superior oblique tenectomy in Brown's syndrome. *Ophthalmology.* 1982;89:303–309.
30. Parks MM, Eustis HS. Simultaneous superior oblique tenotomy and inferior oblique recession in Brown's syndrome. *Ophthalmology.* 1987;94:1043–1048.
31. Wright KW, Byung-Moo M, Park C. Comparison of superior oblique tendon expander to superior oblique tenotomy for the management of superior oblique overaction and Brown syndrome. *J Pediatr Ophthalmol Strabismus.* 1992;29:92–97.
32. Khodadoust AA, von Noorden GK. Bilateral vertical retraction syndrome. *Arch Ophthalmol.* 1967;78:606–612.
33. Leone CR, Weinstein GW. Orbital fibrosis with enophthalmos. *Ophthal Surg.* 1972;3:71–75.
34. von Noorden GK. Congenital hereditary ptosis with inferior rectus fibrosis. *Arch Ophthalmol.* 1970;83:378–380.
35. Matsuo T, Ohtsuk H, Sogabe Y, et al. Vertical abnormal retinal correspondence in three patients with congenital absence of the superior oblique muscle. *Am J Ophthalmol.* 1988;106:341–345.

36. Helveston EM, Giangiacomo JG, Ellis FD. Congenital absence of the superior oblique tendon. *Trans Am Ophthalmol Soc.* 1981;79;123–135.

37. Cuttone JM. Absence of the superior rectus muscle in Apert's syndrome. *J Pediatr Ophthalmol Strabismus.* 1979;16:349–354.

38. Mets MB, Parks MM, Freeley DA, et al. Congenital absence of the inferior rectus muscle: A report of three cases and their management. *Binocular Vision.* 1987;2(2):77–86.

39. Pinchoff BS, Sandall G. Congenital absence of the superior oblique tendon in craniofacial dysostosis. *Ophthal Surg.* 1985;16:375–377.

40. Traboulsi EI, Maumenee IH. Extraocular muscle aplasia in Moebius syndrome. *J Pediatr Ophthalmol Strabismus.* 1986;23(3):120–122.

41. Mather TR, Saunders RA. Congenital absence of the superior rectus muscle: a case report. *J Pediatr Ophthalmol Strabismus.* 1987;24(6):291–295.

42. Sandall GS, Morrison JW. Congenital absence of lateral rectus muscle. *J Pediatr Ophthalmol Strabismus.* 1979;16:35–39.

43. von Noorden GK, Murray E. Up- and downshoot in Duane's retraction syndrome. *J Pediatr Ophthalmol Strabismus.* 1986;23:212–215.

44. Rogers GL, Bremer DL. Surgical treatment of the upshoot and downshoot in Duane's retraction syndrome. *Ophthalmology.* 1984;91(11):1380–1383.

45. Bleeker GM, Lyle TK. *Fractures of the Orbit.* Baltimore, MD, Williams & Wilkins; 1970.

46. Kushner BL. Paresis and restriction of the inferior rectus muscle after orbital floor fracture. *Am J Ophthalmol.* 1982;94;81–86.

47. Saunders RA. Incomitant vertical strabismus. *Arch Ophthalmol.* 1984;102(8):1174–1177.

48. Pratt-Johnson JA, Tillson G. *Management of Strabismus and Amblyopia: A Practical Guide.* New York, NY: Thieme Medical Publishers; 1994.

49. Parks MM, Mitchell PR. Oblique muscle dysfunctions. In: Duane TD, Jaeger EA, eds. *Clinical Ophthalmology.* Philadelphia, PA: Harper & Row; 1987:chap. 17.

50. Parks MM. The overacting inferior oblique muscle. *Am J Ophthalmol.* 1974;77:787–797.

51. Wilson ME, Parks MM. Primary inferior oblique overaction in congenital esotropia, accommodative esotropia and intermittent exotropia. *Opthalmol.* 1989; 96:950–957.

52. von Noorden GK. *Burian-von Noorden's Binocular Vision and Ocular Motility.* 3rd ed. St. Louis, MO: Mosby; 1985.

53. Fink WH. *Surgery of the Oblique Muscles of the Eye.* St. Louis, MO: Mosby; 1951.

54. Apt L, Call B. Inferior oblique muscle recession. *Am J Ophthalmol.* 1978;85:95–100.

55. Helveston EM. Dissociated vertical deviation: a clinical and laboratory study. *Trans Am Ophthalmol Soc.* 1980; 78:734–779.

56. Sprague JB, Moore S, Egges H, et al. Dissociated vertical deviation, treatment with the Faden operation of Cupper's. *Arch Ophthalmol.* 1980;98:465–468.

57. Mims JL, Wood RC. Bilateral anterior transposition of the inferior obliques. *Arch Ophthalmol.* 1989;107:41–44.

Pediatric Ophthalmology
Edited by P. F. Gallin
Thieme Medical Publishers, Inc.
New York © 2000

14
∎∎∎

Horizontal Strabismus Surgery

MARSHALL M. PARKS

This chapter is written with the assumption that the patient is in need of surgery on the horizontal rectus muscles to treat esotropia or exotropia. The selection of surgery for treating the esotropia may be recession of the medial rectus muscles of each eye, or only one eye, or possibly a recession of the medial rectus and resection of the lateral rectus muscles of the same eye. For exotropia the recession may be of the lateral rectus in either one or both eyes, or it could be a recession of the lateral rectus combined with a resection of the medial rectus on the same eye. These procedures, the most common and straightforward extraocular muscle surgery procedures, will be illustrated in this chapter.[1]

∎ Preoperative Preparation

The patient is positioned at the end of the operating table. The patient's chin is elevated throughout the surgery, which is accomplished best by having a shoulder roll under the patient's upper chest and shoulder. This assures that the neck will be extended, keeping the face in a 20- to 30-degree chin-up position, which makes it easier for the sitting surgeon and assistant to do the surgery. If the surgeon and assistant stand, it probably is not important to place the head in a chin-up position. However, most

ophthalmic surgeons sit because this position offers better control for fine hand movements because it allows them to anchor their elbows against their rib cage.

The face is prepped with Betadine solution, and a half concentration of Betadine is irrigated into the eyes followed by an irrigation of sterile saline solution. The patient is draped, the eyelid speculum is placed, and surgery is ready to begin.

∎ The Incision

Access to the extraocular muscles is through the 10-mm area that extends between the limbus and conjunctival cul de sac behind the eyelids. The eye speculum exposes this access zone very well. All four rectus muscles insert within the surgical access zone. The first objective of the surgeon is to make an incision through the conjunctiva, Tenons, and intermuscular septum down to the sclera so that a muscle hook can be introduced under the muscle to engage the tendon at its insertion.

The surgeon has only two options in choosing the site for making the incision. The incision should be either limbal or in the fornix. Never place the incision over the surface of the rectus muscle because incised tissue heals by scarring to its surrounds. An incision made over the surface of the rectus muscle results in adherence of the overlying Tenons and conjunctiva to the underlying capsule of the rectus muscle. With time, the scar cicatrizes, pulling the eye out of the desired alignment and restricting the full duction amplitude that the muscle is capable of delivering. Moreover, if secondary surgery is required, the separation of the scarred conjunctiva, Tenons, and muscle capsule requires sharp dissection, which is bloody because the muscle bleeds profusely as soon as its capsule is nicked. After the secondary surgery the same undesirable scarring of the muscle to the same surrounding tissues will recur, and the process is destined to repeat itself. To avoid this chain of events, the incision must be placed away from the rectus muscle at the initial surgery. By placing the incision at the limbus or in the fornix between neighboring rectus muscles, the undesirable scarring process is avoided.

The advantage of the limbal incision (Figs. 14–1 through 14–3) is that it offers a direct route to the muscle. Its main disadvantage is the discomfort the patient experiences from the incision adjacent to the copious corneal nerves.

Other disadvantages include the formation of a circumlimbal mound of tissue, from the edematous conjunctiva adjacent to the cornea, that can interfere with covering of the neighboring corneal epithelium by the tear film, resulting in a dellen, and a visible incisional scar.

The advantages of the fornix incision (Figs. 14–4 through 14–6) are that it is hidden behind the lower eyelid, the patient is comfortable, and the potential complication of a dellen is eliminated. The disadvantage is that the surgeon must first slide the conjunctiva and Tenons over the rectus muscle before it is visualized, and these layers of tissue must be retracted while suturing the muscle onto the sclera. For the inexperienced strabismus surgeon, anatomic landmarks are often "misplaced" while recessing the muscle.

The two incisions are illustrated in Figures 14–1 through 14–6. To demonstrate the incisions, surgery on the right medial rectus muscle has been chosen. The eye speculum is a Lancaster (Storz E-4056). For a small child a better speculum is the Barraquer child size (Storz E-4107). While the assistant positions the eye with Lester fixation forceps (Storz E-1656), either incision is made with the Westcott tenotomy scissors (Storz E-3321).

LIMBUS INCISION

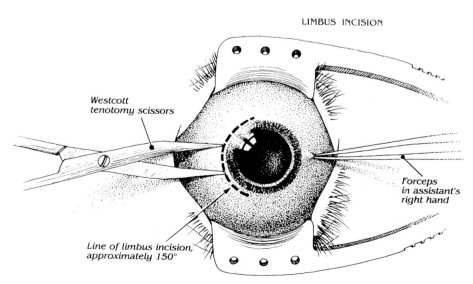

FIGURE 14–1. The limbal incision. The assistant positions the eye in 10-degree abduction with a Lester fixation forceps. (Parks MM. *Atlas of Strabismus Surgery*. Philadelphia: Harper & Row; 1983:79.)

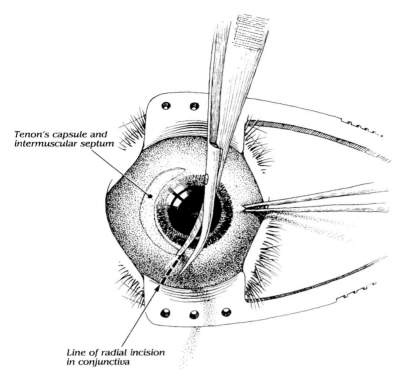

Tenon's capsule and
intermuscular septum

Line of radial incision
in conjunctiva

FIGURE 14–2. The conjunctival incision is enlarged by an 8-mm radial cut from the superior end of the limbal portion of the conjunctival incision. (Parks MM. *Atlas of Strabismus Surgery*. Philadelphia: Harper & Row; 1983:82.)

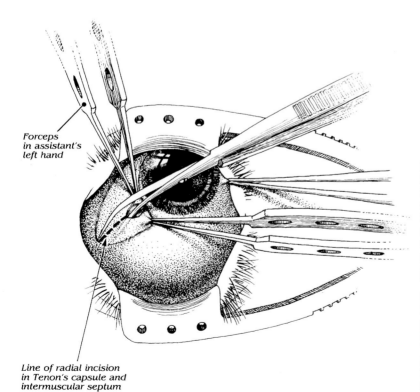

Forceps
in assistant's
left hand

Line of radial incision
in Tenon's capsule and
intermuscular septum

FIGURE 14–3. The radial cut is through Tenons and intermuscular septum, which exposes the sclera between the medial and superior rectus muscles. The eye is displaced inferiorly by the assistant while both the assistant and surgeon elevate Tenons and intermuscular septum with Bishop-Harmon forceps (Parks MM. *Atlas of Strabismus Surgery*. Philadelphia: Harper & Row; 1983:83.) This may be repeated routinely in the inferior medial quadrant by the same surgeons.

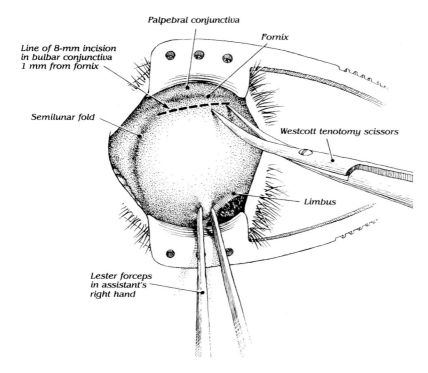

Line of 8-mm incision
in bulbar conjunctiva
1 mm from fornix

Palpebral conjunctiva

Fornix

Semilunar fold

Westcott tenotomy scissors

Limbus

Lester forceps
in assistant's
right hand

FIGURE 14–4. The fornix incision is not literally in the fornix; it is 2 mm above the fornix in the bulbar conjunctiva. It is 8 mm long with the nasal terminus for the inferomedial incision at the semilunar fold (plica). The tips of the open scissors are gently pushed perpendicularly into the conjunctiva, closed, which incises the conjunctiva for 3 mm. This maneuver is repeated in approximately three steps completing the conjunctival incision. (Parks MM. *Atlas of Strabismus Surgery*. Philadelphia: Harper & Row; 1983:71.)

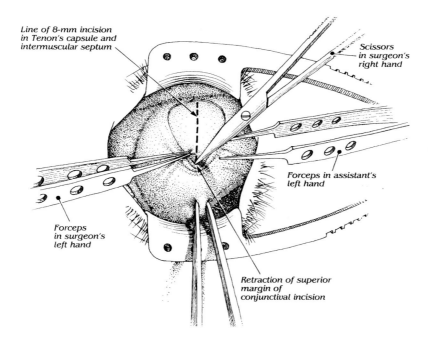

Line of 8-mm incision
in Tenon's capsule and
intermuscular septum

Scissors
in surgeon's
right hand

Forceps in assistant's
left hand

Forceps
in surgeon's
left hand

Retraction of superior
margin of
conjunctival incision

FIGURE 14–5. While the eye is held upward and abducted by the assistant, the surgeon using the closed scissors retracts upward the superior margin of the conjunctival incision. Both the assistant and the surgeon with their free hand grasp and raise the combined Tenons and intermuscular septum with forceps, which is incised by the surgeon, revealing the sclera. (Parks MM. *Atlas of Strabismus Surgery*. Philadelphia: Harper & Row; 1983:74.)

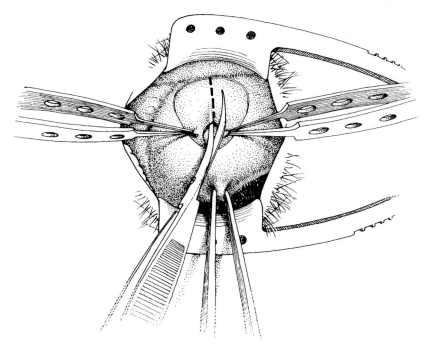

FIGURE 14–6. The incision of Tenons and intermuscular septum is completed. The incision should never go beyond the fornix; otherwise, bleeding will be profuse as the very vascular extraconal fat is incised. (Parks MM. *Atlas of Strabismus Surgery.* Philadelphia: Harper & Row; 1983:76.)

■ The Dissection of the Muscle

Having completed the incisions and being able to visualize the sclera, the surgeon now turns to dissecting the horizontal rectus muscle. A Stevens tenotomy hook (Storz E-600) is slipped under the insertion of the right medial muscle in a manner that does not traumatize it (Fig. 14–7). For hooking the medial rectus the assistant uses the Lester forceps to abduct and elevate the eye for the surgeon. Once the Stevens hook engages the lower half of the horizontal rectus muscle at its insertion, the surgeon can control the position of the eye, so the assistant removes the Lester forceps. The large Green strabismus hook (Storz E-588) replaces the Stevens hook, capturing the entire muscle width on the hook (Fig. 14–8).

However, the muscle still is not visualized at this point. The Stevens hook then is introduced under the combined layers of conjunctiva and Tenons, sweeping and lifting the upper side of the incision over the toe of the Green hook to expose the muscle (Fig. 14–9). This maneuver is facilitated by infraplacing the suspended medial rectus muscle on the Green hook (Fig. 14–10) toward the inferior fornix incision. The intermuscular septum superior to the Green hook is exposed by the former step. It must be opened to visualize the superior pole of the muscle (Fig. 14–11). The intermuscular septum tissue extending toward the limbus from the tendon capsule must be cleared away to visualize the tendon insertion site to the sclera prior to preplacing the suture (Fig. 14–12).

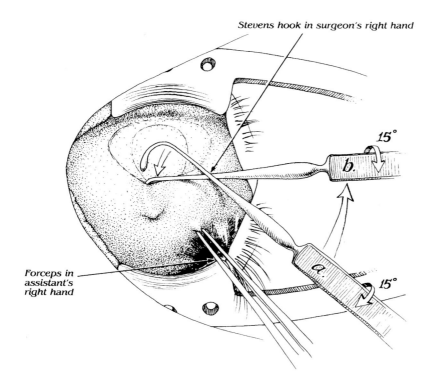

Stevens hook in surgeon's right hand

Forceps in assistant's right hand

FIGURE 14–7. The Stevens hook is flat against face with the handle lying across the nasal bridge when hooking the medial rectus and (not shown here) across the lateral orbital rim when hooking the lateral rectus. The toe of the hook rotated inward 15 degrees depresses the sclera away from the undersurface of the muscle. The hook is then swept upward from position *a* to position *b,* sliding beneath the medial rectus as it moves. (Parks MM. *Atlas of Strabismus Surgery.* Philadelphia: Harper & Row; 1983:92.)

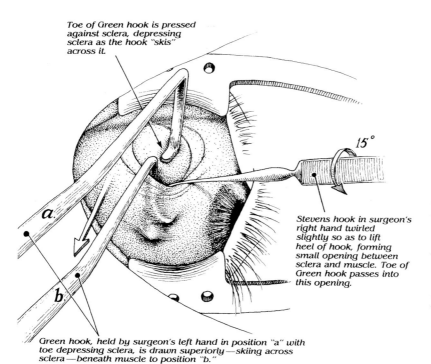

Toe of Green hook is pressed against sclera, depressing sclera as the hook "skis" across it.

Stevens hook in surgeon's right hand twirled slightly so as to lift heel of hook, forming small opening between sclera and muscle. Toe of Green hook passes into this opening.

Green hook, held by surgeon's left hand in position "a" with toe depressing sclera, is drawn superiorly—skiing across sclera—beneath muscle to position "b."

FIGURE 14–8. With the eye maintained in the abducted position by tension on the Stevens tenotomy hook, the Green muscle hook is introduced in a plane perpendicular to the sclera. As it skids across the sclera, the entire rectus muscle is engaged on the hook, and the Stevens hook is removed. (Parks MM. *Atlas of Strabismus Surgery.* Philadelphia: Harper & Row; 1983:93.)

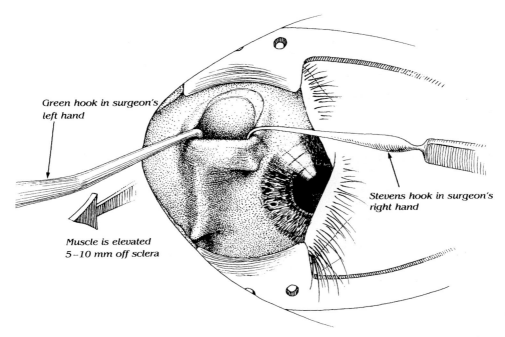

*Green hook in surgeon's
left hand*

*Muscle is elevated
5–10 mm off sclera*

*Stevens hook in surgeon's
right hand*

FIGURE 14–9. The Stevens hook retracts the conjunctiva, Tenons, and intermuscular septum layers over the taut rectus muscle on the Green hook. (Parks MM. *Atlas of Strabismus Surgery*. Philadelphia: Harper & Row; 1983:97.)

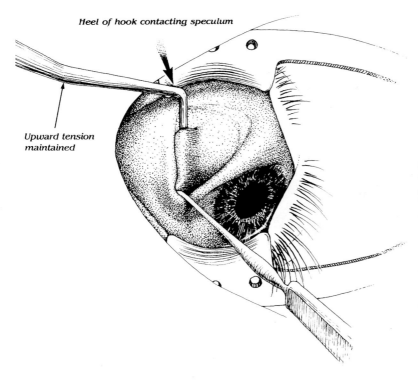

Heel of hook contacting speculum

*Upward tension
maintained*

FIGURE 14–10. Uncovering the toe of the Green hook suspending the muscle involves a two-handed maneuver by the surgeon. First, the Green hook is lowered to bring the muscle inferiorly to the incision, and, secondly, the Stevens hook brings the tissues it is retracting upward to clear the toe of the Green hook. (Parks MM. *Atlas of Strabismus Surgery*. Philadelphia: Harper & Row; 1983:98.)

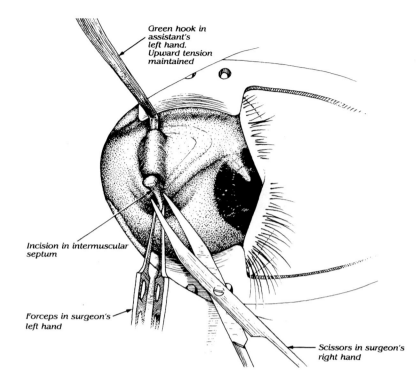

Green hook in
assistant's
left hand.
Upward tension
maintained

Incision in intermuscular
septum

Forceps in surgeon's
left hand

Scissors in surgeon's
right hand

FIGURE 14–11. Opening the intermuscular septum attached to the superior border of the rectus muscle. (Parks MM. *Atlas of Strabismus Surgery.* Philadelphia: Harper & Row; 1983:99.)

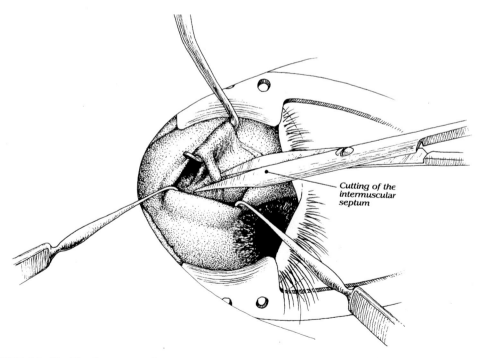

Cutting of the
intermuscular
septum

FIGURE 14–12. The intermuscular septum tissue that extends between the tendon capsule and limbus must be cut away to visualize the insertion prior to preplacing the suture. The assistant, with two Stevens hooks, exposes the superior pole of the tendon and the intermuscular septal tissue for the surgeon. (Parks MM. *Atlas of Strabismus Surgery.* Philadelphia: Harper & Row; 1983:102.)

■ The Recession Procedure

Absorbable synthetic sutures of 6-0 size with double arm spatulated needles are used (Vicryl No. J-555G with S-29 needles or Dexon No. 7529-13 with SLO-1 needles). The preplaced suture is passed into the tendon fibers 1 mm from the sclera along the full tendon width, and a locking bite is placed on each end [Fig. 14–13; the needle holder depicted in this figure is a Barraquer curved-jaw with lock (Storz E-3843)]. The tendon is disinserted with Manson-Aebli corneal section scissors (Storz right E-3289-M, left E-3290-M). To obtain a flush cut from the sclera, which is required to avoid leaving an undesirable cosmetic ridge of tendon, the deep

scissors blade must be introduced under the tendon as depicted in Figure 14–14. Consequently, right and left scissors are required, depending on which eye is being operated.

In reattaching the muscle the assistant positions and immobilizes the globe for the surgeon by grasping the sclera with Stern-Castroviejo forceps with lock (Storz E-1789-S) at the superior and inferior poles of the disinserted tendon's insertion site. The scleral needle entry site is measured in increments of 0.5 mm with the Castroviejo caliper (Storz E-2404), as shown in Figure 14–15. A long tunnel with the "crossed swords" is shown in Figure 14–16. The muscle is pulled up and tied (Fig. 14–17). The long scleral tunnel through which the sutures

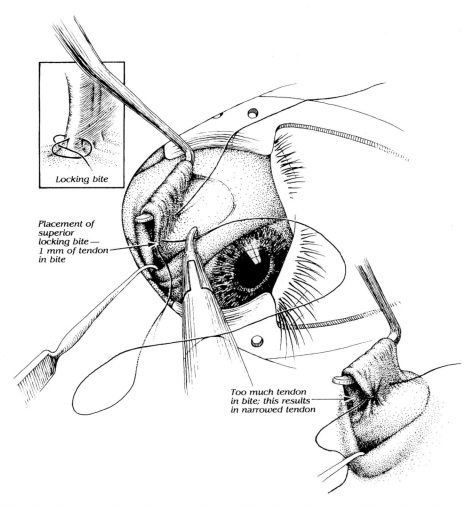

Locking bite

Placement of superior locking bite— 1 mm of tendon in bite

Too much tendon in bite; this results in narrowed tendon

FIGURE 14–13. Preplacing the suture in the tendon 1 mm from the sclera. (Parks MM. *Atlas of Strabismus Surgery.* Philadelphia: Harper & Row; 1983:107.)

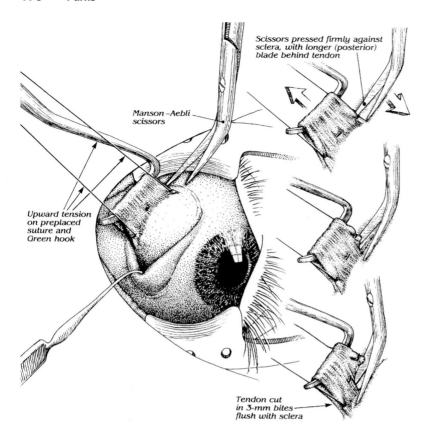

Scissors pressed firmly against
sclera, with longer (posterior)
blade behind tendon

Manson–Aebli
scissors

Upward tension
on preplaced
suture and
Green hook

Tendon cut
in 3-mm bites
flush with sclera

FIGURE 14–14.
Disinserting the tendon.
The flat surfaces of the
scissors blades are flush
with the scleral surface.
Several small cuts with the
scissors are made for
safety in avoiding excising
a segment of sclera. (Parks
MM. *Atlas of Strabismus
Surgery*. Philadelphia:
Harper & Row; 1983:109.)

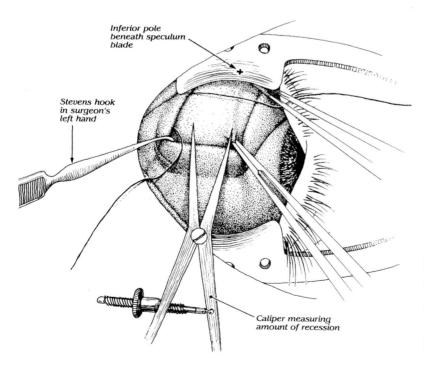

Inferior pole
beneath speculum
blade

Stevens hook
in surgeon's
left hand

Caliper measuring
amount of recession

FIGURE 14–15. Scleral
marking with the caliper the
site the needle will enter to
complete the upper 6 mm
scleral tunnel. (Parks MM.
*Atlas of Strabismus
Surgery*. Philadelphia:
Harper & Row; 1983:111.)

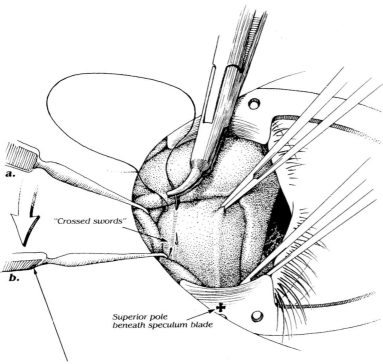

a.

"Crossed swords"

b.

Superior pole
beneath speculum blade

*As the needle is advanced in the scleral tunnel, the surgeon
advances the Stevens hook from a to b.*

FIGURE 14–16. The completion of the lower 6-mm scleral tunnel, giving a 10-mm-long tunnel with 2-mm distance between the overlapping "crossed swords" needle exiting sites from the sclera. (Parks MM. *Atlas of Strabismus Surgery*. Philadelphia: Harper & Row; 1983:113.)

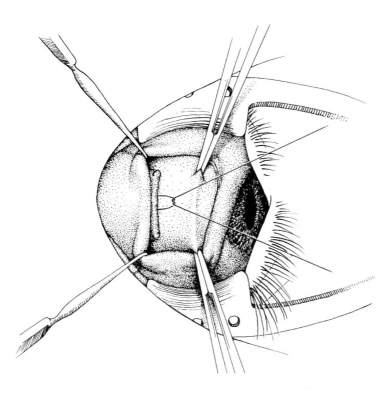

FIGURE 14–17. The muscle is pulled up and tied. Its postoperative width is comparable with its preoperative width. (Parks MM. *Atlas of Strabismus Surgery*. Philadelphia: Harper & Row; 1983:114.)

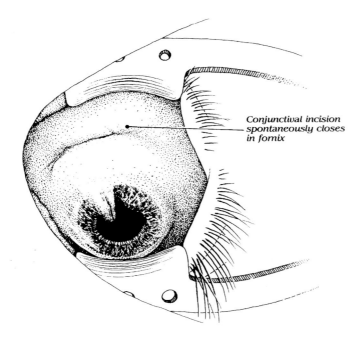

Conjunctival incision
spontaneously closes
in fornix

FIGURE 14–18. The retracted intermuscular septum, Tenons, and conjunctiva fall back into the fornix. (Parks MM. *Atlas of Strabismus Surgery*. Philadelphia: Harper & Row; 1983:115.)

pass insures that the normal width of the recessed muscle is retained. At the conclusion of the surgery the incised tissue falls back into the fornix, and the surgeon determines whether a suture is required to coapt the sides of the conjunctival incisions (Fig. 14–18). Often it is not necessary to close the fornix incision if it is well opposed at the conclusion of the case. If a limbal incision was used, closure requires a stitch at the site where the radial cut was started at the limbus. The same suture for the muscle surgery is also used as an interrupted suture(s) to close the conjunctival incision, whether it be limbal or fornix.

■ The Resection Procedure

The resection procedure is slightly more complex for the surgeon and more uncomfortable for the patient because it tightens the muscle tissue as opposed to the recession procedure, which loosens the muscle tissue. The horizontal rectus is dissected more extensively for the resection than the recession by cutting the intermuscular septum back further along the sides of the muscle and cutting the check ligaments over the surface of the muscle. Two Green muscle hooks are introduced under the muscle, and the quantity of resection is measured (Fig. 14–19). Two double arm 6-0 sutures are used for the resection compared with only one for the recession. Because the muscle is tightened and the substance through which the sutures are passed is more apt to be soft muscle fibers than firm tendon fibers, there is greater concern that the sutures may cut through the tissue, which would result in a slipped muscle. Keeping the sutures orderly and under control is best accomplished by taping them to the drapes (Fig. 14–20). A Hartman hemostatic mosquito forceps (Storz E-3915) is clamped across the muscle just anterior to the preplaced sutures, and the muscle is disinserted (Fig. 14–21). The redundant muscle tissue distal to the clamp is

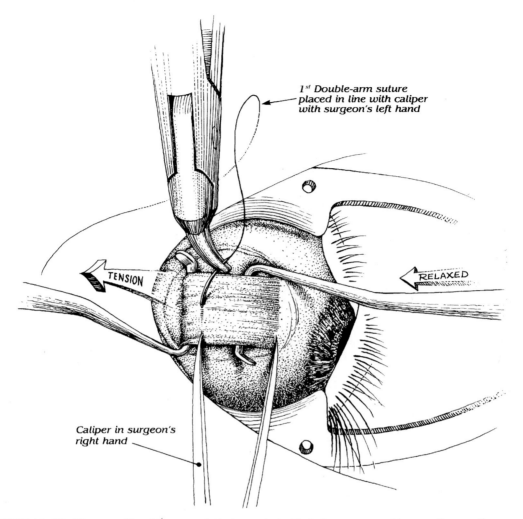

FIGURE 14–19. The quantity of the muscle to be resected is being measured by a caliper as the surgeon is preplacing the needle of the superior double-arm suture into the muscle fibers. (Parks MM. *Atlas of Strabismus Surgery*. Philadelphia: Harper & Row; 1983:121.)

excised (Fig. 14–22) with a scalpel (Storz Bard-Parker blade No. 15E-338-15 and Bard-Parker handle No. 9 Storz E-334). The Hartman is left clamped to the muscle to prevent bleeding, and the sutures are passed through the sclera in a "crossed swords" manner (Fig. 14–23). The clamp is removed and, if done carefully, and if the resected end of the muscle is not touched,

bleeding usually does not occur. Pull the sutures up. The muscle is snug against the old insertion site and spread out to its preoperative dimension. Tie the sutures down (Fig. 14–24) and replace the incised tissue back into the fornix. Closure of the conjunctival incision may require an interrupted suture or two regardless of whether a fornix or limbal incision was used.

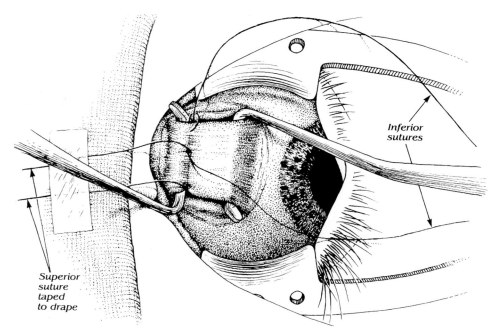

Inferior
sutures

Superior
suture
taped
to drape

FIGURE 14–20. The two double-arm preplaced sutures are taped to the drapes. (Parks MM. *Atlas of Strabismus Surgery*. Philadelphia: Harper & Row; 1983:123.)

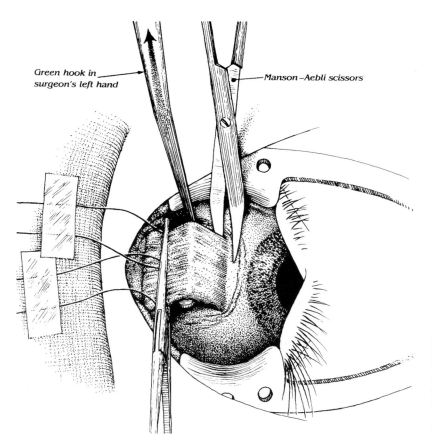

Green hook in
surgeon's left hand

Manson–Aebli scissors

FIGURE 14–21.
Disinserting the muscle
with a Hartman clamp
anterior to the preplaced
sutures. (Parks MM. *Atlas
of Strabismus Surgery*.
Philadelphia: Harper &
Row; 1983:125.)

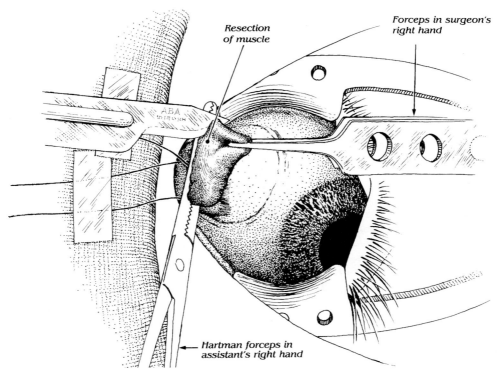

FIGURE 14–22. The redundant muscle is resected distal to the clamped muscle. (Parks MM. *Atlas of Strabismus Surgery*. Philadelphia: Harper & Row; 1983:126.)

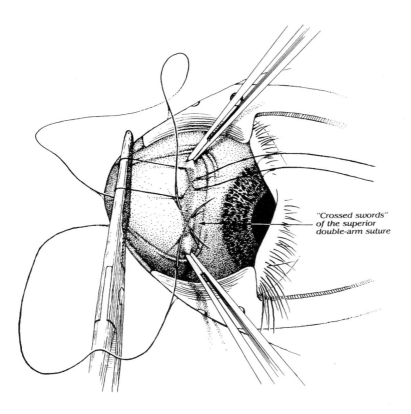

FIGURE 14–23. The two double-arm sutures are passed through the sclera. Bleeding from the resected muscle is controlled by retaining the Hartman clamp on the muscle. Cautery should not be used on the resected end of the muscle because of the risk that it would burn the sutures. (Parks MM. *Atlas of Strabismus Surgery*. Philadelphia: Harper & Row; 1983:129.)

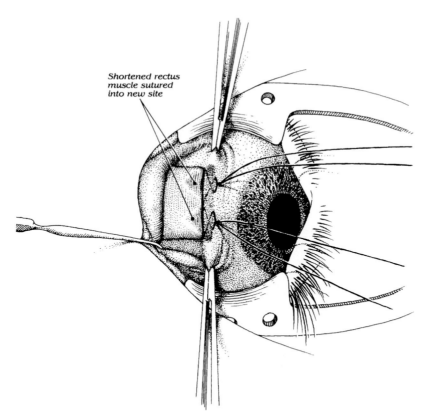

Shortened rectus muscle sutured into new site

FIGURE 14–24. The clamp has been removed, the muscle is pulled up to the original insertion, and the sutures are tied. The conjunctiva will fall into the inferior fornix naturally. One or two interrupted sutures may be necessary to close the conjunctival incision. (Parks MM. *Atlas of Strabismus Surgery.* Philadelphia: Harper & Row; 1983:131.)

■ The Quantity of Surgery

The amount of recession and resection is titrated according to the quantity of the eye deviation determined by prism and alternate cover tests or by corneal light reflex. For esotropia the initial surgery is usually a recession of the medial rectus muscles. Occasionally, surgery is performed on only one eye, for example, a recession of the medial rectus and resection of the lateral rectus muscle. Secondary surgery for residual esotropia usually is a resection of the lateral rectus muscles. Table 14–1 provides the quantity of surgery recommended by the author for esotropia, and Table 14–2 for exotropia.[2] Generally, for exotropia, the initial surgery is recession of the lateral rectus muscles, but in some cases it is unilateral surgery, requiring recession of the lateral rectus and resection of the medial rectus. Secondary surgery consists most frequently of resections of the medial rectus muscles.

Some surgeons[3] modify the quantity of surgery by adjusting the amount that the muscle is advanced or retroplaced (adjustable suture technique), according to the patient's finding some hours or a day after the initial surgery. The technique was not described here because I consider it to be more complicated and more fraught with complications than the standard techniques just described. Certainly, one should learn the standard techniques first.

■ Postoperative Care

During the first several hours after recovery from anesthesia, patients appreciate the soothing effect that continuous cold wet compresses to the eyes provide. Soaked turkish wash cloths

TABLE 14–1. Surgery for Esotropia

Angle of Dev (Δ)	Rec MROU (mm)
15	3.0
20	3.5
25	4.0
30	4.5
35	5.0
40	5.5
50	6.0
60 or >	7.0

Angle of Dev (Δ)	Rec MR (mm)	Res LR (mm)
15	3.0	4
20	3.5	5
25	4.0	6
30	4.5	7
35	5.0	8
40	5.5	9
50	6.0	10
60 or >	7.0	11

Angle of Dev (Δ)	Res LROU (mm)
15	4
20	5
25	6
30	7
35	8
40	9
50	10
60 or >	11

Dev, deviation; MR, medial rectus; LR, lateral rectus;
OU, both eyes; Rec, recession; Res, resection; Δ, diopters.

TABLE 14–2. Surgery for Exotropia

Angle of Dev (Δ)	Rec LROU (mm)
15	4
20	5
25	6
30	7
40 or >	8

Angle of Dev (Δ)	Rec LR (mm)	Res MR (mm)
15	4	3
20	5	4
25	6	5
30	7	6
40	8	7
50	9	8
60	10	9
80	11	10

Angle of Dev (Δ)	Res MROU (mm)
15	3
20	4
25	5
30	6
40 or >	7

Dev, deviation; MR, medial rectus; LR, lateral rectus;
OU, both eyes; Rec, recession; Res, resection; Δ, diopters.

are the best thing to use as compresses. A combined antibiotic–steroid drop is instilled prior to the patient's departure from the operating room and continued for 10 days at the dosage of q.i.d. Do not use an ointment because it obscures vision. No bandages are necessary. The need to administer systemic antibiotics postoperatively is controversial. Unfortunately, during the second to fourth postoperative days the operative reaction can mask the early signs of infection. It is comforting to the surgeon to already have a blood-level of antibiotic in the patient at the time this differential presents. This frequent occurrence tips the controversy, in my opinion, to routinely using systemic antibiotics. Staphylococcal infections account for almost all reported postoperative infections. Rhinorrhea is probably the most common source. Upper respiratory infections that become manifest in the immediate postoperative period are always possible. It is impractical

to see the patient daily during the first 5 days after surgery. Therefore, with this potential risk I have become a convert to using a systemic antibiotic that is maximally effective against the staphylococcus for the first 5 postoperative days, starting the medication per eye on the morning of the day after surgery. Dicloxacillin is the least expensive and best but can be taken only in pill form and only if the patient is not allergic to penicillin. If allergic to penicillin, the patient is given erythromycin. For children who refuse or are unable to take pills, the appropriate pediatric dosage (according to the weight of the patient as listed in the Physicians' Desk Reference) of an antibiotic suspension, such as Lorabid, is prescribed.

Usually nothing is needed for discomfort other than extra-strength Tylenol for the first day or two after surgery. No limitations on using the eyes after surgery are imposed on the patient. Most patients resume full visual activity in the range of 3 to 5 days after surgery. If possible, the first postoperative visit occurs at approximately 3 days. The alignment and ductions can usually be investigated at that time.

The final outcome of the surgery is not declared until the 6-week postoperative visit. In some cases the change between 3 days and 6 weeks is striking. This is especially evident in exotropia surgery following recessions of the lateral rectus muscles. Usually, postoperative esotropia of 15 to 20 diopters lasts for 7 to 21 days before reducing to near orthophoria. During this period diplopia is expected. However, in all muscle surgery for whatever the deviation, transient diplopia is very common until muscle function returns to normal, when the postoperative inflammation and edema in the operated muscles subside. The patient/parent must be informed about this prior to surgery and given reassurance after the surgery.

REFERENCES

1. Parks MM. *Atlas of Strabismus Surgery.* Philadelphia: Harper & Row; 1983.
2. Parks MM. *Duane's Clinical Ophthalmology.* Tasman W, Jaeger EA, eds. Philadelphia: Lippincott-Raven; 1995;1;12:10, 1;13:11–12.
3. Wright KW. *Color Atlas of Ophthalmic Surgery Strabismus.* Philadelphia: Lippincott; 1991;7:87–124.

Pediatric Ophthalmology
Edited by P. F. Gallin
Thieme Medical Publishers, Inc.
New York © 2000

15

Ocular Trauma

ERIC KRUGER, B. DAVID GORMAN,
HERMANN D. SCHUBERT, AND SAN DEEP JAIN

Each year an estimated 1.3 million Americans suffer eye injuries. A disproportionate share of ocular and orbital injuries occur in children.[1] The population-based estimate of the incidence of ocular trauma in children is 15.2 per 100,000 per year.[2] Ocular injuries in children over 10 years of age are most commonly sports related, whereas injuries in the home account for the majority of trauma in children younger than 10 years of age.[3] The majority of pediatric eye injuries are preventable. Visual disability in children that is secondary to eye injuries can be greatly reduced by the implementation of well-established safety precautions and supervision.

Appropriate and timely management of eye trauma is essential to ensuring optimal outcome for the child. As many of the cases are initially managed by pediatric practitioners, the child with eye trauma should be promptly referred to an ophthalmologist. A 3-year survey conducted at the Wills Eye Hospital revealed that approximately 22% of all ocular injuries in children required hospital admissions.[4] Only admissions for strabismus account for more pediatric hospitalizations than for eye injuries.

In this chapter we will discuss the standardized classification of ocular trauma and the major causes of pediatric eye trauma and its management.

■ Classification of Ocular Trauma

A classification of ocular trauma (Table 15–1) has been developed by Kuhn et al.[5] This classification has been endorsed by the International Society of Ocular Trauma, United States Eye Injury Registry, and American Academy of Ophthalmology. At the time of initial presentation, an attempt should be made to classify the injured eye based on this classification system.

■ Management of Pediatric Ocular Trauma

The key to proper management of pediatric ocular trauma is a systematic approach including a thorough history and a methodical examination. Unfortunately, this evaluation may be hampered by inadequate instrumentation, an uncooperative patient, or fear of causing further damage to the eye.

The time of examination should be documented. An external exam should be performed first to look for eyelid lacerations. Visual function should be estimated (best corrected visual acuity, color vision, confrontation visual field, presence of relative afferent pupillary defect), followed by a slit lamp biomicroscopic exam to evaluate for signs of conjunctival tears, corneal fluorescein stain, depth of anterior

TABLE 15–1. Definitions of the Proposed Ocular Traumatology Terms

Term	Definition	Remarks
Eyewall	Sclera and cornea	Technically, the wall of the eye has three tunics (coats) posterior to the limbus; therefore, for clinical purposes, it is best to restrict the term *eyewall* to the rigid stuctures of the sclera and cornea
Closed-globe injury	The eyewall does not have a full-thickness wound	Either there is no corneal or scleral wound at all (contusion) or it is only of partial thickness (lamellar laceration); rarely, a contusion and a lamellar laceration may coexist*
Open-globe injury	The eyewall has a full-thickness wound	The cornea and/or the sclera sustained a through-through injury; depending on the inciting object's characteristics and the injury's circumstances, ruptures and lacerations are distinguished; the choroid and the retina may be intact, prolapsed, or damaged
Rupture	Full-thickness wound of the eyewall, caused by a blunt object; the impact results in momentary increase of the IOP and an inside-out injury mechanism	The eye is a ball filled with incompressible liquid: a blunt object with sufficient momentum creates energy transfer over a large surface area, greatly increasing the IOP; the eyewall gives way at its weakest point which may or may not be at the impact site; the actual wound is produced by an inside-out force; consequently, tissue herniation is very frequent and can be substantial
Laceration	Full-thickness wound of the eyewall, usually caused by a sharp object; the wound occurs at the impact site by an outside-in mechanism	Further classification is based on whether an exit wound or an IOFB is also present; occasionally, an object may create a posterior (exit) wound while remaining, at least partially, intraocular (IOFB)*
Penetrating injury	Single laceration of the eyewall, usually caused by a sharp object	No exit wound has occurred; if more than one *entrance* wound is present, each must have been caused by a different agent
Intraocular foreign body injury	Retained foreign object(s) causing entrance laceration(s)	An IOFB is technically a penetrating injury but is grouped separately because of different clinical implications (treatment modality, timing, endophthalmitis rate, etc.)
Perforating injury	Two full-thickness lacerations (entrance + exit) of the eyewall, usually caused by a sharp object or missile	The 2 wounds must have been caused by the same agent

IOP = intraocular pressure; IOFB = intraocular foreign body.

*Rarely, the injury is so atypical that characterization is very difficult; the clinician should use his or her best judgment, based on the information provided here.

chamber, anterior chamber activity, hyphema, iridodialysis, iridodonesis, and phacodonesis.

A dilated fundus exam also should be performed. Retinal pathology should be carefully drawn. The initial exam may well be the only opportunity to visualize the retina. If there is a vitreous hemorrhage, the retinal view may be lost during subsequent exams.

Ultrasound biomicroscopy should be performed carefully without applying undue manipulation of and pressure on the globe. It is a safe and effective adjunctive tool for the clinical assessment and management of ocular trauma, especially when visualization is limited and multiple traumatic injuries are involved. Eyes with angle recession, iridodialysis, cyclodialysis, hyphema, intraocular foreign body, scleral laceration, and subluxed crystalline lens have been imaged without complication. Ultrasound biomicroscopy aids in the diagnosis when visualization is limited by media opacities or distorted anterior segment anatomy.

Plain radiographs of the orbit help to localize metallic foreign bodies. Caldwell view, Water's view, and lateral views should be requested to identify orbital foreign bodies and orbital bony fractures.

Computed tomography scans are extremely helpful in identifying retrobulbar hemorrhage, differentiating between intraocular and orbital foreign bodies, and identifying orbital bony fractures and extraocular muscle entrapment.

Intravenous antibiotics and tetanus toxoid injection should be administered when open globe injury is suspected. Treatment of corneal abrasions, hyphema, traumatic optic neuropathy, and other sequelae of closed globe injuries is according to the standard of care.

Surgical Intervention and Exploration under General Anesthesia

If an open globe injury is suspected, only minimal ocular examination and manipulations should be performed. After radiological investigations to rule out an intraocular foreign body, surgical intervention should be urgently performed under general anesthesia to repair or explore the globe. The threshold for exploration should be low whenever a penetrating or perforating injury or rupture of the globe is suspected. In addition, the globe should be explored under general anesthesia if an examination is not possible because the child is combative.

Examination under anesthesia often allows for careful indirect ophthalmoscopy if no intraocular hemorrhage is present. If the view of the fundus is unobscured, a subsequent surgical exploration may not be necessary. On the other hand, the optic disc and the macula can be carefully assessed for prognostication and medical/legal sequelae.

An adequate view of the fundus might not be possible due to corneal laceration, hyphema, cataract, or vitreous hemorrhage. If a laceration of the cornea is present this should be closed, approximating the limbus first. The conjunctiva should be incised to expose the course of the laceration. As the laceration is seen, it should be closed step by step. The laceration should be closed anteriorly prior to further posterior exploration to prevent extrusion of intraocular tissues.

Lacerations can be found anywhere on the globe. Ruptures are often at the limbus and at the muscle insertions. If the penetrating injury crosses the muscle insertion, the vitreous base may be involved. The suture material is then changed to absorbable suture material to allow for placement of a scleral buckle. The wound at, and posterior to, the muscle insertion is closed and placed on a radial or circumferential buckle.

If vitreous hemorrhage is present, a foreign body may be present. The foreign body is removed using an external or internal magnet according to the principles of foreign body vitreous surgery. If vitreous hemorrhage is present without a foreign body, it should be observed for infection and clearing. Ultrasound is used to monitor the eye. If vitreous hemorrhage does not clear, and amblyopia is a concern, vitreous surgery is undertaken to clear and remove the blood and reattach the retina as indicated.

■ Major Causes of Pediatric Ocular Trauma

Child Abuse (See also Chapter 7, Child Maltreatment.)

There are an estimated 2 million victims of child abuse in the United States per year. Physical abuse is the leading cause of serious head injury in infants. Although physical abuse has in the past been a diagnosis of exclusion, data regarding the nature and frequency of head trauma consistently support a medical presumption of child abuse when a child younger than 1 year of age has intracranial injury.[6] **Any physician who suspects child abuse is required by U.S. law to report the incident to a designated governmental agency for appropriate investigation.**

The presenting sign of child abuse involves the eye in 5% of cases. Forty percent of physically abused children will present with ocular and periocular findings. Blunt trauma inflicted with fingers, fist, belts, or straps is the usual mechanism of injury. Typical anterior segment findings include periorbital ecchymosis, subconjunctival hemorrhage, hyphema, and subluxated lenses. Posterior segment findings include retinal hemorrhages, retinal tears, and rhegmatogenous retinal detachments. The optic nerve can show papilledema or atrophy (see Chapter 21).

Certain diagnostic findings are also highly suggestive of child abuse such as the pattern of two or three parallel bruises on the face as in a slap, the paired semicircular bruises of the human bite, or bruises on the thorax or upper arm.[16] Furthermore, some general findings that lead to suspicion include several sites of soft tissue or bony injuries that are in different stages of healing, when multiple hospital admissions to different hospitals are reported in the history, when the guardian's report regarding the injury does not match the extent or location of findings, or when the reported events are inconsistent with the child's likely behavior at that age.

Conceptually, alcohol and drug abuse during pregnancy may be considered a form of "child abuse" as the effects last through childhood and beyond. The ophthalmic findings of fetal-alcohol syndrome have been well described and include craniofacial abnormalities, lid shortening, cataract, increased tortuosity of the retinal vessels, optic nerve hypoplasia, and learning disabilities.[7] Although clinical and experimental evidence of retinal vascular abnormalities with retinal hemorrhages has been reported from maternal use of cocaine,[8] not all studies have confirmed the clinical significance of this abuse.[9] More work in this area is needed to fully elucidate the relationship between drug abuse and congenital ocular disease.

Accidental Injury

There are reports of association of ocular injury with infant walker use.[10] Penetrating ocular injury has been reported after a minor fall with some designs of rigid infant pacifiers.[11] Corneal abrasion secondary to accidental trauma should be considered in an inconsolably crying otherwise asymptomatic infant.[12]

Accidental Blows and Falls
The most common cause of pediatric ocular trauma is accidental blows and falls.[2] Injuries

include orbital contusions and hematomas, facial hypesthesia, eyelid lacerations, subconjunctival hemorrhages, corneal edema and abrasion, hyphemas, traumatic iritis, iris sphincter ruptures, iris atrophy, angle recession, iridodialyses, traumatic cataract, vitreous hemorrhages, retinal hemorrhages, macular hole formation, optic atrophy, and bony orbital wall fractures.

Bungee cords,[13] merchandise display hooks,[14] and water balloon slingshots[15] have also been associated with accidental ocular trauma.

In accidental trauma the most frequent sites of injury include the forehead, anterior tibia, and other bony protuberances such as the chin. Injury to the face, trunk, buttocks, and genital area may suggest deliberate or malicious injury.

Sports and Recreational Activities
Sports trauma is a leading cause of permanent vision loss in the United States irrespective of age. The type of sport and the mechanism most frequently responsible for injuries are, respectively, outdoor and indoor soccer and ball trauma.[17] Basketball, baseball, and the racquet sports are other leading causes of ocular trauma.[18] Common injuries include corneal abrasion, traumatic iritis, lid or orbital contusions, and conjunctival hemorrhages. **The great majority of injuries could have been prevented if adequate protective eyewear had been worn.** Eye care practitioners should advocate the use of protective eyewear for patients who participate in sports activities (see position paper by American Academy of Ophthalmology and Pediatrics).

Bungee jumping is a recreational sport that has gained worldwide popularity. The injuries and deaths that have occurred have made safety an integral issue in the practice of the sport. Although early reports of significant injuries are infrequent, more recent investigations have indicated severe sequelae, including ocular hemorrhage.[19]

Pets
Tarantulas have become increasingly popular pets.[20] Typically, owners are unaware of the potential risk of ocular injury from the barbed urticating hairs found on the dorsal aspect of a tarantula's abdomen. Patients who manifest red

eye and pain after handling a tarantula should be examined to determine if offending barbed hairs are present in the cornea and conjunctiva.

Automobile Accidents

The effectiveness of air bags as a safety device in decreasing fatalities and reducing morbidity in frontal impact motor vehicle accidents has been well established. However, ocular injuries can occur due to air bag inflation, particularly when seatbelts are not worn properly.[21] Hyphema and corneal abrasions are the most common injuries related to air bag inflation. Several serious cases of vision-threatening injuries, including retinal detachment, retinal dialysis, scleral rupture, and dislocated lens, have also been reported. Eyeglass wear presents an additional risk factor for serious and permanent ocular damage.

Thermal and Chemical Burns

Eye injuries caused by fireworks are often severe and can cause permanently reduced visual acuity or blindness. Approximately 12,000 persons are treated each year in U.S. emergency departments because of fireworks-related injuries; of these, an estimated 20% are eye injuries.[22] In one study 95% of children treated for injuries associated with fireworks were reported to be injured during the 3-week period of June 22 to July 14.[23] Firecrackers are associated with the majority of injuries, followed by bottle rockets, Roman candles, sparklers, fountains, and jumping jacks. Permanent sequelae are more common for eye injuries caused by rockets than eye injuries caused by other types of fireworks. Children and their families should be encouraged to enjoy fireworks at public fireworks displays conducted by professionals.

The most common type of thermal burn to the ocular surface in children is due to contact with the tip of a cigarette. This type of injury typically occurs in children 2 to 4 years of age. It should be noted that these injuries occur frequently. At this age, toddlers frequently run into cigarettes inadvertently held by an adult at the child's eye level. When the cigarette burn is accidental, the corneal abrasion is usually in conjunction with a lid burn as well; the child's lids began to close from the blink reflex. When

the injury is purposeful and is child abuse, the lids have been forcibly held open and there is a discrete corneal burn only.

Chemical burns in children are often due to household products kept on low shelves. These include various organic solvents, soaps, drain cleaners, and household cleaning agents. They are some of the strongest acidic and alkaline substances known to cause ocular injury.

A high index of suspicion is in order when a child presents for evaluation of a red eye with a corneal or conjunctival abrasion. Very often in the pediatric age group, the traumatic event is not witnessed, and the parent may not be aware of the fact that the eye has been exposed to a caustic agent. A piece of pH paper briefly inserted into the inferior conjunctival fornix may provide an indication of the acidic or alkaline nature of the offending agent and serve to help guide further management. As in adults, acid burns may initially cause severe damage upon contact; however this is usually self-limited due to the rapid production of a coagulum that limits further damage. Alternatively, alkali burns may reveal a less impressive initial presentation. However, due to the fact that alkaline substances result in the saponification of fatty acids in the cornea, alkali burns may actually "melt" the cornea and gain access to the internal structures of the eye with disastrous consequences. **When it comes to management, copious irrigation is the rule, irrespective of the nature of the offending agent.** This often involves several liters of normal saline and should be continued for at least 30 minutes. The pH should then be checked again to ensure neutrality. Irrigation should be followed by the meticulous removal of any particulate matter with specific attention paid to the upper and lower conjunctival fornices. Particulate matter often contains small amounts of the culpable agent in addition to necrotic debris. Limbal vasculature blanching, also known as marblization, is a warning sign of ocular ischemia, and therefore its presence is a poor prognostic indicator.

Although almost all chemical injuries will reveal significant loss of corneal and conjunctival epithelium, if the limbal stem cell population has not been damaged, these injuries typically heal well with a topical antibiotic, cycloplegic, and lubricant. In the setting of an alkaline burn, a topical steroid may be added during the initial portion of therapy. For burns of the ocular surface recalcitrant to conventional therapeutic modalities, newer therapies have yielded promising results, such as limbal autograft transplantation. In this procedure, portions of the limbus and adjacent conjunctival tissue are harvested from the healthy fellow eye and transplanted to the injured eye, thus repopulating the injured eye with the limbal stem cells needed for wound repair. Results of this technique have been encouraging.

Overall, children should be re-evaluated frequently to confirm compliance with the prescribed regimen, an often difficult prospect for both the child and the parent. Furthermore, frequent re-examination is necessary to monitor for failure to heal. It should be noted that, in addition to observing the cornea and conjunctiva for healing, specific attention should be paid to the conjunctival fornices, often the site of insidiously developing symblepharon.

Self-Mutilation

Self-inflicted injury to the eyes is an extremely uncommon form of behavior. Intentional, severe, self-inflicted eye injuries may be seen in patients with organic disabilities, either autism, dementia, or severe mental retardation, where a lack of impulse control and preexisting eye irritation or surgical operation may contribute to the act.[24] Severe ocular injuries due to self-mutilation include retinal detachment resulting in visual loss and self-enucleation.[25] Active vigilance from caretakers and psychiatrists is essential as the majority of the patients are confined at the time of the act. Trichitellemania is an entity whereby children, usually adolescents, pull out their lashes continually until none remain. This is treated with counseling and antidepressive agents; however, it is quite difficult to cure.

■ Types of Ocular Trauma

Birth Trauma

Trauma secondary to childbirth is usually due to traumatic vaginal delivery or application of obstetric forceps. The frequency of sight threatening complications in instrumental deliveries is, however, low. The injuries are generally superficial, and include periorbital ecchymosis and lid edema, conjunctival chemosis, subconjunctival hemorrhage, corneal abrasion or corneal edema, and obliquely oriented Descemet's tears.

Scrolls of Descemet's membrane are usually present at each margin of the break. Obstetric forceps pressure strong enough to cause corneal injury usually leaves an occipital depression from the opposite forceps blade[26] (Fig. 15–1).

Posterior segment findings are usually limited to flame-shaped retinal hemorrhages. The anatomic location and appearance of retinal hemorrhages in infants provide important clues in the diagnosis of underlying disorders. Although neonatal retinal hemorrhages related to birth trauma are common, benign, and self-limited, retinal hemorrhages may also be caused by a variety of ocular (e.g., PHPV, ROP) or systemic diseases (e.g., hematological or cardiovascular disorders and infections).[27] Prompt diagnosis of retinal hemorrhages in infants is crucial because treatment may be required to prevent amblyopia and blindness. Birth weight is likewise a factor as fetal macrosomia has been associated with increased risk of birth trauma in vaginal deliveries.[28] However, low birth weight is also a factor predisposing to some types of injuries. Hypoxia, coagulation dysfunction, and neonatal vascular fragility are mentioned as mechanisms in these instances.[29]

Orbital Fracture

Blunt impact in the region of the eye may produce orbital bone fractures. Fractures of the orbital floor or "blowout fractures" are common in children when objects larger than the orbital rim strike the eye. In children, these commonly include projectile injuries such as those due to balls and rocks. Examination often reveals limitation of ocular motility frequently associated with restriction of ocular motility on attempted upgaze, although downgaze may be affected as well. These restrictions may be manifest only as diplopia on extreme upgaze or downgaze. Restrictions in other fields of muscular action may occur as well. Other signs of orbital floor fracture include orbital emphysema, subconjunctival emphysema, epistaxis, and hypesthesia

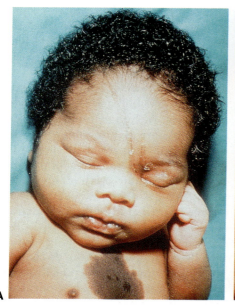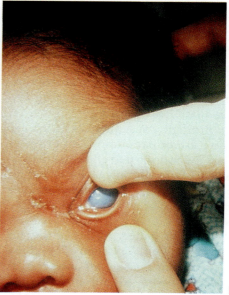

A   B

FIGURE 15–1. (A) Neonate with evidence of forceps-related birth trauma on forehead and eyelid of left eye. **(B)** Same child with corneal edema secondary to rupture of Descemet's membrane.

of the ipsilateral cheek and upper lip. Management considerations of orbital floor fractures are similar to those for adults and are beyond the scope of this text.

Fracture of the medial wall of the orbit may occur via the same forces that produce orbital floor fracture and the two are often seen simultaneously. Signs of medial wall fracture include orbital emphysema, epistaxis, and enophthalmos. Medial canthal tendon injury may be associated with a medial wall fracture and often results in an increased intercanthal tendon distance. Furthermore, the nasolacrimal drainage apparatus may be damaged, resulting in a variety of complications including epiphora.

Although rare in adults, isolated fracture of the orbital roof is the most common type of fracture of the orbit encountered in early childhood.[30] It is thought that differences in early anatomy may help to explain this discrepancy. In adults, the relatively thicker superior orbital rim and the fully developed frontal sinus might limit deflection of the orbital roof and prevent fracture. However, in young children, the superior orbital rim is considerably less well developed, and the lack of frontal

sinus pneumatization potentially allows for momentary deflections of the orbital roof large enough to rupture adjacent blood vessels and fracture bone.

The clinical presentation of orbital roof fracture in children is quite characteristic. The history often involves a blunt impact to the brow or forehead. A periorbital hematoma may develop after a few hours as blood from disrupted vessels of the superior orbit migrates to the more dependent upper lid and possibly to the lower lid as well. The time course and distribution of this periorbital hematoma help to identify orbital roof fracture and to distinguish it from the myriad of other causes of lid swelling and ecchymosis. Orbital roof fracture is not likely to result in concurrent globe injury. This differs from orbital floor fracture and is thought to be due to the fact that orbital roof fractures do not involve the same force transmission patterns through the soft tissues of the orbit as those that occur in orbital floor fracture. Although an inferiorly displaced globe with variable degrees of axial proptosis may be seen, persistent abnormality of ocular motility is not often encountered with roof fractures. Furthermore, in spite of the fact that the levator is anatomically located in the vicinity of the fracture site, ptosis is unusual. It is thought that entrapment of orbital soft tissues between fracture fragments is prevented by the normal pressure gradient between the anterior cranial fossa and the orbit. For similar reasons, displacement of bony fragments is more frequently downward than upward.

Acute neurologic consequences of orbital roof fracture are of paramount importance; however, it is noteworthy that enduring deficits do not usually occur. Chronic changes that do occur are a direct result of distortion of the normal anatomy. The most severe chronic complications occur when there is disruption of both bone and the dura mater. In this setting an encephalocele may form. **Pulsation of the globe occurring with transmission of intracranial pulse pressure is an identifying sign of encephalocele formation**. Again variable inferior displacement and axial proptosis of the globe may be seen. Encephalocele formation seems to occur more frequently when there is a comminuted fracture with inferiorly displaced bone fragments. Other potential complications of orbital roof fracture with dural penetration include an accumulation of cerebrospinal fluid in the orbit or lid and the drainage of cerebrospinal fluid from around the globe simulating the appearance of lacrimal epiphora.

In conclusion, orbital roof fracture should be suspected in any child presenting with blunt injury to the brow or forehead region with the subsequent development of a hematoma of the upper lid in the hours following injury. All such patients should be studied radiologically with high-resolution CT including coronal imaging. When an orbital roof fracture is found, neurosurgical input must be obtained immediately. Frequent follow-up is in order so that the signs and symptoms of chronic complications may be identified early.

Eyelid Abrasions and Lacerations

Eyelid trauma in children ranges from superficial abrasions to near or total avulsion of the lid. Eyelid abrasions are a frequent finding concurrent with a variety of traumatic insults. Superficial abrasions can be treated with local debridement, which can often be accomplished with vigorous irrigation alone. A topical antibiotic ointment may then be used to prevent infection. Tetanus history should be obtained from the parent or guardian and appropriate prophylaxis administered.

Surgical closure of full-thickness eyelid lacerations should be carried out under general anesthesia. Although older children may be able to tolerate closure under local anesthesia, this decision must be made on an individual basis. Complications of inadequate lid margin restoration include epithora and dry eye. Like adults, surgical reapproximation often utilizing a three-layered closure is recommended.

Canalicular lacerations are particularly important in children as the long-term sequelae include epiphora, irritation, discharge, and dry eye with its attendant potential for corneal damage. The most common cause of canalicular lacerations in the pediatric age group is dog bites and scratches, comprising approximately 33% of canalicular lacerations in children less than 15 years of age, twice that of any other cause.[31] The bite of a dog can exert a force of 200 to 450 psi, sufficient to penetrate sheet metal.[32] In turn, damage typically includes a combination of lacerations, puncture wounds, and crush injuries (Fig. 15–2). All dog bite injuries must be reported to the appropriate health authorities and rabies prophylaxis considered. Dog saliva contains 10^6 organisms/ml, and reported rates of infection from dog bites when the entire body is considered range from 0.5% to 50%.[33] Most infections are mixed, with organisms including *Staphylococcus aureus*, *Pasteurella multocida*, *Pseudomonas aeruginosa*, and anaerobic cocci. Forceful hydraulic debridement with a large syringe and cannula has been shown to most effectively decrease the microbial inoculum. Choice of antibiotics in this setting should include coverage for the less typically encountered bacterial contaminants that may be found in dog bite wounds such as *Bacteroides fragilis*. Antibiotic therapy should be tailored to the individual case but will often consist of a penicillinase-resistant penicillin, amoxicillin/clavulanic acid, cephalexin, cefuroxime, or erythromycin.

Other frequent causes of canalicular lacerations in children include falls and contact with immobile objects. When all age groups are considered, approximately 8% of canalicular lacer-

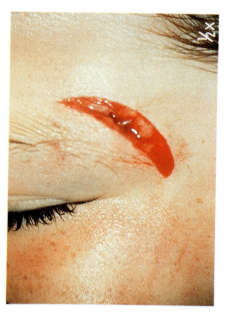

FIGURE 15–2. 17-year-old female with dog bit injury to left upper lid.

ations occur during sports activities, most frequently during basketball. Canalicular lacerations represent one of the few instances in pediatric ocular trauma where the incidence is higher in girls than in boys. The percentage of canalicular lacerations occurring in females less than 15 years of age is 44.6%, whereas the percentage occurring in males less than 15 years of age is 27.7%.[31] When a canalicular laceration is encountered, a vigorous search for concurrent ocular trauma will often be revealing. Macular or peripheral retinal edema will be found in 12% of patients, corneal abrasions in 11%, orbital fracture in 71%, and hyphema in 7%.

Most canalicular lacerations in children are preventable. Due to their small stature, children are especially vulnerable to animal bites even from well-intentioned house pets. Children participating in sports activities should be required to wear protective eyewear (see Chapter 5).

Corneal and Conjunctival Foreign Bodies

The treatment of corneal foreign bodies in children is quite similar to that in adults. Emphasis must be placed on a complete slit lamp examination to inspect for damage not immediately obvious upon presentation. Adequate topical anesthetic assists in the thorough inspection and removal process. Upon ensuring limitation of injury to the cornea, removal of a foreign body in a child should be attempted at the slit lamp. Beware of corneal perforation with a needle in a squirming child. Care must be taken to monitor for atypical infections that can be encountered with foreign bodies. If removal at the slit lamp is not feasible due to poor cooperation or significant penetration of the foreign body, consideration must be given to removal in the operating room under general anesthesia.

Conjunctival foreign bodies should be suspected in children presenting with pain, redness, and a foreign body sensation. A thorough inspection of the bulbar and palpebral conjunctiva should be conducted. A high index of suspicion must be maintained upon encountering a bulbar conjunctival foreign body. The child should be presumed to have a scleral perforation until proven otherwise. If the conjunctiva, as well as the retained foreign body, is not freely mobile over the underlying sclera or if the foreign body appears tethered to the subconjunctival structures, an accompanying scleral injury should be suspected and further manipulation deferred to the more controlled setting of the operating room. An X-ray can determine if there is an intraocular foreign body.

Intraorbital Foreign Bodies

Approximately 32,000 nonpowder firearm injuries are reported annually with more than 60% occurring in the pediatric population.[34]

Air guns associated with BB gun pellets (BB guns) can cause serious ocular injury. In one report, 66% of air gun injury victims had permanent visual loss, and 39% of these were blinded.[35]

Intraorbital foreign bodies are often due to projectiles such as BBs, and metallic fragments, however, they may also be due to organic materials, such as wood, that have become projectile. Initial evaluation of the child with a suspected intraorbital foreign body should involve primarily a multisystem trauma evaluation to rule out the possibility of nonocular trauma including intracranial injury. This should be followed by a complete ocular examination to search for associated occult ocular injuries.

Findings such as sectoral cataract, vitreous hemorrhage, conjunctival or scleral injection, perforation of the iris, or hyphema may indicate that an intraorbital foreign body has passed through some portion of the globe. Furthermore, even if the globe has not been violated by an intraocular foreign body, shock waves liberated by a high-velocity missile may produce a concussive injury to the posterior eye in a process termed retinitis sclopetaria (Fig. 15–3). In retinitis sclopeteria, the choroid and retina are ruptured in an area adjacent to the missile's path. Extension into the macula and concussive nerve injury occur frequently as well. Extensive intraocular hemorrhage is followed by retinal destruction and proliferation, and resulting visual acuity is usually poor.

Having excluded the possibility of associated ocular injury, one may next focus on the accurate localization of the foreign body based on clinical and radiologic information. Although a plain film "foreign body series" may serve to reveal the size and number of metallic foreign bodies, it often does not adequately reveal nonmetallic foreign bodies, and it does not determine the exact three-dimensional orientation of the foreign body with respect to the globe. Furthermore, plain films are not adequate for the full evaluation of adjacent bony structures, sinuses, and soft tissues. It is therefore recommended that patients with suspected intraorbital foreign bodies be evaluated with CT employing high-resolution axial as well as coronal images of the orbit with 1.5- to 3.0-mm cuts. Magnetic resonance imaging (MRI) should be deferred in the setting of intraorbital foreign bodies as the possibility of a metallic component to an intraorbital foreign body usually cannot be completely excluded.

Air gun BBs, bullets, and metallic fragments are the most common types of intraorbital foreign bodies, although other materials such as wood, glass, plastic, and stone may become intraorbital as well in the right setting. The kinetic energy ($\frac{1}{2} mv^2$) of a material correlates with its ability to penetrate. A recent study by Finkelstein et al[36] analyzed the kinetics of projectile foreign bodies and revealed the following information. Most BB pellets are approximately 4.5 mm in diameter, weigh 5.4 grains (1 grain = 0.0648 grams), and are fired at velocities of 250 to 750 ft/s. They will therefore usually only have sufficient energy to penetrate the orbit and not the more distal structures such as the intracranial vault. Metallic fragments tend to be lighter and travel with less velocity and hence tend to penetrate less than BBs. This is also the case with nonmetallic foreign bodies. On the other hand, bullets are generally larger structures, weigh 3.2 to 16.0 grains, and travel with exit velocities of 733 to 3250 ft/s. They therefore have sufficient kinetic energy to penetrate deeper into the orbit and therefore a greater chance of involving adjacent structures, including bone, sinus, and brain.

For most intraorbital foreign bodies, management is dictated by the nature of the material, the location of the foreign body, and associated functional deficits. Commercially manufactured BBs in the United States are steel, coated with a zinc or copper alloy. Although these are well tolerated by the intraorbital structures in general, previous oxidation or exposure to foreign material may render the BB infectious or inflammatory.

Finkelstein et al[36] detail an algorithm for management based on location and functional deficits. For anterior orbital foreign bodies that are palpable, surgical removal is recommended. The potential complications of not removing the foreign body, including fistula formation and the inability to undergo MRI in the future

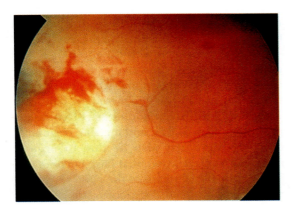

FIGURE 15–3. 14-year-old male with intraorbital foreign body that resulted in retinitis sclopetaria and a retinal tear during intraorbital passage. (Photo courtesy of Dr. Richard B. Rosen.)

for other potential systemic pathology, were thought to be more significant than the risks of removal. In the setting of nonpalpable anterior orbital foreign bodies, careful observation is recommended with removal at the first signs of infection, inflammation, motility disturbance, or ptosis. In contrast to anterior orbital foreign bodies, in most situations it is recommended that posteriorly located foreign bodies not be removed. This is due to the rigors of exploration deep within the confines of the orbit as well as the fact that the location of the foreign body may be elusive even with adequate radiologic imaging. However, in the setting of radiologic or clinical evidence of optic nerve involvement, surgical removal is recommended. Surgery may also be considered if infection or excessive inflammation is suspected. The appropriate use of antibiotics and steroids remains somewhat unclear, and decisions should be made on a case-by-case basis. The factors most closely associated with good final visual acuity after injury has resulted in an intraorbital foreign body are anterior location of the foreign body within the orbit and good visual acuity on presentation.

Air guns are a significant cause of ocular morbidity in childhood. **The percentage of severe eye injuries in children caused by air guns has been reported to be in the range of 4 to 15%.** In a recent study of risk factors for ocular injuries associated with air gun use, it was found that, of those children using air guns, injuries were 24 times more likely to occur when there was no adult supervision at the time of injury, 12 times more likely to occur at a friend's home, and 5 times more likely to occur when air guns were used indoors.[37] Furthermore, injury is 6 times more likely to occur when air guns are used for any purpose other than target practice. Overall, it is clear that unsupervised access to air guns and unstructured air gun use are the principal risk factors for air gun–associated ocular injury.

Corneal Abrasions

Corneal abrasions are one of the most common ocular injuries of childhood. When the corneal epithelium is scratched, abraded, or denuded of its epithelium, a significant amount of pain may result. In turn, the child with a corneal abrasion can be difficult to examine. Instillation of Alcaine with symptomatic relief can be diagnostic of the presence of an abrasion in a child. A thorough slit lamp examination should be attempted. The presence of stromal infiltration or anterior chamber inflammation should alert the examiner to the possibility of infection. If slit lamp examination is not possible due to the patient's age or poor cooperation, fluorescein instilled into the conjunctival fornices can be viewed with a Wood's light or via a cobalt filter, such as that available on many indirect ophthalmoscopes.

The treatment of corneal abrasions in children is similar to that in adults. Paramount issues are to relieve pain and to promote rapid healing. A pressure patch is the preferred treatment. However, children will often attempt removal of the patch. Many very small corneal abrasions will usually heal in young children within 1 to 2 days without a patch. Use of a topical cycloplegic and a broad-spectrum topical antibiotic ointment relieves pain resulting from ciliary spasm and provides for a lubricated antibacterial interface between the corneal surface and the palpebral conjunctiva thereby reducing irritation and decreasing the risk of infection. **Topical anesthetics should never be prescribed as they delay wound healing and may cause a secondary keratitis.** Patients should be re-examined in 24 hours to assess the progress of healing and to ensure that an infection has not developed.

Corneal/Scleral Lacerations

Penetrating eye injury remains one of the most important topics in pediatric ocular trauma. Up to 50% of all penetrating injuries of the eye occur in children, and 3.9 per 100,000 children suffer penetrating eye injuries each year (Fig. 15–4).[2] Management of this formidable problem in children requires attention to details less relevant in similar adult injuries. The initial examination is often hindered by poor historical accounts of the events surrounding the injury as well as the child's emotional reaction

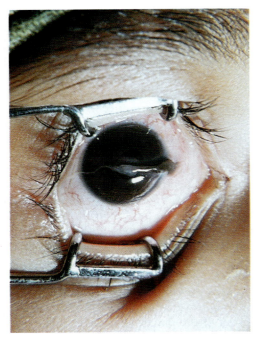

FIGURE 15–4. 11-year-old male with corneoscleral laceration with iris prolapse through the wound.

to a distressing situation. Therefore, suspicion of a penetrating injury justifies an evaluation under anesthesia in the operating room where the nature and extent of the injury may be adequately addressed (Fig. 15–5).

Corneal lacerations may be full or partial thickness. As in adults, the examination consists primarily of determining whether the cornea has been violated. The presence of a positive Siedl test is, of course, a reliable indicator of a full-thickness penetrating injury. More subtle changes are often the only available clues to the severe extent of injury. Small distortions in anterior chamber structures may serve to increase the clinician's index of suspicion. Often the pupillary margin or other portions of the iris are drawn anteriorly up to, or into, a penetrating wound (Fig. 15–6). Furthermore, due to the continuity between the iris and the rest of the uveal tract, a tented iris may be an indicator of a distant scleral rupture in the absence of corneal rupture. In this setting, the iris is typically tented in the meridian of the scleral laceration. These features are reliable indicators of penetration when they are present, but their absence does not rule out a penetrating injury, particularly in children. The lack of a positive Siedl test may simply be the result of a self-sealing wound, particularly if there has been a delay from the time of injury to the time of presentation. Often, children have been evaluated by nonophthalmic personnel for a red eye and the diagnosis of a penetrating wound has been overlooked, resulting in delayed ophthalmologic evaluation. In this circumstance, the corneal epithelium may actually close the defect.

The essential principles of primary surgical repair of a corneal or scleral wound in children are the same as those for adults. However, the pediatric cornea and sclera necessitate specific management considerations. The laxity of the corneoscleral tissue and the swift and exuberant

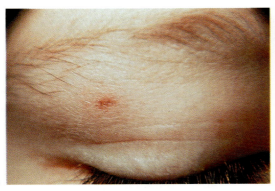
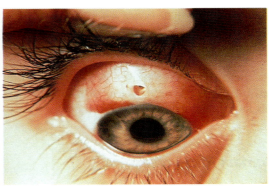

A   B

FIGURE 15–5. 15-year old male with arrow-head injury to upper lid with occult scleral penetration. (Photo courtesy of Dr. Richard B. Rosen.)

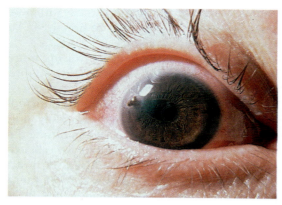

FIGURE 15–6. Perforating corneal injury with iris tenting in the 9 o'clock meridian.

inflammatory response of youth pose unique problems. Moreover, the profound wound healing response of childhood may increase the rate of late complications such as irregular astigmatism, ocular surface abnormalities, glaucoma, and persistent intraocular inflammation. Furthermore, difficulties encountered in follow-up examination and the almost inevitable rigors of strict amblyopia therapy pose special problems for the pediatric patient. Due to the complexity of this issue there is considerable debate as to what constitutes appropriate management for the child with a penetrating eye injury.

Primary surgical closure is the rule. Corneal wounds heal relatively rapidly in children, and sutures should be removed earlier than in adults. Amblyopic visual loss contributes significantly to the posttraumatic visual acuity, and therefore aggressive visual rehabilitation is indicated.

Overall, penetrating keratoplasty for the treatment of corneal scarring is felt to be effective in the pediatric population, with approximately 75% of children showing visual improvement.[38] Postoperative amblyopia therapy is a crucial component of the therapeutic regimen and serves to maintain any improvement in visual acuity.

Traumatic Iritis, Iridodialysis, and Cyclodialysis

Blunt ocular injury may result in damage to the anterior intraocular structures including the iris and ciliary body. Patients with iritis typically present with pain, significant photophobia, and conjunctival injection, often in a perilimbal distribution. Slit lamp examination reveals inflammatory and pigmented cells in the anterior chamber often associated with flare. A history of blunt trauma should prompt a full examination of the pupillary margin, which may reveal small sphincter tears, often manifest as anisocoria. Other potential causes of traumatic anisocoria including optic nerve injury must be ruled out. The treatment of traumatic iritis in children is similar to that in adults and consists mainly of topical cycloplegia combined with a topical steroid. In children, instillation of a longer acting cycloplegic should be considered to maximize the dosing interval if compliance is questionable. Rapid cycloplegic and steroid taper is initiated within several days.

Disinsertion of the iris root at its insertion is termed iridodialysis. Iridodialysis is often manifest as polycoria in association with photophobia, glare, and possibly diplopia. Frequently, other associated ocular pathology coexists including hyphema, lens dislocation, and cataract. Detailed notes of any iris abnormality should be made and communicated to the parent to prevent future confusion by other physicians. Slit lamp photographs are helpful for this purpose.

A cyclodialysis cleft is a disruption of the circumferential attachment of the fibers of the meridional ciliary muscle to the scleral spur that results in a direct communication between the anterior chamber and the suprachoroidal space. **Cyclodialysis clefts occur in 1 to 11% of all blunt ocular trauma and are often underdiagnosed.** The most common presenting symptom is a decrease in visual acuity, often to the 20/200 level or worse. Additionally, patients may complain of chronic or intermittent redness, pain, and tearing. Examination may reveal a shallowing of the anterior chamber, mild inflammation, and a chronically low intraocular pressure (IOP) with its attendant complications including corneal edema, Descemet's folds, and choroidal and retinal folds. It should be noted that a hyperopic shift may also be present due to anterior rotation of the lens–iris diaphragm. The etiology of the decrease in IOP associated with a cyclodialysis cleft is poorly understood but is believed to be secondary either to decreased aqueous humor production or to increased uveoscleral outflow. IOP usually stabilizes within several weeks after formation of the cyclodialysis cleft; however, delayed development of hypotony has been reported up to 5 years after injury.

Hyphema

Hyphema represents a significant source of ocular morbidity in children. **One third to one half of all hospital admissions following eye trauma in children are due to hyphema. Of all hyphemas, 70% occur in people less than 20 years of age.**[39] As the child is often a poor informant, the exact etiology of the injury is frequently difficult to determine. However, an attempt should be made to document the time of injury as this information will help guide management and predict the time course for potential complications. Furthermore, the history should include the recent use of all medications, including aspirin or related compounds. The anticoagulant properties of these drugs may have profound effects on the course of healing.

When a clear history of events surrounding the injury is lacking, the possibility of child abuse or a nontraumatic etiology must be considered. Several disease processes may masquerade as traumatic hyphema including retinoblastoma, juvenile xanthogranuloma, leukemia, and other blood dyscrasias such as Hermansky-Pudlak. Management should therefore always include a complete blood count and basic coagulation studies. Moreover, if extensive hyphema precludes a thorough evaluation of the ocular structures, radiologic studies such as ultrasound or CT should be considered to rule out the possibility of an intraocular neoplasm. Obtain a sickle cell prep on all non-Caucasian children presenting with hyphema. Traumatic hyphemas in children in the setting of sickle cell disease are managed differently from those occurring in children without sickle cell disease.

Most hyphemas (71 to 94%) result from disruption of the anterior ciliary face including the major arterial circle and its branches, recurrent choroidal arteries, or ciliary body veins.[40] The remainder result from ruptured iris vessels, cyclodialysis, or iridodialysis. Penetrating trauma may cause a hyphema directly with penetrating rupture of vessels or indirectly via an acute decrease in intraocular pressure.

In general, those hyphemas involving more than half of the anterior chamber are more likely to be associated with delayed clearing of blood and its attendant complications, including glaucoma, blood staining, rebleeding, and poor visual outcome. Hospitalization during the first 5 days, the most common time for rebleeding, remains justifiable in children. Furthermore, hospitalization allows for frequent monitoring of the child's progress and reduces the possibility of strenuous physical activity.

Intraocular pressure often guides the course of therapeutic decision making, and therefore frequent measurement of IOP is required. However, accurate measurement of IOP in children can be significantly more complicated than in adults. Applanation tonometry at the slit lamp is often impossible. The use of a tonopen with a topical anesthetic often provides an excellent alternative. Care must be taken to avoid errors in measurement of IOP; in young children even gentle pressure on the globe will produce large IOP inaccuracies. In addition, crying can produce IOP inaccuracies due to valsalva maneuvers. Surprisingly, IOP can often be measured in the very young child with a tonopen while the child is asleep.

Medical management of hyphema varies from one institution to another but should follow certain basic tenents. The reported rate of rebleeding has varied from approximately 7 to 20%, depending on the population studied. In one study of hyphema in children 91% of children with non-rebleeding hyphemas achieved a final visual acuity of 20/30 or better compared with 77% of those with a secondary hemorrhage.[41] Therefore, one of the goals of therapy is to prevent rebleeding. The use of a topical cycloplegic agent as well as a topical cortico-steroid is recommended. These agents serve to improve comfort and reduce inflammation and possibly to reduce the likelihood of rebleeding. The use of oral corticosteroids (prednisone) and antifibrinolytic agents (aminocaproic acid and transexamic acid) in the management of traumatic hyphema is common and varies from one institution to another.

Use of topical IOP-lowering medications is recommended when IOP is elevated. The time course for surgical evacuation of a clot should follow guidelines comparable to those in adults. These include an IOP of 50mm Hg for 5 days, 35mm Hg for 7 days, and 25mm Hg for 6 days when blood is in direct apposition with the endothelium (blood staining). Vigilant monitoring of the cornea must be maintained to prevent the development of corneal blood staining and its main attendant complication in the young, amblyopia. Therefore, total or "eight-ball" hyphemas should be evacuated on the fourth or fifth day postinjury. Children with hemoglobinopathies may require earlier intervention.

In the weeks following resolution of the hyphema, children should have a gonioscopic exam to examine the anterior chamber angle for the presence of angle recession, iridodialysis, and cyclodialysis. If there is angle pathology, the parent should be informed of the future risk for elevated IOP over the child's lifetime and the need for follow-up examinations.

Lens Dislocation

The rapid equatorial expansion that occurs with traumatic anteroposterior compression may produce disruption of the zonules and result in partial or total dislocation of the lens. The extent of lens dislocation is dictated by the completeness of zonular dehiscence. When only a partial rupture exists, the lens will be drawn to the side opposite the zonular rupture, whereas total zonular dehiscence may allow for complete dislocation of the lens. A minimally dislocated lens may manifest only as sudden induced myopia or astigmatism. Progressing along a spectrum of severity, if the edge of the lens encroaches on the visual axis, monocular diplopia is often the result.

On examination, the traumatized eye with a dislocated lens may reveal a deepened anterior chamber relative to the uninvolved eye, iridodonesis, or phacodonesis. Zonular disruption can be visualized gonioscopically in the older child. If the lens is completely dislocated and moves anteriorly, the pupillary aperture may be obscured, predisposing the eye to relative pupillary block glaucoma. Further anterior movement of the lens into the anterior chamber may produce contact between the lens and the corneal endothelium, disrupting the ability of the endothelium to maintain a state of corneal deturgescence. If the lens is completely dislocated posteriorly, a dilated fundus examination may reveal the lens in the vitreous.

Although emergent surgical removal of the lens may only be necessary in the adult population with a relative pupillary block or dislocation into the anterior chamber, the necessity of maintaining visual acuity and preventing amblyopia must be of regard in the pediatric population. Therefore, uncorrectable induced myopia, astigmatism, or monocular diplopia may be sufficient rationale in children for lens extraction followed by visual rehabilitation.

Choroidal and Retinal Injury

Injuries to the choroid and retina are often found in association with various types of ocular trauma. When there is a strong suspicion of severe posterior segment pathology such as a scleral perforation or retinal tear, an examination under anesthesia must be considered.

Vitreous hemorrhage following blunt ocular trauma can prevent adequate examination of the posterior structures of the eye and mandates ultrasound examination. It should be seen as a warning sign of occult pathology such as a retinal tear, choroidal rupture, intraocular or intraorbital foreign body, or damage to the optic nerve. If a posterior view is possible and a scleral or corneal perforation has been completely ruled out, examination of the peripheral retina with scleral depression may reveal covert pathology, such as a retinal tear, as the source of the vitreous hemorrhage. However, it is often wise to defer scleral depression as an occult or posteriorly located perforation may be difficult to detect during the primary examination, and scleral depression in the context of a scleral discontinuity could have disastrous consequences.

The choroid is particularly vulnerable to the anteroposterior compression of the globe, which is often associated with an anterior blunt injury. The sudden horizontal, equatorial expansion of the globe associated with anteroposterior compression tends to tear the relatively inelastic choroid, resulting in choroidal rupture. Although hemorrhage may initially obscure the view, the typical appearance is of

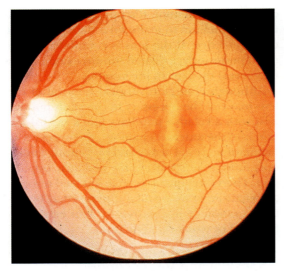

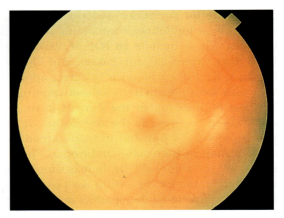

FIGURE 15–8. 9-year-old male with diffuse commotio retinae due to blunt injury.

FIGURE 15–7. 12-year-old male with blunt injury to globe resulting in choroidal rupture. (Photo courtesy of Dr. Richard B. Rosen.)

crescent-shaped, yellow to white curvilinear streaks usually concentric with the optic disc. The macula is often involved (Fig. 15–7). Occasionally, radially oriented or multiple ruptures may occur. Visual acuity loss is rapid and profound, often to 20/200 or less depending on the exact location of the rupture. Although no adequate treatment for choroidal rupture is available, children must be monitored lifelong for the development of subretinal neovascularization, a potential complication of choroidal rupture that can produce further visual loss.

Commotio retinae, also known as Berlin's edema, is typically a contrecoup injury manifested posteriorly after a blunt anterior impact. Usually developing minutes to hours after the injury, commotio retinae is a creamy opacification of the outer retinal layers. It tends to have a geographic pattern with poorly defined edges (Fig. 15–8). The fundoscopic appearance depends on the distribution of forces imparted by trauma, although there is a tendency toward macular involvement. When the macula is involved, visual acuity can be drastically reduced, whereas if it is not involved visual acuity may remain normal. During the first few weeks after injury, the opacification usually clears, and visual acuity returns to the preinjury level. Occasionally, however, there is a perma-

nent decrease in visual acuity.

The same anteroposterior compression and attendant horizontal expansion of the globe that results in choroidal rupture may result in retinal damage as well. During this horizontal expansion, the vitreous base exerts tractional forces upon the peripheral retina, potentially resulting in a number of injuries, depending on the exact localization of the forces involved. Possibilities include retinal dialysis, peripheral retinal tears and holes, and avulsion of the vitreous base. Examination of the traumatized eye, and in particular the traumatized myopic eye, may reveal a giant retinal tear. Giant retinal tears occur at the border of the vitreous base and extend circumferentially for more than 90 degrees, or 1 quadrant, of the globe. They often present with overt symptomatology, including photopsias, floaters, and reduced vision. Approximately 50% of all traumatic retinal detachments will become manifest during the first month following injury. As with vitreous hemorrhage, the presence of symptoms and signs referable to the retina warrants a complete retinal exam; however, scleral depression should be deferred until the possibility of a penetrating scleral injury has been ruled out.

Similar blunt traumatic forces can result in a traumatic macular hole. The strong adherence of the vitreous to the macula combined with the acceleration and sudden deceleration typical of blunt trauma can result in a partial- or full-thickness hole. Traumatic macular holes may also be found as sequelae of commotio retinae, subretinal hemorrhage, or choroidal rupture. Visual acuity is variable. However, with a full-thickness hole, vision is most often reduced below the 20/80 level. Treatment initially consists of conservative observation unless evidence of progressive detachment develops. If this occurs, vitrectomy, scleral buckling, and laser photocoagulation may be considered in an attempt to salvage remaining vision.

Pediatric patients with a variety of traumatic ocular injuries may have concurrent damage to the optic nerve, including laceration or avulsion. Historical information is important when one is suspicious of optic nerve injury. Of foremost importance is the rapidity with which vision was lost, often occurring immediately with optic nerve trauma. This history can be difficult to obtain in a child. Therefore, signs such as an afferent pupillary defect and hemorrhage emanating from the optic nerve head should be sought after and should increase the clinical suspicion of optic nerve trauma.

Penetrating orbital trauma may result in the direct laceration or avulsion of the optic nerve. In addition, blunt trauma may produce bone fragments within the optic canal, which can lacerate the nerve. Moreover, blunt forces can disrupt the vascular supply to the nerve resulting in ischemic compromise.

Traumatic optic neuropathy should be suspected when the patient has loss of vision that cannot be explained by injury to the globe, intraorbital optic nerve, or posterior visual pathways. Typically an afferent pupillary defect will be present. A paucity of information exists for the proper management of traumatic optic neuropathy in adults, and the issue is nebulous in children. Treatment options include conservative observation, very high dose steroids, and surgical decompression of the optic canal.

Traumatic Cataracts

Lenticular damage is the most common cause of decreased visual acuity following ocular trauma in children. Any blunt or penetrating injury to the anterior surface of the eye may be complicated by damage to the lens. Alterations in lens structure can range from a small rent in the anterior lens capsule, leading to a small localized cataract, to total disruption of the lens with flocculent cortical material filling the anterior chamber. Intralenticular foreign bodies may occur (Fig. 15–9).

Blunt trauma to the eye produces coup and contrecoup forces that may result in a contusion cataract (Fig. 15–10). Contusion cataracts frequently progress and completely obscure the visual axis; however, contusion cataracts are not universally progressive and may be localized to a small sector of lens. Therefore, when a cataract is nonprogressive, the examiner needs to determine whether the cataract is visually significant enough to produce a significant amblyopia. Traumatic cataracts resulting from

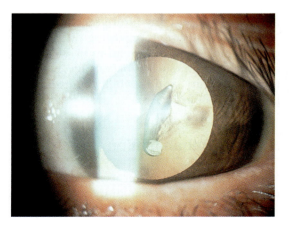

FIGURE 15–9. 16-year-old male with intralenticular foreign body due to nail injury. (Photo courtesy of Dr. Richard Rosen.)

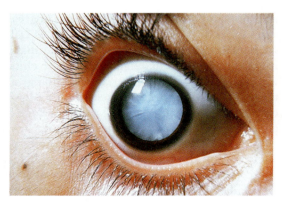

FIGURE 15–10. 16-year-old female with traumatic cataract due to blunt injury.

penetrating eye injury are typically more rapidly progressive than contusion cataracts. Furthermore, they generally reduce visual acuity to a greater extent and may result in lens-induced glaucoma or inflammation.

The appropriate management of traumatic cataracts in the pediatric population remains the subject of debate.

Following corneal penetration, fibrin clots often form rapidly in the anterior chamber. These clots are reminiscent of cataractous lens cortex, and the import of distinguishing the two cannot be overemphasized.

Whether a cataractous lens is removed at the time of primary wound closure or as a secondary procedure is a source of disagreement and is ultimately determined by the operating surgeon. Visual rehabilitation for the now aphakic child becomes the preeminent issue. Options available for the correction of aphakic refractive error include epikeratophakia, aphakic spectacle correction, contact lens fitting, and implantation of an intraocular lens (see Chapter 20).

Epikeratophakia may be difficult to apply in the setting of a corneal scar or wound, and time lost waiting for the epilenticule to achieve clarity is important from a deprivational standpoint.

Although aphakic spectacles may be a suitable choice for the binocularly aphakic child, in the setting of a monocular traumatic cataract they probably represent a poor choice. The significant anisokonia produced is beyond the limits of tolerability and carries its own complications, including loss of stereopsis.

Contact lens fitting remains a viable alternative in many instances. Silicone lenses with high oxygen permeability may allow for less frequent insertion and removal, which are times of great stress for both child and parent. However, social, economic, and environmental factors may make it quite difficult to manage the aphakic child with a contact lens. Moreover, the psychological trauma of injury superimposed upon a physically damaged ocular surface may produce a child who is intolerant of contact lens use.

The fourth, and probably most controversial, alternative in the rehabilitation of the aphakic child is the implantation of an intraocular lens (IOL). The IOL provides a constant, high-quality optical image of similar magnification to the natural lens. The avoidance of anisokonia in the

child is crucial and serves to maintain binocularity. Furthermore, the IOL may provide an excellent alternative to contact lens therapy in the pediatric patient with corneal scarring and ocular sensitivity. However, several theoretical and practical concerns regarding the use of IOLs in children remain. One of the foremost issues is that of ocular growth. There is a paucity of information on how aphakia or pseudophakia affect subsequent growth of the eye. Another challenging issue is that of selection of lens power.

Management of the posterior capsule during and after intraocular lens insertion remains challenging in the child. The intact posterior capsule in the pseudophakic child less than 12 years of age will opacify nearly 100% of the time due to the vigorous growth of residual lens epithelial cells.[42] This can occur quite rapidly over weeks to months in children. In fact, the posterior capsule is often one of the most significant impediments to visual rehabilitation after IOL insertion. The incidence of secondary surgery for pediatric IOLs has been high in the past, with over 60% of patients requiring discission of the posterior capsule.

Recently, several potential advances have come to light to address the issue of the posterior capsule. Nd:YAG laser posterior capsulotomy has been used with some success. If a surgical posterior capsulotomy is going to be performed at the time of cataract surgery, a peripheral rim of anterior and posterior capsule should be left behind. The anterior and posterior leaflets fuse together and will serve to guide and support any future secondary IOL. Management decisions regarding the posterior capsule must be made on an individual basis, addressing factors such as patient age, nature of traumatic injury, and feasibility and timing of laser capsulotomy.

■ Visual Rehabilitation

Visual rehabilitation is a crucial component in the management of ocular injury and is vital to a successful outcome. It has clearly been shown in studies of all types of ocular trauma that even the best medical and surgical management will fail if appropriate amblyopia therapy is not employed.

REFERENCES

1. Morris RE, Witherspoon CD, Helms HA Jr, Feist RM, Byrne JB. Eye Injury Registry of Alabama (preliminary report): demographics and prognosis of severe eye injury. *South Med J.* 1987;80(7):810–816.

2. Strahlman E, Elman M, Daub E, Baker S. Causes of pediatric eye injuries: a population-based study. *Arch Ophthalmol.* 1990;108(4):603–606.

3. DeRespinis PA, Caputo AR, Fiore PM, Wagner RS. A survey of severe eye injuries in children. *Am J Dis Child.* 1989;143(6):711–716.

4. Grin TR, Nelson LB, Jeffers JB. Eye injuries in childhood. *Pediatrics.* 1987;80(1):13–17.

5. Kuhn F, Morris R, Witherspoon CD, Heimann K, Jeffers JB, Treister G. A standardized classification of ocular trauma. *Ophthalmology.* 1996;103(2):240–243.

6. Committee on Child Abuse and Neglect, 1993–1994. Shaken baby syndrome: inflicted cerebral trauma. *Del Med J.* 1997;69(7):365–370.

7. Stromland M, Sundelin K. Paediatric and ophthalmologic observations in offspring of alcohol abusing mothers. *Acta Paediatr.* 1996;85:1463–1468.

8. Silva-Araujo A, Tavares MA, Patacao MH, et al. Retinal hemorrhages associated with in utero exposure to cocaine: experimental and clinical findings. *Retina.* 1996;16:411–418.

9. Stafford JR Jr, Rosen TS, Zaider M, Merriam JC. Prenatal cocaine exposure and the development of the human eye. *Ophthalmology.* 1994;101:301–308.

10. Koser M, DeRespinis PA. The association of vision-threatening ocular injury with infant walker use. *Arch Pediatr Adolesc Med.* 1995;149(11):1275–1276.

11. Stubbs AJ, Aburn NS. Penetrating eye injury from a rigid infant pacifier. *Aust NZ J Ophthalmol.* 1996; 24(1): 71–73.

12. Harkness MJ. Corneal abrasion in infancy as a cause of inconsolable crying. *Pediatr Emerg Care.* 1989;5(4): 242–244.

13. Cooney MJ, Pieramici DJ. Eye injuries caused by bungee cords. *Ophthalmology.* 1997;104(10):1644–1647.

14. Fannin LA, Fitch CP, Raymond WR, Flanagan JC, Mazzoli RA. Eye injuries from merchandise display hooks. *Am J Ophthalmol.* 1995;120(3):397–399.

15. Bullock JD, Ballal DR, Johnson DA, Bullock RJ. Ocular and orbital trauma from water balloon slingshots: a clinical, epidemiologic, and experimental study. *Ophthalmology.* 1997;104(5):878–887.

16. Cavanaugh N. Non-accidental injuries. In: Taylor D, ed. *Pediatric Ophthalmology.* Boston: Blackwell; 1990:545–550.

17. Filipe JA, Barros H, Castro-Correia J. Sports-related ocular injuries: a three-year follow-up study. *Ophthalmology.* 1997;104(2):313–318.

18. Orlando RG, Doty JH. Ocular sports trauma: a private practice study. *J Am Optom Assoc.* 1996;67(2):77–80.

19. Vanderford L, Meyers M. Injuries and bungee jumping. *Sports Med.* 1995;20(6):369–374.

20. Waggoner TL, Nishimoto JH, Eng J. Eye injury from tarantula. *J Am Optom Assoc.* 1997;68(3):188–190.

21. Vichnin MC, Jaeger EA, Gault JA, Jeffers JB. Ocular injuries related to air bag inflation. *Ophthalmic Surg Lasers.* 1995;26(6):542–548.

22. United States, 1990–1994. Serious eye injuries associated with fireworks. *MMWR.* 1995;44(24):449–452.

23. Smith GA, Knapp JF, Barnett TM, Shields BJ. The rockets' red glare, the bombs bursting in air: fireworks-related injuries to children. *Pediatrics.* 1996;98(1):1–9.

24. Field HL, Waldfogel S. Severe ocular self-injury. *Gen Hosp Psychiatry.* 1995;17(3):224–227.

25. Ashkenazi I, Shahar E, Brand N, et al. Self-inflicted ocular mutilation in the pediatric age group. *Acta Paediatr.* 1992;81(8):649–651.

26. McDonald MB, Burgess SK. Contralateral occipital depression related to obstetric forceps injury to the eye. *Am J Ophthalmol.* 1992;114(3):318–321.

27. Kaur B, Taylor D. Fundus hemorrhages in infancy. *Surv Ophthalmol.* 1992;37(1):1–17.

28. Mikulandra F, Perisa M, Stojnic E. When is fetal macrosomia (> or = 4500 g) an indication for Caesarean section? *Zentralbl Gynakol.* 1996;118:441–447.

29. Wang F. Perinatal ophthalmology. In: Tasman W, Jaeger EA, eds. *Duane's Clinical Ophthalmology.* Philadelphia, PA: JB Lippincott; 1993;8:8–10.

30. Greenwald M, Boston D, Pensler J, et al. Orbital roof fractures in childhood. *Ophthalmology.* 1989;96:491–497.

31. Kennedy RH, May J, Dalley J, et al. Canalicular laceration: an 11-year epidemiologic and clinical study. *Ophthalmic Plast Reconstr Surg.* 1985;1:185–190.

32. Chambers GH, Payne JF. Treatment of dogbite wounds. *Minn Med* 1969;52:427–430.

33. Edlich RF, Spengler MD, Rodeheaver GT, et al. Emergency department management of mammalian bites. *Emerg Med Clin North Am.* 1986;4:595–604.

34. Scribano PV, Nance M, Reilly P, Sing RF, Selbst SM. Pediatric nonpowder firearm injuries: outcomes in an urban pediatric setting. *Pediatrics.* 1997;100(4):E5.

35. Bratton SL, Dowd MD, Brogan TV, Hegenbarth MA. Serious and fatal air gun injuries: more than meets the eye. *Pediatrics.* 1997;100(4):609–612.

36. Finkelstein M, Legmann A, Rubin P. Projectile metallic foreign bodies in the orbit. *Ophthalmology.* 1997; 104: 96–103.

37. Enger C, Schein O, Tielsch J. Risk factors for ocular injuries caused by air guns. *Arch Ophthalmol.* 1996; 114:469–474.

38. Dana M, Schaumberg D, Moyes A, et al. Outcome of penetrating keratoplasty after ocular trauma in children. *Arch Ophthalmol.* 1995;113:1503–1507.

39. Kennedy RH, Bribaker RF. Traumatic hyphema in a defined population. *Am J Ophthalmol.* 1988; 106: 123–130.

40. Wilson FM. Traumatic hyphema: pathogenesis and management. *Ophthalmology.* 1980;87:910–919.

41. Agapitos PJ, Noel LP, Clarke WN. Traumatic hyphema in children. *Ophthalmology.* 1987;94:1238–1241.

42. Apple DJ, Kincaid MC, Mamalis N, et al. *Intraocular Lenses: Evolution, Designs, Complications, and Pathology.* Baltimore: Williams & Wilkins; 1989.

Pediatric Ophthalmology
Edited by P. F. Gallin
Thieme Medical Publishers, Inc.
New York © 2000

16

The Red Eye

QUAN DONG NGUYEN AND C. STEPHEN FOSTER

The eye, of an adult or of a child, may become red for a variety of reasons; some are trivial and some are vision threatening. There are six major etiologic categories that can cause red eye in infants and children: conjunctivitis, keratitis, uveitis, scleritis, angle closure glaucoma, and malignancy. Detailed discussion about uveitis, scleritis, angle closure glaucoma, and malignancy are given elsewhere in this book. We will thus concentrate on conjunctivitis and keratitis as causes of red eye in this chapter.

■ Conjunctivitis

Neonatal Conjunctivitis

Neonatal conjunctivitis (ophthalmia neonatorum) occurs in early infancy prior to 1 month of age.[1] The most common cause of neonatal conjunctivitis is chemical conjunctivitis, secondary to silver nitrate gonorrhea prophylaxis, which occurs in approximately 90% of infants who receive this treatment.[2]

The conjunctival flora of newborns reflects the exposure during the birth process; 80% of infants delivered by cesarean section within 3 hours of membrane rupture have sterile conjunctiva.[3] Vaginally delivered infants have conjunctival flora similar to that of female genital tract.[3,4] This is obviously important in regard to

sexually transmitted diseases, and hence, in all developed countries, prophylactic treatment is initiated immediately upon delivery.

Infectious neonatal conjunctivitis occurs in about 1 to 12% of infants,[5,6] and can be caused by a number of infectious agents: *Chlamydia trachomatis*, *Streptococcus* species, *Staphylococcus* species, *Escherichia coli*, *Haemophilus* species, *Neisseria gonorrhea*, and herpes simplex virus. The availability and wide application of topical antibiotics or chemical prophylaxis at birth have helped to decrease the incidence of the once vision-threatening epidemic of *N. gonorrhea* ocular infection.

Table 16–1 summarizes the etiology relative to the time of onset and the clinical presentation of various causes of neonatal conjunctivitis. However, because gonococcal infections are rapidly destructive, conjunctivitis in the newborn should be considered an ophthalmic emergency. The physician should not rely exclusively on the timing of the infection or the clinical appearance to make a specific diagnosis. Empiric treatment with topical erythromycin should be begun while awaiting culture results.

Laboratory

Any infant who presents with conjunctivitis must have a very careful evaluation, including conjunctival scraping for Gram- and Giemsa-

TABLE 16–1. Neonatal Conjunctivitis

Etiology	Onset	Presentation	Findings on conjunctival scraping
Silver nitrate	Within 24 h	Lid edema, watery discharge	None to few polymorphonuclear leukocyte
Neisseria gonorrhea	2–4 d	Severe, purulent discharge, with lid edema	Gram-negative intracellular diplococci
Chlamydia trachomatis	4–10 d	Lid edema and pseudomembrane formation	Giemsa stain for basophilic cytoplasmic inclusion bodies; positive direct immunofluorescent assay
Other bacteria	4–7 d	Severe inflammation and mucopurulent discharge	Gram stain positive for specific organism
Herpes simplex	7–14 d	Unilateral injection and discharge, with concurrent keratitis	Gram stain for multinucleated giant cells

stained smear and for culture on chocolate agar or Thayer-Martin for *N. gonorrhea* and culture on blood agar for other bacteria. Chlamydial infection can be assessed by a Giemsa stain of the conjunctival scraping for intracytoplasmic inclusion bodies, which can often be done immediately by the physician in the emergency room, or direct immunofluorescence antibody assay. If a corneal epithelial defect is present, culture for herpes simplex virus is indicated.

The physicians should initiate treatment of neonatal conjunctivitis immediately prior to laboratory results, as certain organisms can penetrate an intact corneal epithelium. Empirical antibiotic coverage may include topical erythromycin ointment and intravenous or intramuscular third-generation cephalosporin (Ceftriaxone, 30 to 50 mm/kg/d).[2] Therapy can then be altered based on laboratory results.

Types of Conjunctivitis

Chemical Conjunctivitis
Chemical conjunctivitis occurs within the first 24 hours of the infant's delivery and is usually bilateral. There is often watery discharge and bulbar conjunctival injection. This conjunctivitis is caused by silver nitrate 1% drop prophylaxis. Fortunately, chemical conjunctivitis generally resolves spontaneously within 2 to 3 days.[2]

Chlamydial Conjunctivitis
Chlamydial conjunctivitis is the second most common type of neonatal conjunctivitis in devel-

oped countries, following chemical conjunctivitis.[7] It has an onset later than that of gonococcal conjunctivitis, usually 4 to 7 days after birth. Chlamydial conjunctivitis is more indolent and less severe than gonococcal conjunctivitis. There may be significant lid swelling, conjunctival hemorrhage (Fig. 16–1), and pseudomembrane formation. The physician can make the diagnosis by observing intracytoplasmic inclusion bodies by Giemsa stain. Giemsa stain of chlamydial conjunctivitis will demonstrate basophilic cytoplasmic inclusion bodies in epithelial cells in 50 to 90% of culture-proven cases.[8] However, currently, the diagnostic method of choice is the direct immunofluorescent monoclonal antibody stain (e.g. MicroTrak), which has 87 to 100%

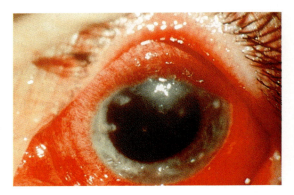

FIGURE 16–1. Conjunctivitis caused by *Chlamydia trachomatis* with marked conjunctival injection and hemorrhage.

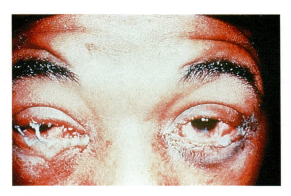

FIGURE 16–2. Conjunctivitis caused by *Neisseria gonorrhea* with severe purulent, serosanguineous discharge, and lid edema and chemosis.

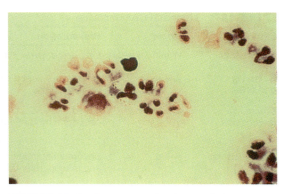

FIGURE 16–3. Gram negative intracellular diplococci from conjunctival scrapings, diagnostic of *Neisseria gonorrhea*.

sensitivity,[9] enzyme immunoassay (e.g., Chlamydiazyme), or DNA probe. McCoy cell cultures are the standard for culturing *Chlamydia*.[8]

Chlamydial neonatal conjunctivitis may resolve spontaneously over several weeks. However, active treatment is indicated to prevent late onset pneumonitis, rhinitis, or otitis.[10] Therapy includes topical eythromycin or tetracyclyine ointment and oral erythromycin 30 to 50 mg/kg/d in four divided doses for 2 to 3 weeks. Both parents should also be treated with oral erythromycin or doxycycline for 2 to 3 weeks.[2]

Gonococcal Conjunctivitis

Effective prophylaxis programs have helped to decrease the incidence of gonococcal neonatal conjunctivitis in the United States and all other developed countries.[7] Gonococcal conjunctivitis typically presents as severe, purulent conjunctivitis with lid edema and chemosis and serosanguineous discharge (Fig. 16–2). The conjunctivitis usually occurs approximately 48 to 72 hours after birth; however, if there is a premature rupture of amnionic membrane, the conjunctivitis may have an earlier onset.[2]

In addition to the conjunctivitis, *N. gonorrhea* can also cause severe keratitis, with corneal ulcer and perforation. Thus, the physician must always use fluorescein staining in evaluating the cornea.

As gonococcal conjunctivitis can lead to devastating sequelae, its diagnosis and treatment must be made promptly. Immediate Gram stain of conjunctival scraping is critical because it will often reveal typical Gram-negative intracellular diplococci (Fig. 16–3), which is virtually diagnostic of *N. gonorrhea*. Chocolate agar-plated cultures in a CO_2 enriched atmosphere or Thayer-Martin media placed in a 37°C incubator should be used for definitive gonococcal cultured isolation.

Appropriate therapy for *N. gonorrhea* conjunctivitis is topical eythromycin ointment and systemic third-generation cephalosporin (Ceftriaxone, administered either intravenously or intramuscularly, 30 to 50 mg/kg/d in divided doses).[2] Some authors have reported effective treatment with a single dose of 1 gram of Ceftriaxone.[11] Intravenous penicillin G 50,000 units/kg/d every 12 hours for 7 days is an alternative treatment[2] but one must be aware that resistant *N. gonorrhea* exists. In addition, the physician must consider concurrent infection with *Chlamydia* or syphilis whenever gonorrhea infection exists. Syphilis infection will require a much-prolonged course of treatment. Coexistent chlamydial infection will necessitate therapy for mother, father, and in some cases, sexual partners.

Herpes Simplex Conjunctivitis

Approximately 70% of cases of herpes simplex neonatal conjunctivitis are secondary to type II herpes simplex virus (HSV).[2] The conjunctivitis often occurs later than does gonococcal or chlamydia conjunctivitis, between 1 and 2 weeks postpartum.[2] Many cases are unilateral, with conjunctival injection and discharge. A concurrent keratitis is often present, with positive typical dendritic fluorescein staining of the corneal epithelial defect. One should request viral cultures of conjunctival scraping to obtain the diagnosis. However, viral cultures may take 7 to 10 days to become positive; treatment should be initiated immediately if there is sufficient clinical suspicion and should include topical trifluorothymidine (Viroptic) drops nine times daily or vidarabine (Vira-A) ointment five times daily and systemic acyclovir.

Prophylaxis

In 1881, Crede first used 2% silver nitrate for prophylaxis against neonatal conjunctivitis caused by *N. gonorrhea*.[12] Prior to that time, gonococcal conjunctivitis was a leading cause of blindness, occurring in 10% of newborns. Prophylaxis with silver nitrate and other agents has greatly decreased the incidence of gonococcal conjunctivitis to approximately 0.06%.[6] In recent years, the administration of silver nitrate to the eyes of neonates is no longer popular for two reasons. First, silver nitrate may cause a chemical conjunctivitis that may masquerade the diagnosis. Second, with the declining incidence of gonococcal conjunctivitis worldwide, *C. trachomatis* is now the leading cause of neonatal conjunctivitis, and silver nitrate does not provide prophylaxis against *Chlamydia*.[6] In 1980 and again in 1986, the American Academy of Pediatrics endorsed the use of 1% tetracycline or 0.5% erythromycin ointment as prophylaxis against neonatal gonococcal conjunctivitis. Currently, there are three accepted forms of neonatal conjunctivitis prophylaxis: 1% silver nitrate, 0.5% erythromycin ointment, and 1% tetracycline ointment; all three seem to have similar efficacy.[6,13] Recently, 2.5% povidone–iodine has been used for ophthalmia neonatum prophylaxis, and this has been shown to be superior to silver nitrate and erythromycin.[14] Povidone–iodine is effective against a broad spectrum of pathogens, including viruses such as human immunodeficiency virus and herpes, and may thus become the gold standard for prophylaxis of neonatal conjunctivitis.[14]

Pediatric Conjunctivitis

Conjunctival inflammation in a child is a nonspecific finding and can be secondary to a variety of disease processes. Infantile glaucoma, bacterial conjunctivitis, infectious keratitis, and uveitis all may share similar signs and symptoms. It is obviously important that the correct diagnosis be established for proper management. It may be necessary to restrain the child or to perform examination under anesthesia so that careful examination (by standard or handheld slit lamp) can be done, including checking intraocular pressure, looking for anterior chamber cells, and staining of the conjunctival and corneal epithelium.

The common causes of pediatric conjunctivitis are listed in Table 16–2. Approximately 50% of acute conjunctivitis in children is secondary to bacterial infection, 20% is caused by adenovirus, and 30% is culture negative.[15] Acute hemorrhagic conjunctivitis is most often caused by *Haemophilus influenzae* and adenovirus,[2] whereas chronic conjunctivitis in childhood is most commonly caused by chronic blepharitis and allergic conjunctivitis.

TABLE 16–2. Common Causes of Pediatric Conjunctivitis

Bacterial
  Staphylococcus species
  Haemophilus species
  Pneumococcus species
  Streptococcus species
  Chlamydia trachomatis
  Bartonella henselae

Viral
  Adenoviruses type 3, 7, 8, and 19
  Molluscum contagiosum
  Human papillomavirus

Noninfectious
  Allergic
    Hay fever conjunctivitis
    Vernal conjunctivitis
    Giant papillary conjunctivitis
  Meibomian gland dysfunction
  Conjunctivitis associated with systemic diseases
    Stevens-Johnson syndrome
    Graft-versus-host disease

Bacterial Conjunctivitis

Distinguishing features of bacterial conjunctivitis are acute purulent inflammation of the bulbar tarsal conjunctiva and mucopurulent

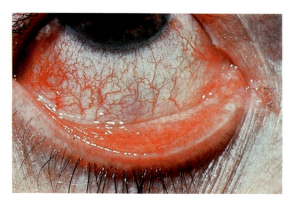

FIGURE 16–4. Staphylococcal conjunctivitis.

discharge. The most common pathogens include species of *Staphylococcus* (Fig. 16–4), *Haemophilus, Pneumococcus,* and *Streptococcus.*[15,16] In many cases, patients are treated empirically with broad-spectrum antibiotics without obtaining a culture. Treatment of acute nonspecific conjunctivitis in children with a broad-spectrum topical antibiotic (polymixin and bacitracin) has been shown to shorten the natural course of the conjunctivitis. A study of 158 patients aged 21 years or less showed similar clinical efficacy for three popular topical antibiotics (gentamycin, sodium sulfacetamide, and trimethoprim and polymixin B) against culture positive *H. influenzae* or *S. pneumoniae* conjunctivitis.[17]

Haemophilus influenzae presents with hemorrhagic conjunctivitis, occurs in children under 4 years of age, and is often associated with concomitant otitis media.[18] In addition to the conjunctivitis, the patient may present with a violaceous hue to the lid skin secondary to a small subcutaneous hemorrhage.[2] *Haemophilus influenzae* vaccination does not protect against untyped *H. influenza* that is responsible for hemorrhagic conjunctivitis.

Adolescent chlamydial conjunctivitis is usually associated with an acute purulent infection or a more indolent chronic conjunctivitis.[2] There are large follicles of the upper and lower tarsal conjunctiva. In adolescents and adults, chlamydial conjunctivitis is sexually transmitted. The patient and the sexual partner should be treated with oral tetracycline (Doxycycline 100 mg oral twice daily) or oral erythromycin 500 mg 4 times daily for 3 weeks. Topical tetracycline (Terak) or erythromycin may be added. It is important to realize, however, that not all cases of chlamydial conjunctivitis are sexually transmitted. In women, sharing of makeup, such as in commercial beauty salons, can also cause transmission of this organism.

Parinaud's oculoglandular syndrome is a unilateral conjunctivitis associated with a nodule of the tarsal conjunctiva, causing a local swelling and ptosis. Cat scratch disease (CSD) is the most common cause of oculoglandular syndrome. The causative organism in CSD is *Bartonella henselae,* a pleomorphic Gram-negative bacillus. The physician should evert the eyelid to look for follicular conjunctival reaction with nodule formation. Typically, the lid mass is associated with ipsilateral adenopathy of the preauricular or submandibular lymph nodes. A rare ocular manifestation of CSD is optic neuritis and macular stellate neuroretinitis. The neuroretinitis can present as stellate maculopathy with macular edema and exudates scattered like a star around the fovea. Fluorescein angiography shows permeability of deep disc capillaries and typically normal retinal vasculature. The patient, with or without an actual cat scratch, usually has a medical history that is positive for cats being in the immediate family or neighborhood. A positive skin test to cat scratch antigen supports the diagnosis. Treatment of CSD is controversial. Some researchers state that antibiotics are not useful.[19] Others have shown resolution in treating CSD with antibiotics, including tetracycline 250 mg q.i.d. for 2 weeks in older children[2]; trimethoprim–sulfamethoxazole (Bactrim) and the fluoroquinolones may also be effective. The prognosis is excellent, and there are usually no sequelae.[19] Bacterial adenitis secondary to *Staphylococcus aureus* or group A β-hemolytic *streptococcus,* atypical microbacteria, tuberculosis, and tularemia can also present as oculoglandular syndrome.[20]

Viral Conjunctivitis

Children with viral conjunctivitis usually present with a history of recent upper respiratory tract infection or contact with someone with red eye. It generally starts in one eye and a few days later involves the contralateral eye. There may be watery mucus discharge, red and edematous eyelids, subconjunctival hemorrhages, palpable preauricular node (PAN), and membrane/pseudomembrane. Subepithelial infiltrates may develop several weeks after the onset of the conjunctivitis.

Epidemic keratoconjunctivitis (EKC) begins as an acute conjunctivitis in one eye and 2 to 7 days later affects the fellow eye. The lids are swollen, the conjunctiva is injected, and subconjunctival hemorrhages are present.[2] Patients begin to complain of photophobia once the cornea becomes involved; mild anterior uveitis may occur once keratitis begins. There may be anterior chamber cells and flare. Acute symptoms can last for up to 3 weeks. EKC is most often associated with adenovirus serotypes 8 and 19. It poses an important public health hazard as it is extremely contagious, hence the word *epidemic*. Health care professionals should wash their hands and all ophthalmic equipment after examining a patient with any type of suspected infection, and parents or others who take care of children with EKC should be *very* careful in cleaning their hands after patient contact to avoid transmitting the virus to others. Towels, swimming pools, and other fomites used or contacted by the patient should be considered contaminated and should be treated as contagious sources and objects. Patients should not be

allowed to return to school for at least 1 week after the resolution of EKC. EKC is best managed conservatively, with application of cold compresses and use of preservative-free artificial tears, without the all-too-prevalent practice of indiscriminate prescribing of antibiotics. In the postacute phase, there may be subepithelial infiltrates (Fig. 16–5), which can cause severe photophobia; this may last several months. Topical steroid may be necessary in severe cases of keratopathy; however, recurrence of infiltrates may occur after discontinuation of steroids.

Pharyngeal conjunctival fever (PCF) is also caused by an adenovirus infection. However, unlike EKC, serotypes 3 and 7 are most common. The patient presents with fever, pharyngitis, and keratoconjunctivitis. Similar to EKC, PCF is highly contagious; patients should be isolated from schoolmates for approximately 2 weeks after onset. The treatment, like in EKC, is conservative, with application of cold compresses and use of artificial tears.

Molluscum contagiosum presents as small cutaneous papules or warts with umbilicated centers that occur along the eyelid margin (Fig. 16–6). It is caused by a pox virus. If these lesions are on the eyelid margin, they can cause a chronic follicular conjunctivitis. The most effective treatment is to excise at the apex of the lesion and to apply pressure to pinch and expulse the central core of the lesion.

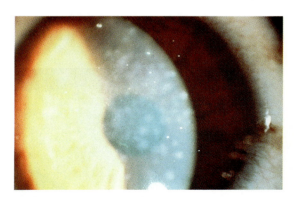

FIGURE 16–5. Subepithelial infiltrates in adenovirus keratoconjunctivitis. These infiltrates are small and uniform in size and shape and are located in the anterior stroma.

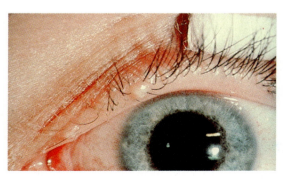

FIGURE 16–6. Molluscum contagiosum presents as small cutaneous papules or warts with umbilicated centers that occur along the eyelid margin.

Papilloma viral conjunctivitis is caused by human papillomavirus. Patients present with multiple papillomas of the conjunctiva and lid. These lesions tend to be recurrent in children and may be very difficult to eradicate. Cryotherapy, cautery, and carbon dioxide laser may be tried. Interferon therapy has been reported.[21]

Allergic Conjunctivitis

Allergic conjunctivitis is caused by immediate hypersensitivity type I reactions due to granulation of mast cells. The mechanism of type I reactions involves the binding of antigen (dust, pollens, danders, microbes, and drugs) to two adjacent IgE molecules already attached to the cell membrane of either a mast cell or a circulating basophil. Antigen binding to immunoglobulin E (IgE) affixed to the mast cell membrane results in increased cyclic adenosine monophosphate (cAMP) levels intracellularly. Tubulin subunits aggregate into microtubules, with degranulation of vasoactive amines as the end results. Mast cell degranulation causes release of histamine, leukotrienes, and other local mediators. This reaction causes hyperemia, vasodilatation, itching, and chemosis. Thus, the hallmark of an allergic or IgE-mediated conjunctivitis is itching and hyperemia.

Mast cell stabilizers such as lodoxamide (Alomide), cromolyn sodium (Opticrom or Crolom), and olopatadine (Patanol) can be used prophylactically for the prevention of degranulation of mast cells. Corticosteroids, because they act directly on the inflammation and hyperemia, can be used in the acute inflammatory response secondary to mediators that have already been released. Prostaglandins are also well-known mediators of ocular inflammation. Thus, nonsteroidal antiinflammatory drugs (NSAIDs), as cyclooxygenase enzyme inhibitors, can be used to reduce some of the symptoms of allergic conjunctivitis.

Hay Fever Conjunctivitis (Seasonal Allergic)

Patients with hay fever conjunctivitis typically present with mild to moderate symptoms of itching, tearing, and photophobia. Ocular signs of inflammation are minimal in comparison to patients' complaints.[2] Often, there is only minimal injection of the conjunctiva. The symptoms are usually seasonal, with exacerbation during the spring. Airborne antigens such as pollens, molds, dander, and dust cause an IgE-mediated reaction that causes degranulation of mast cells. Hay fever conjunctivitis can usually be managed through allergen avoidance and as-needed topical antihistamine use of olopatadine (Patanol) or levocabastine (Livostin). In more severe and prolonged cases, topical mast cell stabilizers such as lodoxamide (Alomide), cromolyn sodium (Opticrom or Crolom), or olopatadine (Patanol) can be used during allergy season. Topical steroids should be reserved for extremely severe cases.

Vernal Conjunctivitis

Vernal conjunctivitis, a severe form of IgE-mediated mast cell-dependent hypersensitivity reaction (type I) and delayed hypersensitivity reaction (type IV), results in giant papillae resembling cobblestones in the upper tarsus (Fig. 16–7). Severe itching is the hallmark of the disease. In advanced vernal conjunctivitis, the upper lid becomes thickened as the giant papillae enlarge, and vision-threatening keratitis can occur. Vernal conjunctivitis is a potentially blinding disease.

The onset is usually between 3 and 6 years of age, and vernal conjunctivitis can last from 4 to 20 years. The disease is termed vernal because it tends to be worse in the spring; however, symptoms may occur anytime of the year. The diagnosis is made on clinical signs and symptoms. Conjunctival scrapings from the upper tarsal conjunctiva reveal eosinophils and high density of mast cells (normally, there are no mast cells).[22] Keratitis occurs secondary to the release

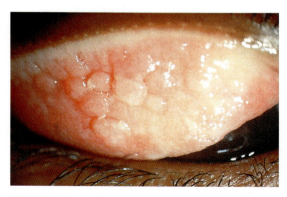

FIGURE 16–7. Giant papillae resembling cobblestones in vernal conjunctivitis.

of major basic protein and cationic protein from eosinophils. Limbal vernal conjunctivitis is associated with papillae that develop along the upper limbus. Dense collections of eosinophils in these papillae appear as white limbal spots called *Trantas dots*. Severe inflammation leads to punctate keratopathy, corneal ulcer, and ptosis.

Management of vernal conjunctivitis can be difficult. The patient should be placed on topical mast cell stabilizer chronically to prevent symptoms. Cromolyn sodium is the traditional choice. The introduction of Iodoxamide (Alomide), a mast cell–eosinophil inhibitor, and olopatadine (Patanol), a combination of antihistamine and mast cell stabilizer, applied twice daily, have brought much relief to patients with vernal conjunctivitis. Intermittent use of topical steroids is usually necessary to relieve acute symptoms of itching and to calm the inflammation. However, chronic use of steroids should be avoided, especially in children, to prevent complications such as cataracts and glaucoma. Topical steroid-sparing agents such as cyclosporin A have recently been tried in patients with vernal conjunctivitis.

Blepharitis and Meibomian Gland Dysfunction

Blepharitis is another common cause of pediatric conjunctivitis. Chronic *Staphylococcus* blepharitis often presents with chronic bilateral ocular irritation, burning, and conjunctival injection. There are dilated blood vessels, scales, and collarettes (a scale centered around an eyelash) on lid margin anterior to the gray line (Fig. 16–8) and, in severe cases, vascular-ization of the anterior lid margin and loss of lashes (madarosis). Staphyloccocal exotoxins induce a delayed or cell-mediated hypersensitivity reaction. The treatment of staphylococcal blepharitis includes lid hygiene, topical antibiotics (erythromycin, tetracycline, bacitracin, and sulfacetamide ointments), and, if sufficiently severe, the addition of topical steroids.

Meibomian gland dysfunction (MGD) is also a common cause of pediatric conjunctivitis. Ocular examination reveals oil goblets at the orifices of meibomian glands with foamy tears along the lower lid (Fig. 16–9). When the lipid within the meibomian gland orifices solidifies, the duct becomes obstructed and the glands dilate. Management of MGD is most effective with lid scrubs and hygiene. Mechanical expression of the lipid from the glands is also helpful to prevent chalazion formation.

Miscellaneous

There are other types of pediatric conjunctivitis, which may include giant papillary conjunctivitis, ligneous conjunctivitis, folliculosis, and conjunctivitis associated with systemic diseases such as Stevens–Johnson syndrome and graft-versus-host disease. However, these types of conjunctivitis are less frequent. Once the physician at the forefront has diagnosed the conjunctivitis and managed the infant or child with traditional therapy and the patient still has persistent symptoms and signs, it is appropriate and recommended that the patient be referred to a pediatric ophthalmologist or to a cornea specialist.

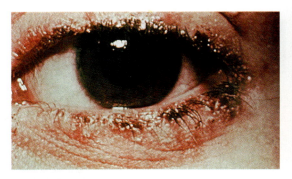

FIGURE 16–8. Staphylococcal blepharitis with madarosis and collarettes on lid margin.

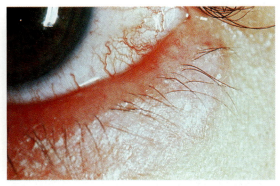

FIGURE 16–9. Meibomian gland dysfunction (meibomianitis).

■ Keratitis

Pediatric keratitis may arise as a result of various factors. Inflammation or infection of the cornea usually causes concurrent inflammation of the conjunctiva, leading to the appearance of a red eye. Any disorder that can cause lid abnormalities and proptosis, such as craniosynostosis or orbital masses, can also induce exposure keratitis. Appropriate treatment is directed at controlling the underlying cause as well as supportive therapy with artificial tears, ointments, and tarsorrhaphy, whenever necessary.

Herpes Simplex Keratitis

Herpes simplex keratitis (HSK) can occur in children of any age. Neonates can become infected as they pass through the birth canal. Eye involvement may occur in as many as 13% of newborns.[2] The pathogen, HSV, is a DNA virus. Infections acquired at birth are usually HSV type 2, whereas herpes contracted later in life is often HSV type 1. The first exposure of herpesvirus to the patient produces "primary" herpes simplex infection. Conjunctivitis is a hallmark sign of primary herpetic infection and is often accompanied by vesicles on eyelids. Preauricular lymph node enlargement is typical.

Corneal involvement in herpes infection of the eye often starts as superficial punctate keratopathy and progresses to classic dendritic keratitis. The epithelium heaps up at the margin of the lesion, and centrally, there is a loss of epithelium. Dendritic lesions stain well with both fluorescein (central ulceration) (Fig. 16–10A) and

Rose Bengal (swollen epithelial cells at the edges of herpetic lesions, which are often heaped up) (Fig. 16–10B). Repeated episodes generally result in corneal hypesthesia. Treatment with topical trifluorothymidine 1% (Viroptic), five times daily is indicated if there is only eyelid or skin involvement and nine times daily after minimal wiping debridement (MWD) if there is corneal epithelial disease. Most patients will heal in 14 to 21 days. MWD is an underrecognized effective treatment, but it obviously may be difficult to perform in young children.[23]

HSK may also manifest as disciform keratitis, which is the cell-mediated immune response to viral antigens.[2] It often develops underneath an intact epithelium. The stroma is edematous and, in severe cases, may become vascularized. There may be keratic precipitates, Descemet's folds, iridocyclitis, and glaucoma. The presence of stromal edema can cause the patient to have tearing, pain, photophobia, and decreased vision. If the visual axis is not involved, topical antivirals can be given; if the visual axis is involved, steroids may be used judiciously.[2] If iridocyclitis is present, in addition to topical steroid, cycloplegia may be used to improve discomfort.[24,25] The blinding complication of HSK results from widespread stromal disease, with subsequent severe vascularization, corneal scarring, and perforation.

Varicella Keratitis

Primary infection with varicella zoster, another member of the herpes virus family, is common among children. Malaise, chills, fever, and vesicular lesions of the skin and mucous membranes are typical systemic findings. The virus resides

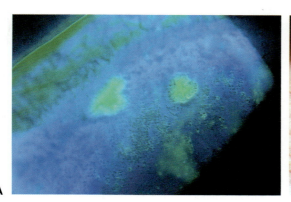
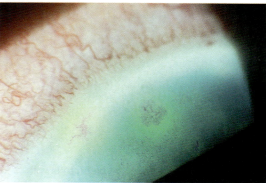

FIGURE 16–10. Herpes simplex dendritic keratitis stained with fluorescein (A) and Rose Bengal (B).

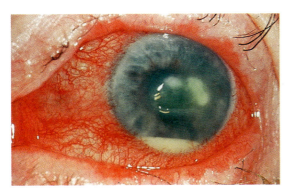

FIGURE 16–11. Herpes zoster keratouveitis and scleritis with corneal epithelial melting and hypopyon.

in the ganglion, which may be the site of latent infection, causing recurrent ocular disease through sensory nerves, such as nasociliary nerve.[26] Corneal disease may follow the acute skin rash by many months to years. Rarely, ocular disease can precede the skin rash.

Zoster ocular infections may present with swelling of the lids, vesicular lesions, and keratoconjunctivitis. Keratitis can result in dendritic lesions, which may be indistinguishable from HSK dendrites. Interstitial keratitis may also occur. Other ocular involvements include chorioretinitis, optic neuritis, uveitis and scleritis (Fig. 16–11), and palsies of extraocular muscles.[27]

Topical antibiotics (erythromycin or bacitracin ointment) may be applied to skin lesions as prophylaxis for bacterial infection. Cycloplegia may be used to reduce pain. If there is any conjunctival (vesicular lesions) or corneal involvement (pseudodendrites or superficial punctate keratitis), cool compresses and erythromycin ointment may be applied to the eye twice daily. In addition, vidarabine 3% (Vira-A) ointment may be applied to the eyelid lesions, conjunctiva, and cornea five times daily. Oral acyclovir (800 mg five times daily) or oral famciclovir (500 mg three times daily) are clearly very helpful in hastening resolution of the active infection, especially if administered within 3 days of the start of the cutaneous eruption.[28]

Bacterial Keratitis

Any bacteria that causes conjunctivitis can also lead to corneal involvement; *Staphylococcus aureus*, *Streptococcus pneumoniae*, *Streptococcus pyo-genes*, and *Haemophilus influenzae* are common bacteria that can cause upper respiratory infections and conjunctivitis in children, and can also lead to keratopathy—superficial punctate keratitis or ulcer. An ulcer must be scraped for smears and culture to identify the causative organisms for proper therapy. Obviously, this will usually require brief general anesthesia. *Neisseria gonorrhea*, a common cause of infantile conjunctivitis, can also cause corneal ulceration and rapid progression to perforation.[29] *N. gonorrhea* is quite unique as it is one of the few bacteria that can cause conjunctivitis and corneal ulceration and may present with an enlarged preauricular lymph node.[2]

Broad-spectrum therapy with fortified antibiotics (tobramycin, vancomycin, fluoroquinolone, or cephazolin) should be initiated as soon as scrapings of lesions have been performed. Subconjunctival antibiotic injection therapy during brief examination under anesthesia every 24 to 48 hours is probably an underutilized but highly effective approach to microbial corneal ulcer therapy of uncooperative children whose excessive tearing results in suboptimal antibiotic topical delivery. As children are not reliable in expressing their symptoms, they should be followed daily during the active phase of the ulcer to avoid occurrence of corneal perforation

Chlamydia Trachomatis

Every physician should always consider *Chlamydia trachomatis* as a cause of "red eye." Although it is a rare cause of blindness in the United States, *Chlamydia* is now the leading cause of blindness worldwide. Regrettably, however, the bacterium is epidemic throughout the United States and the leading cause of sterility in women because it causes "silent," chronic pelvic inflammatory disease. Unfortunately, sexual abuse of a child by an adult must also be considered in a case of pediatric chlamydial conjunctivitis or keratitis. *Chlamydia* can cause acute purulent or papillary conjunctivitis, which if not properly treated will progress to chronic follicular conjunctivitis, cicatrizing conjunctival and corneal changes, and eventual corneal opacification and blindness. Proper therapy for ocular chlamydia in children is with topical tetracycline four times daily and oral erythromycin 30 to 50 mg/kg/d in four divided doses for 14 days.[29,30] Systemic tetracycline should be avoided as it can cause staining of teeth, hypoplasia of dental enamel, and abnormal bone growth in children less than 8 years of age.

Vernal Keratoconjunctivitis

Vernal conjunctivitis has been described previously. Corneal involvement in vernal disease includes superficial punctate keratopathy and shield ulcer (Fig. 16–12) in up to 5% of patients with vernal conjunctivitis in the superior half of the cornea.[2] The shield ulcer may result in stromal opacity. Because vernal keratoconjunctivitis is associated with a high incidence of keratoconus, physicians should look for evidence of keratoconus—paracentral thinning and bulging of the cornea, Fleischer's ring (epithelial iron deposits at the base of the cone), Munson's sign (bulging of the lower eyelid when looking downward), and corneal hydrops (sudden development of corneal edema resulting from a rupture in Descemet's membrane).

Interstitial Keratitis

Interstitial keratitis (IK), another possible cause of red eye, is a nonsuppurative inflammation of the corneal stroma, without involvement of other layers of the cornea, which can be caused by herpes simplex virus, congenital syphilis, tuberculosis, Cogan's disease, mumps, herpes zoster virus, rubeola, sarcoidosis, leprosy, onchocerciasis, and lymphogranuloma venereum. In general, systemic therapy of the underlying disease is indicated when IK is diagnosed.

Miscellaneous

Other causes of keratitis that may produce a red eye include superficial punctate keratopathy caused by adenoviruses, influenza viruses, and paramyxoviruses (rubeola, mumps); acanthamoeba; fungi; toxic keratopathy secondary to chronic use of topical antibiotics (tobramycin or gentamycin), antivirals, preservatives (benzalkonium chloride), and topical anesthetics; avitaminosis A; and neurotropic keratitis sec-

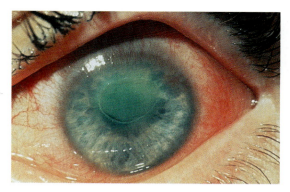

FIGURE 16–12. Corneal shield ulcer in vernal keratoconjunctivitis.

ondary to fifth nerve damage associated with herpes zoster, herpes simplex, trauma, intercranial tumors, and oculofacial syndromes.

■ Summary

There are six major categories of ocular disorders that can manifest as "red eye" in infants and children. In this chapter, we have discussed two: conjunctivitis and keratitis; the others are described elsewhere in this volume. Conjunctivitis and keratitis have numerous potential etiologies, many of which have potentially blinding consequences. In addition, managing infants and children may be technically challenging, as the patients often do not clearly express their symptoms and cannot cooperate with a complete ocular exam. Thus, it is important that the physician spend adequate time obtaining a detailed history from the parents or caretakers and performing a thorough examination with the same careful ophthalmic ritual every time, even if sedation or anesthesia is required to do so.

A final word of caution: there exist subgroups of red eye that respond exceptionally well to topical steroid therapy. In such cases, steroids are very attractive to both physicians and patients. However, a competent ophthalmologist will realize that topical steroids may not directly control the underlying problem and that chronic use of steroids may produce the appearance of a quiet, comfortable eye while inducing glaucoma, cataract, or corneal perforation. Therefore, for every patient, every attempt should be made to identify the underlying disorder so that appropriate therapy can be initiated.

REFERENCES

1. Grosskreutz C, Smith L. Neonatal conjunctivitis. *Int Ophthalmol Clin.* 1992;32:71–79.
2. Wright K. Conjunctivitis. In: Wright K, ed. *Pediatric Ophthalmology and Strabismus.* St. Louis, MO: Mosby; 1995; 1: 279–292.
3. Isenberg S, et al. Source of the conjunctival bacterial flora at birth and implications for ophthalmia neonatorum prophylaxis. *Am J Ophthalmol.* 1988;106:458–462.
4. Isenberg S, et al. Bacterial flora of the conjunctiva at birth. *J Pediatr Ophthalmol Strabismus.* 1986;23:284–286.
5. Armstrong J, et al. Ophthalmia neonatorum: a chart review. *Pediatrics.* 1976;57:884–892.
6. Hammerschlag M, et al. Efficacy of neonatal ocular prophylaxis of the prevention of chlamydia and gonoccocal conjunctivitis. *N Engl J Med.* 1989;320:769–772.
7. Rapoza P. Epidemiology of neonatal conjunctivitis. *Ophthalmology.* 1986;93:456–461.
8. Fraioli A. Conjunctivitis and orbital cellulitis in childhood. In: Albert O, Jakobicc F, eds. *Principles and Practice of Ophthalmology.* Philadelphia, PA: WB Saunders; 1994;4:2827–2835.
9. Rapoza P, et al. Assessment of neonatal conjunctivitis with a direct immunofluorescent monoclonal antibody stain for *Chlamydia. JAMA.* 1986;255:3369.
10. Harrison J. Chlamydia trachomatis infant pneumonitis. *N Engl J Med.* 1978;298:702–708.
11. Haimovici R, Roussel T. Treatment of gonococcal conjunctivitis with single dose intermuscular Ceftriaxone. *Am J Ophthalmol.* 1989;107:511–514.
12. Crede K. Die Verhütung der Augenentzündung der Neugeborenen. *Arch Gynakol.* 1881;17:50–53.
13. Laga J, et al. Prophylaxis of gonococcal and chlamydial ophthalmia neonatorum. *N Engl J Med.* 1988; 318: 653–657.
14. Isenberg S, et al. A controlled trial of povidone-iodine as prophylaxis against ophthalmia neonatorum. *N Engl J Med.* 1995;332:562–566.
15. Gigliotti F. Etiology of acute conjunctivitis in children. *J Pediatrics.* 1981;98:531–536.
16. Seal D, et al. Etiology and treatment of acute bacterial infection of the eye. *Br J Ophthalmol.* 1982;66:357–360.
17. Lohr J. Comparison of three topical antimicrobials for acute bacterial conjunctivitis. *Pediatr Infect Dis J.* 1988;7:626–629.
18. Bodor F. Bacterial etiology of conjunctivitis otitis syndrome. *Pediatrics.* 1985;76:26–28.
19. Moriarty R. Cat scratch disease. *Infect Dis Clin North Am.* 1987;1:575–590.
20. Martin X, et al. Ophthalmia nodosum and the oculoglandular syndrome of Perinaud. *Br J Ophthalmol.* 1986;70:536–542.
21. Lass J, et al. Interferon-alpha therapy of recurrent conjunctival papillomas. *Am J Ophthalmol.* 1987; 103: 294–301.
22. Alansmith M, et al. (1978). Number of inflammatory cells in normal conjunctiva. *Am J Ophthalmol.* 1978; 86:250–259.
23. Pavan L. Diagnosis and management of herpes simplex ocular infection. *Int Ophthalmol Clin.* 1975;15(5):19–35.
24. Nahmias A, Roizman B. Infection with herpes simplex viruses 1 and 2. *N Engl J Med.* 1973;289:781–789.
25. Nahmias A, Norrild B. Herpes simplex viruses 1 and 2—basic and clinical aspects. *Dis Mon.* 1979;25:1–49.
26. Wilhelmus K, et al. Varicella disciform stromal keratitis. *Am J Ophthalmol.* 1991;111:575–580.
27. Weinhoff M. Herpes zoster ophthalmicus. *Ophthalmic Semin.* 1976;1:227–252.
28. Reuler J, Chang M. Herpes zoster: epidemiology, clinical features, and management. *South Med J.* 1984; 77:1149–1156.
29. Fransen L, Klauss V. Neonatal ophthalmia in the developing world: epidemiology, etiology, management and control. *Int Ophthalmol.* 1988;11(3):189–196.
30. Thylefors B. A simple system for the assessment of trachoma and its complication. *Bull WHO.* 1987;65: 477–483.

Pediatric Ophthalmology
Edited by P. F. Gallin
Thieme Medical Publishers, Inc.
New York © 2000

17

Uveitis

MICHAEL J. WEISS AND ALBERT J. HOFELDT

The blood–aqueous and blood–retinal barriers are designed to prevent inflammatory components from entering the eye. When these barriers break down, regardless of the mechanism involved (infectious, autoimmune, etc.), uveitis ensues. Ocular inflammation may occur with or without an accompanying systemic illness. The diagnostic evaluation of uveitis in children therefore involves (1) a careful and detailed ocular and medical history, (2) ocular and systemic examination, and (3) appropriate laboratory tests tailored to the pertinent uveitis history and findings on examination.

■ History

The relevant history is best understood if one is thoroughly familiar with all the potential diagnostic possibilities.[1-4] The reader is encouraged to refer to the specific uveitis syndromes to further understand the relevance of each part of the history taking. The list below outlines all pertinent history that should be obtained.

Obtaining Patient History

Demographics: Establish the age, gender, and ethnicity of the patient.

Present illness: Presenting symptoms (if any) such as pain, redness, photophobia, floaters, and decreased vision are established. Determine the onset time and whether the disease is unilateral or bilateral. Of note,

although some uveitides may have bilateral involvement, only one eye may be affected during any single inflammatory episode. Preceding events (e.g., trauma, viral illness, or recent immunization) should be determined. What has been the course of the disease including response to anti-inflammatory therapy? Establish the treatment regimens previously used and the degree of patient compliance to determine if previous attempts at treatment were adequate to justify using alternative anti-inflammatory medicines.

Ocular history: A history of previous eye disease should be ascertained.

Medical history: Is there a history of arthritis or joint pain [juvenile rheumatoid arthritis (JRA), sarcoid, ankylosing spondylitis]? Any history of gastrointestinal symptoms such as abdominal pains, bloody stool, or chronic diarrhea [Inflammatory bowel disease (IBD), Reiters]? Any history of skin disease [Vogt-Koyanagi-Haradas (VKH), psoriatic arthritis, sarcoid, Bechets]? History of exposure to tuberculosis? History of tick bite or hiking in wooded areas (Lyme)? History of any neurological symptoms (VKH, sarcoid, Bechets, multiple sclerosis)? History of urethral discharge (Reiters)?

Travel and geographic history: Lyme disease is most common in the mid-Atlantic, New England area. Histoplasmosis is endemic in the Ohio–Missisippi–Missouri Valley region, and Coccidiomycosis-related uveitis is primarily seen in the San Joaquin Valley in California. Cysticercosis, amebiasis, and onchocerciasis are primarily found in Central and South America and Africa.

Pet history: Did patient's mother have exposure to cats or cat feces during pregnancy (toxoplasmosis)? Did patient have any exposure to dogs or dog feces [e.g., contaminated sandboxes (toxocariasis)]? History of pica?

Dietary history: Did patient's mother ingest undercooked meat during her pregnancy (toxoplasmosis)?

Sexual history: Is the patient sexually active? What is the number of sexual contacts? Sexual orientation of the patient? Any penile or vaginal sores? Is there a history of venereal disease?

Drug history: Is there a history of maternal intravenous drug use (HIV, fungal infection, CMV retinitis)?

Family history: Does mother of patient have a history of active syphilis or HIV infection during pregnancy? Although uveitis is generally not inherited, a family history of uveitis should be sought because certain uveitides have strong HLA associations.

■ Examination

External examination should be tailored to the elicited history. The joints should be examined for evidence of joint swelling. Look for cutaneous manifestations such as rash, erythema nodosum (subcutaneous erythematous tender nodules most commonly in the anterior tibial region), mucocutaneous lesions, psoriatic lesions, vitiligo, poliosis, alopecia, nail pitting, and onychyolysis. Is seventh nerve function intact (sarcoid or Lyme disease)? The lids and periorbital region should be examined for lacrimal, salivary, or parotid gland swelling and lid margin granulomas. The conjunctiva should be inspected for evidence of sarcoid granulomas, ciliary flush (perilimbal injection), episcleritis, or scleritis. (In scleritis the vascular congestion is localized in the deep episcleral network and does not vasoconstrict with 10% neosynephrine drops.)

Slit Lamp Examination

Anterior Segment Evaluation

Examine the cornea for evidence of dendritic keratitis and check for normal corneal sensation (herpes simplex or herpes zoster–related uveitis). The presence of band keratopathy should be noted. The endothelium should be examined for the presence of keratic precipitates (KPs), which are the most common corneal finding in uveitis patients (Fig. 17–1). The pattern of KP distribution should be noted. KPs usually accumulate in the lower half of the cornea in a base down triangle configuration (Arlt's triangle). Small KPs with distinct margins are classified as nongranulomatous, whereas larger greasy appearing KPs are classified as granulomatous. The anterior chamber should be inspected for the presence of cells and flare

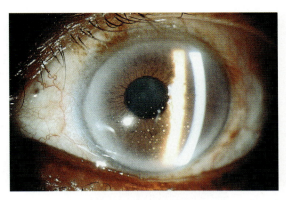

FIGURE 17–1. Slit lamp photograph of granulomatous keratic precipitates in a patient with sarcoidosis.

(protein) and the degree of inflammation carefully graded (Table 17–1). Cells and flare can be identified by shining the slit lamp beam obliquely across the anterior chamber while focusing posterior to the cornea (Fig. 17–2). Anterior chamber cells are more easily seen by tipping the light source housing approximately 10 degrees from its normal vertical position. Of note, because chronic flare is generally felt to be a manifestation of chronic damage to the blood–aqueous barrier (and not a sign of active inflammation), flare alone should not be treated. The iris should be assessed for evidence of stromal atrophy and heterochromia. The iris should also be inspected for the presence of nodules. Koeppe nodules are located at the sphincter margin and may be seen in granulomatous and nongranulomatous inflammatory disorders. Bussaca nodules are located on the iris stroma and are generally seen only in granulomatous inflammatory conditions (Fig. 17–3). Because uveitis can produce ischemia, the examiner should look for signs of iris rubeosis (usually evident at the sphincter margin). The presence or absence of posterior synechiae should be noted. A gonioscope or three-mirror

TABLE 17–1. Grading of Aqueous Cells[a]

No. cells/1 × 1 mm slit beam	Grade
1–2	Rare
3–4	Trace
5–10	1+
10–20	2+
20–50	3+
Over 50	4+

[a] Light intensity and magnification should be maximal.

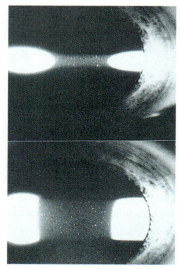

FIGURE 17–2. Slit lamp photograph demonstrating the apprearance of cells and flare.

lens should be used to look for signs of peripheral anterior synechiae. The angle should also be inspected for the presence of rubeosis, occult foreign body, or malignancy. The lens should be evaluated for the presence of cataract formation. Because glaucoma is a common complication of uveitis and/or the use of steroids the intraocular pressures must always be checked. Alternatively ocular hypotony may be present secondary to chronic inflammation leading to ciliary body shutdown.

Vitreous
The vitreous should be inspected for the presence of cells, opacities, snowballs (vitre-

ous cells in clumps), and posterior vitreous separation. Posterior KPs may be seen lining the posterior hyaloid. Cellular activity primarily in the retrolental area (Berger's space) generally signifies ciliary body involvement. To grade the degree of vitreous inflammation a grading scale based on the qualitative view of the optic nerve and posterior retina compared to standard color photographs is felt to be more useful than trying to grade the number of vitreous cells by retroillumination.[5]

Retina and Choroid
The optic nerve should be examined for evidence of hyperemia, papillitis, or papilledema. Of note, granulomas and drusen of the optic nerves can simulate an elevated nerve. The macula is inspected for cystoid macula edema, the most common retinal finding in patients with uveitis (Fig. 17–4). Retinal neovascularization or choroidal neovascularization may occur as a complication of uveitis. The presence of a choroidal neovascular membrane involving the macula is suggested by the finding of subretinal heme lipid or serous detachment. Vascular alterations such as occlusion sheathing, hemorrhages, and cotton wool spots should be noted. Of note, sheathing is more easily seen in the posterior pole compared to the retinal periphery. The retina and choroid are then examined for evidence of focal

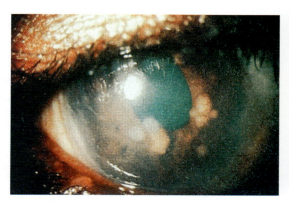

FIGURE 17–3. Slit lamp photograph of Bussaca iris nodules in a patient with sarcoidosis.

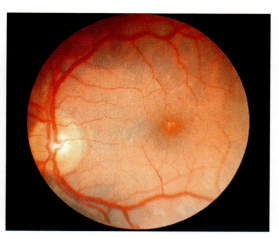

FIGURE 17–4. Fundus photograph demonstrating the appearance of cystoid macula edema.

inflammatory lesions. Exudative nonrhegmatogenous serous retinal detachments may be seen (VKH, scleritis, central serous retinopathy). The retinal periphery should be examined for the presence of a pars plana snowbank, which appears as a white mass usually over the inferior pars plana and adjacent ora serrata region.

■ Classification of Uveitis

Several classification schemes may be used to help classify uveitis.

Duration of Inflammatory Activity

Acute uveitis is defined as inflammatory activity that with appropriate intervention lasts less than 3 months, usually between 2 and 6 weeks. The inflammation may recur (acute recurrent), but between episodes the patient is inflammation free.

Chronic inflammation is defined as inflammatory activity that persists beyond 3 months despite appropriate intervention. Periodic exacerbation of the baseline inflammatory activity may occur (chronic–recurrent). Both acute and chronic inflammation may have a sudden or insidious onset.

Severity of Inflammatory Activity

The severity of disease can be graded according to the extent of visual damage. Severe inflammation is defined as greater than 50% visual loss as assessed by visual acuity or electroretinogram, whereas mild inflammation would represent less than a 50% loss.

Anatomic Region of Involvement

Inflammatory activity confined to the anterior chamber is termed iritis. Iritis plus cells in the retrolental space signifying ciliary body involvement is called iridocyclitis. Intermediate uveitis is characterized by inflammation predominantly involving the vitreous and peripheral retina sometimes associated with a peripheral perivasculitis. Posterior uveitis is characterized by inflammation posterior to the vitreous base. Depending on the site of primary involvement, posterior uveitis may be subclassified as focal,

multifocal, or diffuse choroiditis, retinitis, or chorioretinitis. When inflammatory findings involve the entire uveal tract the term *panuveitis* is used.

Response to Steroid Therapy

Inflammatory activity is either responsive or resistant to steroid therapy. If responsive, the maintenance dose needed to control inflammation should be noted.

■ Masquerade Syndromes of Anterior and Posterior Uveitis

In the pediatric age group masquerade syndromes of anterior and posterior uveitis include rhegmatogenous retinal detachment, intraocular foreign body, and intraocular neoplasm such as retinoblastoma, leukemia, and juvenile xanthogranuloma. Juvenile xanthogranuloma, which may masquerade as anterior uveitis, occurs in children under 15 years of age and is characterized by yellowish-gray iris tumors associated with spontaneous hyphema and anterior segment inflammation. The diagnosis may be established by anterior chamber paracentesis, iris biopsy, and skin examination.

■ Noninfectious Causes of Anterior Uveitis

Juvenile Rheumatoid Arthritis (JRA)

JRA is a rheumatoid factor negative inflammatory arthritis of at least 3 months' duration that develops before age 16. **Approximately 70% of all childhood arthritis is secondary to JRA.** Girls are only slightly more commonly affected than boys, but girls carry a much higher risk of developing uveitis. The peak incidence of JRA occurs between ages 2 and 4, whereas the average age of diagnosis of uveitis is 6 (range 1 to 35 years). If there is no evidence of ocular inflammatory disease within 7 years of the diagnosis of JRA, the subsequent risk of developing uveitis is considered small.[6–8]

Three subgroups of JRA are identified by the extent of joint involvement that occurs during the first 3 months: systemic onset (or Still's disease), polyarticular onset, and pauciarticular onset. The risk of developing uveitis is determined by the extent of joint involvement during the first 3 months of the disease and not by the extent of joint involvement at the time of the patient's first visit.

Systemic onset JRA occurs in approximately 20% of JRA patients. Onset is characterized by fever, lymphadenopathy, hepatosplenomegaly, pericarditis, and a maculopapular rash. Most patients do not develop progressive arthritis. The development of uveitis in this subgroup is so uncommon that annual eye screening for uveitis is adequate.

Polyarticular onset JRA occurs in an estimated 20% of JRA patients. It is characterized by involvement of five or more joints. About one fourth of patients in this subgroup are seropositive for rheumatoid factor. Like adults with rheumatoid arthritis they are not at risk for developing uveitis. The incidence of uveitis ranges between 7 and 14%. Due to the moderate risk of developing uveitis, screening every 6 months is recommended.

Finally, 60% of JRA patients will have pauciarticular onset characterized by involvement of four or fewer joints. The knees and, less frequently, ankles and wrists are most commonly involved. The incidence of uveitis in this subgroup ranges between 78 and 91%. Of note, JRA that is diagnosed as pauciarticular may years later evolve into the polyarticular form. Nevertheless, these patients still carry the risk of developing uveitis associated with the pauciarticular subgroup. Due to the high risk of developing uveitis, eye screening every 3 months is recommended.[9] The presence of circulating antinuclear antibodies (ANAs) is especially common in patients with eye involvement. Therefore, in the setting of pauciarticular ANA-positive JRA, routine eye screening is recommended every 2 months (Table 17–2).

Uveitis in JRA is usually asymptomatic, bilateral, and of the chronic anterior nongranulomatous variety. In eyes with severe anterior segment inflammation, cells may also be seen in the anterior vitreous (iridocyclitis). Common complications of uveitis include band keratopathy, posterior synechiae, cataract (incidence of 28 to 31%) glaucoma (incidence of 14 to 22%), and cystoid macula edema.

The treatment of uveitis is designed to eliminate the cellular component of the inflammation and not necessarily the flare that may also be present. Topical steroids (prednisolone acetate 1%) may initially need to be used up to every hour for several days with gradual tapering thereafter. For patients requiring high-frequency dosing of topical steroids or who have not adequately responded to topical steroids, anterior subtenon injections of methylprednisolone and/or a brief course of systemic steroids may be helpful.[10] The antimetabolite methotrexate, given weekly in low doses, can be a safe and effective alternative to the use of oral steroids. Other immunosuppressive agents to consider in the treatment of JRA include azathioprine, chlorambucil, cyclosporin, and cyclophosphamide. EDTA chelation is used to remove visually significant band keratopathy. To prevent posterior synechiae formation a short-acting mydriatic such as Mydriacyl 1% should be used several times a day. In mild cases one drop at bedtime may be adequate. Cataract surgery should ideally be performed after intraocular inflammation has been controlled for at least 2 to 3 months. In many cases this goal may be difficult to achieve, resulting in a significant delay in surgery, and must be weighed against the possibility of irreversible amblyopia that may develop as a result of the delayed surgery. Lensectomy–vitrectomy through an incision at the limbus or pars plana is the method of choice. Of note implantation of an intraocular lens in JRA patients with chronic uveitis is contraindicated. For control of complicating glaucoma, nonmiotic medical management should initially be employed, although

TABLE 17–2. Juvenile Rheumatoid Arthritis

% of Patients with JRA	No. Joints Involved	Frequency of Uveitis	Frequency of Eye Exam
Systemic onset 20%	Uncommon	Uncommon	q year
Polyarticular 20%	>5	7–14%	q 6 month
Pauciarticular 60%	<4	78–91%	q 3 month[a]

[a] If ANA is positive frequency of exams should be q 2 month.

glaucoma filtering surgery with antimetabolites or trabeculodialysis is often eventually required. Macula edema is often secondary to uncontrolled inflammation and is best treated by controlling intraocular inflammation.

Juvenile Ankylosing Spondylitis (JAS)

Childhood juvenile spondylitis is initially characterized by a peripheral lower limb arthritis, which in 15% of cases may be complicated by acute unilateral nongranulomatous anterior uveitis. Early on there may be no sacroiliac involvement, although eventually sacroiliac and lumbosacral spine involvement occurs. The disease typically affects males approximately 10 years of age who carry the HLA B27 tissue haplotype. Rheumatoid factor and antinuclear antibody are generally negative. As in adult ankylosing spondylitis, there is no correlation between disease activity and uveitis.[11]

Patients are usually symptomatic with blurred vision, pain, and redness. The uveitis is classified as the acute–recurrent type. Although attacks are usually unilateral, both eyes eventually become involved. Signs of acute anterior iritis include nongranulomatous KPs, cells, and flare. Repeated bouts may lead to chronic changes such as band keratopathy, synechiae, and cataract. Treatment involves the use of topical steroids and mydriatics.[7]

Juvenile Psoriatic Arthritis

Definite JPsA is defined as (1) arthritis associated but not necessarily coincident with a typical psoriatic rash or (2) arthritis plus three of four of the following minor criteria: dactylitis (inflammation of fingers), nail pitting, family history of psoriasis, or a nontypical psoriasis-like rash. Onset of the arthritis is usually pauciarticular with a polyarticular course. Both small and large joints may be involved with prominent knee and digital involvement common. Females are twice as likely as males to be affected. ANA positivity is common but rheumatoid factor (RF) is absent. There may be an association with HLA B-7 antigen. The anterior uveitis that occurs in approximately 15% of children is usually bilateral and chronic. Treatment involves the use of topical steroids and cycloplegics.[7,12]

Juvenile Reiter's Syndrome

This syndrome, which is rare in children, includes the triad of arthritis, urethritis, and conjunctivitis.[13] An antecedent history of gastrointestinal tract infection caused by gram-negative organisms such as salmonella, shigella, and yersinia is common. It may also follow a nongonococcal urethritis caused by chlamydia or ureaplasma urealyticum. A strong association with HLA B27 haplotype exists. Approximately 2% of patients will develop an acute anterior uveitis. The conjunctivitis is self-limited. Treatment of the anterior uveitis involves topical steroids and cycloplegics.[7]

Inflammatory Bowel Disease

Inflammatory bowel disease is characterized by a peripheral arthritis in association with regional enteritis (Crohn's) or ulcerative colitis.[14] Ocular findings include episcleritis, scleritis, keratitis, and iritis. The anterior uveitis may be acute or chronic and is more commonly seen with ulcerative colitis (10%) compared to Crohn's (2%).[15] Posterior segment findings may include vitritis, retinal vasculitis, and optic neuritis.

Pediatric Sarcoidosis

Sarcoidosis is a noncaseating granulomatous multisystem disease of unknown etiology usually presenting in adults. Although the disease is considered relatively rare in children, several hundred cases of sarcoid have been documented in children under 15 years of age. Pediatric sarcoid may be divided into two subgroups depending on the age of onset of disease.[16] Most cases of sarcoid occurring between the ages of 8 and 15 years have lung involvement, but joint involvement is rare. In contrast, cases of sarcoid beginning at age 5 or under are characterized by the triad of uveitis, arthropathy, and skin rash with pulmonary involvement in only one third of these cases. The arthritis is usually polyarticular and characterized by nontender effusions of the knees and wrists usually with little limitation of movement. Cutaneous involvement includes sarcoid-specific lesions that on biopsy reveal noncaseating granulomas and nonspecific lesions such as erythema nodosum.

As in adults, anterior uveitis is the most common manifestation of pediatric ocular sarcoid.[8] Posterior uveitis is much less frequently seen. Signs of anterior uveitis include eyelid granulomas, episcleritis, scleritis, conjunctival nodules, band keratopathy, granulomatous or nongranulomatous KPs, cells and flare, iris nodules, posterior synechiae, and cataract. Posterior segment manifestations include vitritis chorioretinal nodules and optic disc edema.

Laboratory tests to establish the diagnosis of sarcoid include (1) biopsy of an appropriate site such as enlarged lymph node, conjuctiva, skin lesion, lung or liver, and synovial fluid; (2) Kveim test (infrequently used because the testing agent is not commercially available); (3) radiologic studies including chest radiograph to identify hilar and/or paratracheal adenopathy, and hand bone radiograph to identify cystic lesions, and Gallium scan of head, neck, and chest to localize areas of active inflammation such as lungs, lacrimal gland, and parotids; and (4) biochemical tests including angiotensin converting enzyme (ACE), serum calcium, and 24-hour urinary calcium excretion. Of note, because ACE levels in normal children are higher than in normal adults, serum ACE activity in children must be compared to normal age-matched controls. Serum lysosyme levels, which generally parallel ACE activity, may also be elevated in patients with sarcoid. (Unlike ACE, lysosyme levels are not elevated in normal children.) Both elevated serum calcium and 24-hour urinary calcium excretion may be found due to increased production of 1,25 dihydroxy Vit-D by macrophages within granulomas.

The differential diagnosis of pediatric sarcoid includes JRA (differentiating features of JRA include usually pauciarticuar arthritis, ANA positivity, skin rash uncommon), juvenile ankylosing spondylitis (predominately involves males, HLA B-27 positive, negative ANA), juvenile psoriatic arthritis, Reiter's (triad of arthritis urethritis and conjunctivitis/iritis), Bechet's (necrotizing occlusive vasculitis characterized by recurrent aphthous ulcers of oral mucous membranes, skin lesions, ocular inflammation, and genital ulcerations), and VKH (ocular inflammation associated with neurological findings and cutaneous changes such as vitiligo alopecia and poliosis).

Treament of anterior uveitis usually involves the use of topical steroids and cycloplegics. Systemic steroids (beginning at a dose of 1 mg/kg/day) and subtenon methyl prednisolone injections are reserved for the more severe cases of anterior uveitis or for patients manifesting posterior segment involvement. For cases that are steroid resistant or require chronic steroid therapy or for patients who are steroid intolerant, other immunosuppressive agents such as cyclosporin chlorambucil or methotrexate have had a positive therapeutic effect. Pediatric sarcoid uveitis is frequently asymptomatic, and therefore minimal follow-up every 3 months is advisable.

Fuchs' Heterochromic Iridocyclitis

Although typically presenting in the 3rd and 4th decades of life, Fuchs' can involve patients of all ages.[17] Cases are typically unilateral, although bilateral cases have been described. Clinical features include an externally quiet eye, nonpigmented diffuse small KPs with fine cotton wisp-like filaments connecting the KPs, mild anterior chamber inflammation, iris heterochromia with the involved eye being lighter in color secondary to stromal iris atrophy, occasional iris nodules, and posterior subcapsular cataract formation. Anterior chamber angle abnormalities include peripheral anterior synechiae, membrane formation, and /or angle neovascularization. Of note, posterior synechiae are generally absent. The fundus is usually normal, although peripheral inactive chorioretinal scars have been described.

The differential diagnosis includes heterochromia and inflammation secondary to a metallic intraocular foreign body, melanoma of the iris, inflammation and stromal atrophy secondary to a herpetic related uveitis, Horner's syndrome, Posner Schlossman syndrome, and pars planitis.

There is no known effective treatment for Fuchs'. Although generally ineffective, a trial of topical steroids may be attempted to control intraocular inflammation. Topical steroids are effective in reducing the density of KPs, which commonly are responsible for decreased vision. Dilation therapy is unnecessary because posterior synechiae generally do not develop. The two main complications of Fuchs' include cataract formation (50%) and secondary open angle glaucoma (15 to 30%). Cataract surgery is generally successful, although an increased rate of postoperative complications including hyphema, refractory glaucoma, and progressive vitreous opacification have been reported. The secondary glaucoma may be medically controlled but ultimately often requires filtration surgery with antimetabolites.

Kawasaki Disease

Kawasaki disease is an idiopathic systemic inflammatory illness of children, characterized by fever, cervical lymphadenopathy, oral mucosal erythema (e.g., strawberry tongue), and a desquamative exanthem of the hands and feet. Anterior ocular manifestations include bilateral bulbar conjunctival injection (found in 90% of cases), subconjunctival hemorrhage, superficial keratitis, and acute nongranulomatous iridocyclitis (66 to 80% of cases).[18,19] Posterior ocular changes include vitreous opacities and papilledema.

The anterior iridocyclitis usually resolves without treatment although in severe cases topical steroids may be used to prevent complications.

Intermediate Uveitis

Intermediate uveitis (formerly known as pars planitis, peripheral uveitis, or chronic cyclitis) represents an anatomic classification of ocular inflammation rather than a distinct clinical entity.[20] Although typically affecting patients in their teens, intermediate uveitis is also a common cause of idiopathic childhood uveitis, accounting for up to 20% of cases.[21] Approximately 70 to 80% of cases are bilateral.[22]

Patients generally present with complaints of floaters and blurred vision. Less characteristic is a presentation characterized by photophobia, pain, tearing, and redness, which may occur when anterior segment inflammation is prominent. Typically the focus of inflammation is in the vitreous and peripheral retina. In adults signs of anterior chamber inflammation are minimal or absent, and the absence of posterior synechiae formation is characteristic. In children, however, anterior segment inflammation is more commonly seen with moderate to severe cells and flare, KPs, band keratopathy, and formation of posterior synechiae. The vitreous demonstrates vitreous cells, debris, and snowballs (aggregates of inflammatory cells) usually more prominent in the anterior and inferior vitreous cavity. As the disease progresses a gelatinous fibroglial mass (snowbank) may be noted over the inferior pars plana, which may extend over the ora serrata and peripheral retina. A snowbank is not required for the clinical diagnosis of intermediate uveitis but is a necessary clinical finding for the subgroup diagnosis of pars planitis. Another fundus finding is a perivasculitis (venules > arterioles), most common in the retinal periphery.

Common complications include cataract formation, cystoid macula edema (most common cause of decreased vision), and neovascularization of the peripheral retina (especially the snowbank) or optic nerve leading to vitreous hemorrhage.

Other uveitis conditions that may present as an intermediate uveitis include sarcoidosis, Lyme, demyelinating disease, Whipple's disease, toxocariasis, IBD, HTLV-1 infection, and intraocular large cell lymphoma.[23] There is no specific diagnostic test to confirm the diagnosis of idiopathic intermediate uveitis. However, to exclude other diagnostic possibilities, an initial workup should include chest radiograph, PPD, ACE, Lyme titer, and VDRL-FTA. A flourescein angiogram may be performed to determine if macula edema is present. Additional studies such as Toxocara titers or a gastrointestinal (IBD) or neurological workup (multiple sclerosis, lymphoma) can be contemplated depending on the elicited history.

Because intermediate uveitis often has a benign course, most experts favor treatment only in eyes with 20/40 or worse vision or in patients who complain of severe floaters. Others favor initiation of antiinflammatory therapy even in eyes with better than 20/40 vision in the belief that early aggressive antiinflammatory therapy improves the long-term visual prognosis. The mainstay of treatment involves the use of systemic or periocular steroids.[24] If the disease is unilateral, injections of subtenon methylprednisolone acetate (40 mg) are recommended every 2 to 4 weeks, depending on the response. In patients with bilateral disease or who are unable to tolerate injections, prednisone is given orally usually starting at a dose of 1 mg/kg. This dosage is continued for 10 to 14 days, at which time a slow taper is begun until the minimum dosage needed to control the inflammation is found. During the slow taper, conversion to alternate day therapy can be attempted to help minimize the undesirable side effects of steroids. If there is either intolerance or inadequate response to steroid therapy, an immunosuppressive drug such as cyclosporin can be added to the antiinflammatory regimen. If medical therapy fails, cryotherapy to the area of pars plana involvement may be attempted.[25] One or two rows of cryotherapy are applied under direct visualization utilizing a single or double freeze-thaw technique (cryotherapy may also be used to treat complicating peripheral retinal neovascularization). In cases resistant to cryotherapy or if the decision is made to bypass cryotherapy (secondary to the reported increased incidence following cryotherapy of proliferative vitreoretinopathy and retinal detachment) a pars plana vitrectomy to remove inflammatory debris should be considered.

■ Noninfectious Causes of Posterior Uveitis

Vogt-Koyanagi Harada Syndrome

VKH is an idiopathic uveomeningeal syndrome characterized by bilateral panuveitis with exudative serous retinal detachments in association with meningeal and cutaneous manifestations.[26] Cutaneous findings that usually occur weeks to months after onset of ocular disease include poliosis vitiligo and alopecia. Neurological findings may precede or occur at the onset of the disease and may include headache, stiff neck, confusion, convulsions, ataxia, cranial nerve palsies, tinnitus, and deafness.

The disease typically affects darkly pigmented races (Asians, Hispanics, American Indians, and blacks). The disease is most common in the 20- to 50-year age group but has been reported in children as young as 7 years of age.

The first stage of the disease, which may last several days, is called the prodromal phase and is characterized by neurological symptoms such as headache, neck pain, vertigo, and dysacousia. The uveitic phase (which may last several weeks) follows shortly thereafter and is manifested by bilateral granulomatous anterior and posterior segment inflammation. The anterior segment findings include cell and flare, mutton fat KPs, iris nodules, and posterior synechiae. A vitritis is almost always present. The fundus shows optic nerve swelling and hyperemia and a diffuse multifocal choroiditis frequently resulting in exudative retinal detachments. The convalescent phase is characterized by depigmentation of the choroid and skin leading to a "sunset glow" fundus appearance and perilimbal vitiligo (Sugiuras sign). Scattered punctate-like areas of chorioretinal atrophy are seen representing regressed Dalen Fuchs nodules. The final phase is called the chronic recurrent phase and is characterized by chronic panuveitis with recurrent exacerbation of anterior segment inflammation. Common complications of VKH include glaucoma, cataract formation, and choroidal neovascularization.

The diagnosis of VKH is primarily clinical and is based on the presence of at least three of the following four clinical criteria: cutaneous findings, neurological findings, anterior uveitis, and posterior uveitis. Laboratory studies to consider include a lumbar puncture, which in over 80% of cases reveals a lymphocytic pleocytosis. A flourescein angiogram can be performed to document the presence of choroiditis and serous retinal detachments. Ultrasonography can be used to demonstrate low to medium reflective thickening of the choroid (in contrast to scleritis where high reflective choroidal thickening is seen).

Treatment of anterior uveitis involves the use of topical steroids and cycloplegics. If necessary periocular and/or systemic steroid therapy can be used to control the anterior segment inflammatory reaction. Posterior uveitis should be treated with oral prednisone in the range of 1 to 2 mg/kg/d followed by a slow taper over several months. Maintenance doses may be required for months to years to prevent recurrences. For steroid-resistant or -intolerant cases, cyclosporin cyclophosphamide or Azathioprin has been utilized to control intraocular inflammation. Laser treatment may be necessary for choroidal neovascularization threatening central vision.

■ Bechets

Bechets is an idiopathic recurrent multisystem inflammatory occlusive vasculitis that has worldwide distribution but is especially common in the Far East and Mediterranean countries. It is an uncommon cause of uveitis in the pediatric-age population.[27] In adults the disease is more common in males with peak onset between ages 20 and 40. Although during the early phases ocular involvement may be unilateral, the disease becomes bilateral in over 90% of patients. The diagnosis is made on the basis of manifesting a certain combination of clinical symptoms, which are classified as either major or minor criteria. The complete Bechet type manifests all four major criteria, which include recurrent aphthous ulcers of oral mucous membranes, skin lesions (e.g., erythema nodosum), ocular inflammation, and genital ulcers (usually affecting the scrotum or vulva). In the incomplete type patients manifest typical ocular disease and one other major criterion or three minor criteria. Minor criteria include arthritis most commonly affecting the knee joint, ileocecal intestinal ulcers, epididymitis, vascular occlusive disease, and neurological symptoms (neuro-Bechets) such as meningoencephalitis, brainstem syndromes, cranial nerve palsies, and pyramidal and extrapyramidal signs.

Ocular involvement is characterized by recurrent attacks of intraocular inflammation, with the majority of patients having either a panuveitis or only posterior segment involvement.[28] Anterior segment findings include nongranulomatous iridocyclitis with fine KPs, flare and cells, transient hypopyon in up to 30% of cases, posterior synechiae, anterior synechiae, and iris atrophy. Trace to mild vitreous inflammation is present. Retinal findings include edema of the optic nerve, localized patches of retinal edema most often in the macula region, whitish retinal infiltrates (pathognomonic), venous dilation, sheathing, yellowish-white exudates, and retinal hemorrhages. Repeated episodes ultimately lead to an atrophic optic nerve and retina with sheathed arteries and veins.

The diagnosis of Bechets disease is primarily clinical and is made on the manifestation of specific clinical criteria. History taking should include ancestry and country of origin due to the high incidence of this disease among patients from the Mediterranean basin and Far East. Also of note is the strong association of the HLA-B5 and HLA -B51 (a subset of B5) haplotype in Japanese patients with Bechets. The pathergy skin test may also be useful because an indurated erythematous lesion occurs in 40% of patients following a needle prick or intradermal injection of saline. Fluorescein angiogram may reveal areas of marked capillary dropout and dye leakage from retinal veins and peripapillary capillaries.

The treatment and its success are difficult to assess due to the natural course of the disease, which is characterized by exacerbations and remissions of varying duration and frequency. The anterior uveitis generally responds to topical steroids and cycloplegics.[29] For posterior segment disease a variety of agents have been employed. Oral prednisone at 1 to 2 mg/kg for 5 to 7 days with a gradual tapering schedule may be used during an acute attack. However, a state of resistance eventually develops, at which time steroids not only lose effectiveness but are felt by some Japanese authorities to cause an actual increase in number and severity of recurrences. Immunosuppressive agents such as cyclosporin, Tacrolimus chlorambucil, azathioprin, and cyclophosphamide have all been used with varying degrees of success. Despite aggressive treatment the long-term prognosis for vision in patients with posterior segment disease is poor.

■ Infectious Etiologies of Pediatric Uveitis

Congenital syphilis is caused by transplacental infection by the spirochete *Treponema pallidum.* A characteristic fundus appearance of a finely pigmented "salt and pepper" retinopathy is seen in the first few months of life. A bilateral interstitial keratitis and anterior uveitis usually occuring between the ages of 5 and 25 years may occur as a late manifestation of congenital disease.[30] Although the optimal treatment regimen is unknown, 10 to 14 days of intravenous aqueous penicillin G 2 to 4 million units every 4 hours is recommended.

Congenital cytomegalovirus is present in up to 0.5% of all live births and presents with either no symptoms or a nonspecific viral syndrome. Systemic features include fever, pneumonitis, and thrombocytopenia. **Central** nervous system involvement may cause cerebral periventricular calcifications, deafness, and seizures. Ocular features include optic nerve atrophy, hypoplasia and coloboma, microphthalmos or anophthalmos, cataracts, and a multifocal **retinochoroiditis** (most common feature) resembling toxoplasmosis.[31,32]

Congenital rubella syndrome is extremely uncommon in the United States because of the widespread use of the rubella vaccine. Systemic features include congenital heart disease, deafness, microcephaly, and mental retardation. The most common ocular feature is the retinopathy characterized by a salt and pepper fundus appearance. Other ocular features include corneal edema, cataract, glaucoma, and microphthalmos.[33] The diagnosis in neonates can be established by the presence of IgM antibodies to the rubella virus.

Mumps is caused by a paramyxovirus and is primarily a disease of childhood. Common systemic features include swelling of the parotid glands (parotitis), orchitis, and meningitis. Ocular findings include a dacryoadenitis (most common ocular feature), conjunctivitis, keratitis, anterior uveitis, and optic neuritis.[34] The anterior uveitis generally responds to treatment with topical steroids and cycloplegics.

Viral infections with measles, influenza, and Epstein-Barr (infectious mononucleosis) may be complicated by a transient mild anterior uveitis. Topical steroids are generally unnecessary, although for severe inflammation topical steroids may be required.

Subacute sclerosing panencephalitis is a rare complication of measles virus infection. The systemic disease is characterized by behavioral changes, declining mental capabilities, and myoclonic seizures. The most common ocular feature involves either pigmentary changes or a focal retinitis involving the macula, papilledema, and optic atrophy.[35] The disease is invariably fatal.

Tuberculosis is a chronic granulomatous infection caused by *Mycobacterium tuberculosis*. In developing countries, up to 32% of uveitis in children may be due to tuberculosis. Ocular tuberculosis usually presents as a granulomatous or less commonly nongranulomatous iridocyclitis, choroiditis, or retinal periphlebitis.[36–40] The diagnosis is usually presumptive (due to the lack of histological or microbiologic confirmation) and is based on a positive PPD skin test and/or chest X-ray consistent with exposure to *M. tuberculosis*. The therapy of uveitis secondary to ocular tuberculosis is systemic and involves the use of at least three antituberculous drugs such as INH, rifampin, and pyrazinamide. Systemic steroids prolong the disease course and should not be used in treating ocular tuberculosis.

Ocular Lyme borreliosis is caused by infection with the spirochete *Borrelia burgdorferi*.[41] The vector is the deer tick Ixodes. Relevant history includes hiking in wooded areas (endemic for Lyme) with high grass, tick bite, or characteristic skin rash (erythema migrans). Systemic findings include erythema migrans, cardiac conduction abnormalities, neurological complications, especially seventh nerve palsies, and arthritis.[42,43] Ocular findings may include conjuctivitis, episcleritis, keratitis, iridocyclitis, pars planitis, intermediate uveitis, and retinal vasculitis.[44] The diagnosis is presumed and is made on the basis of compatible history, clinical findings, and positive antibody titers to *B. burgdorferi*. Antibody testing has a high rate of false-positives due to common cross-reacting bacterial and spirochete antigens. To increase specificity, positive specimens should also be tested by a Western immunoblot. Treatment of mild ocular disease may respond to oral amoxicillin, but definitive treatment involves intravenous ceftriaxone.

Keratouveitis caused by herpes simplex is diagnosed by characteristic corneal dendrites or more commonly a stromal or disciform keratitis associated with anterior chamber inflammation.[45,46] Of note, uveitis may also occur without evidence of concomitant active corneal disease. Herpetic keratouveitis is commonly complicated by posterior synechiae, hyphema, and hypopyon. Secondary glaucoma is common and may prove refractory to medical management.[47] Treatment of keratouveitis involves topical antiviral therapy with trifluidine (viroptic), topical steroids, and cycloplegic agents to prevent posterior synechiae formation.

Varicella-zoster virus (VZV) in children may cause a keratouveitis in the setting of a chickenpox infection or herpes zoster ophthalmicus (HZO).[48] HZO in childhood probably represents reactivation of latent VZV acquired transplacentally from varicella infection of the mother during pregnancy. As in adults ocular involvement is uncommon unless the nasociliary branch is involved (manifested by vesicles affecting the tip or side of the nose). Ocular manifestations include dendritic stromal or disciform keratitis, mild to severe iritis with medium to large KPs, "moth eaten" iris stromal atrophy, hyphema, and hypopyon.[49] Anterior vitreous cells may be present, but the fundus is usually normal. The anterior uveitis occurs from ischemia secondary to vascular occlusion. HZO uveitis may be complicated by posterior synechiae formation cataract and glaucoma. Topical steroids should be used to control the anterior uveitis with slow taper to prevent rebound inflammation.[50] Low-dose chronic topical steroids may occasionally be necessary to prevent recurrent inflammation. Cycloplegics should be used to prevent posterior synechiae formation. Currently there are no definitive data regarding the value of using systemic acyclovir to prevent or mitigate the severity of the ocular disease.

Ocular Toxoplasmosis

Toxoplasmosis is caused by the cat parasite *Toxoplasma gondii* and represents the most common cause of posterior uveitis in children. Ocular toxoplasmosis is almost always congenital (an uninfected seronegative female seroconverts during pregnancy and passes the infection transplacentally to the fetus).[51] Maternal infection is caused by exposure to cat feces or by the ingestion of undercooked meat contaminated with tissue cysts. The severity of fetal involvement depends on when during pregnancy the infection occurs. Although early infection may result in severe central nervous system disease,

infection acquired during the third trimester may lead only to healed chorioretinal lesions at birth and unless there is macula involvement generally goes undetected. Patients become symptomatic due to recurrences that appear in the form of an active satellite lesion adjacent to an old chorioretinal scar.

Toxoplasmosis usually becomes active in only one eye at a time. During a recurrence of ocular toxoplasmosis the anterior segment may demonstrate Kps cells and flare, all due to spillover from the posterior segment.[52] The classic fundus lesion is a focal area of exudative retinitis usually greater than 1DD adjacent to an old chorioretinal scar with overlying vitritis (headlight in the fog). Sheathing of retinal vessels may be seen in the area of an active lesion. Less commonly serous retinal elevation may be seen associated with large active lesions. Papillitis may also occur due to retinitis in the papillary or juxtapapillary area. A deep outer retinal form of ocular toxoplasmosis with minimal or no vitreal reaction and small multifocal outer retinal lesions usually in the paramacular area has also been described.[53]

The diagnosis of ocular toxoplasmosis is made by serologic evidence of previous exposure to toxoplasmosis and a characteristic fundus lesion. Any titer even in undiluted serum is significant.[54] Because treatment may involve the use of systemic steroids a chest X-ray, PPD should be obtained to exclude tuberculosis.

In immunocompetent patients, recurrences are self-limited and may not require any therapeutic intervention. Treatment is needed only for lesions that threaten the macula, involve the optic nerve or papillomacular bundle, or have an associated severe vitritis.[55] Treatment continues for 4 to 6 weeks and includes pyrimethamine (1 mg/kg/d up to a maximum dose of 25 mg/d) or clindamycin (15 mg/kg/d up to a maximum dose of 1200 mg/d in four divided doses) used in combination with sulfadiazine (100 mg/kg/d up to a maximum dose of 4 g/d in four divided doses). If sulfadiazine cannot be obtained bactrim is an effective substitute. If pyrimethamine is used folinic acid must be given to prevent bone marrow depression. In addition pretreatment and weekly complete blood count with platelets should be drawn. Pyrimethamine should be discontinued if any drop in blood cell or platelet count is noted. Prednisone beginning with 1 mg/kg should be used for 7 to 10 days with gradual tapering to 30 mg every other day by 1 month. This dose is maintained until cessation of treatment at 6 weeks. Of note steroids should never be used without the use of concomitant antiparasitic therapy.

Ocular Toxocariasis

Ocular toxocariasis is caused by hematogenous invasion of the eye by the larva of the intestinal roundworm of dogs, *Toxocara canis*, and occasionally by the feline, *T. cati*. Transmission to humans occurs by ingestion of soil or food contaminated with ova shed in dog or cat feces. Ova hatch in the small intestine, penetrate the small intestine, and reach various organs such as the liver, brain, lung, and eyes. *T. canis* is present in more than 80% of puppies, and 10 to 30% of soil samples from playgrounds are contaminated with *Toxocara* eggs. Thus, risk factors for infection include contact with dogs and ingestion of soil or dirt. Ocular toxocariasis is typically found in children (mean age 7.5 years) and is almost always unilateral.

At least three distinct clinical presentations are recognized: endophthalmitis (most common form), posterior pole retinochoroidal granuloma, and peripheral retinochoroidal granuloma (simulating pars planitis).[56] In the endophthalmitis form the presenting sign is often leukocoria.[57] Granulomatous anterior segment inflammation is seen. The anterior vitreous demonstrates a dense vitritis. A peripheral or posterior pole granuloma may occasionally be seen through the dense vitreous haze. Complications of the endophthalmitis form include cataract, cyclitic membrane formation, and retinal detachment. In the posterior pole and peripheral granuloma presentations, minimal inflammation may be seen overlying a round, elevated, yellow–white solitary granuloma (0.5 to 4 disc diameters in size). In the later stages, traction bands extending from the granuloma to the posterior pole develop producing retinal folds, macula heterotopia, and occasionally retinal detachment. Ocular toxocariasis should be considered in the differential diagnosis of leukocoria. Other disease entities to consider include retinoblastoma, Coats' disease, persistent hypertrophic primary vitreous (PHPV), retinopathy of prematurity (ROP), pars planitis, toxoplasmosis, and familial exudative vitreoretinopathy (FEV). Retinoblastoma patients are usually diagnosed before the age of 2 years and have no inflammation, cataract, or cyclitic membrane. Coats' is a retinal vascular disease characterized by retinal telangiectasis associated with intraretinal exudation and, like retinoblastoma, has no associated inflammation. PHPV is usually diagnosed during the first few weeks of life and is associated with microphthalmia and prominent ciliary processes that are pulled into a retrolental mass. ROP is almost always bilateral and associated with a history of prematurity, low birth weight, and the use of supplemental oxygen. Pars planitis is usually bilateral and, although associated with inflammation and a snowbank, does not develop a distinct retinochoroidal mass. Toxoplasmosis patients will typically have inactive chorioretinal scars adjacent to an active satellite of acute retinitis. In addition healed toxoplasmosis scars are flat or depressed in contrast to the slightly elevated lesions of *Toxocara*. Finally FEV is usually bilateral, typically has no associated inflammation, and because of its autosomal dominant inheritance will frequently affect other family members.

The definitive diagnosis of *Toxocara* requires the demonstration of *Toxocara* larvae in the eye. This criterion for diagnosis is rarely satisfied. Typically, a history of pica and contact with puppies is elicited. An ELISA test for evidence of exposure to *Toxocara* should be performed. A titer of 1 : 8 is considered positive, but lower titers may also be significant. In atypical cases when the diagnosis is in question due to negative serum titers, aqueous or vitreous samples can also be checked for antibody titers. The demonstration of eosinophils in the aqueous or vitreous helps confirm the diagnosis. Ultrasound is helpful to exclude retinoblastoma and PHPV. Stool for ova and parasites is not useful because the larvae do not mature in the human intestine.

In patients with minimal to absent inflammation, no treatment is required. For anterior segment inflammation, topical prednisolone acetate and cycloplegics should be used as necessary. For inflammation involving the pars plana and posterior segment, subtenon injections of methylprednisolone can be given. Alternatively oral prednisone can be administered with gradual tapering. The role of antihelminthic agents such as thiabendazole and diethylcarbamazine is unclear. They should be used only in conjunction with oral corticosteroids. Pars plana vitrectomy may be used for severe intraocular inflammation unresponsive to medical management. Pars plana vitrectomy and/or scleral buckling may be necessary to repair *Toxocara*-related tractional or rhegmatogenous retinal detachment.

Ocular Complications in AIDS Patients

In the pediatric age group, AIDS most commonly occurs in newborns of affected mothers and in patients with hemophilia who have received tainted blood transfusions. Common ocular complications include HIV retinopathy (manifested by cotton wool spots and occasionally intraretinal hemorrhages), cytomegalovirus (CMV) retinitis, and toxoplasmosis retinochoroiditis.[58,59] In addition, acute retinal necrosis (which typically affects adults) has been reported in patients as young as 9 years of age.[60]

CMV retinitis is generally accompanied with only minimal anterior segment and vitreous inflammation. The characteristic CMV lesion is a granular or fluffy whitish-yellow retinal lesion with or without associated retinal hemorrhage.[61] The disease tends to progress in a perivascular distribution. Older lesions spread to involve previously normal retina leading to a "brushfire" appearance with retinal pigment epithelium (RPE) stippling centrally surrounded by the advancing edges of the lesion, which are white with associated retinal hemorrhages. When the disease reaches end stage the fundus is characterized by a pale optic nerve, atrophic retina, and narrow sheathed retinal vessels.

Treatment of CMV retinitis involves antiviral therapy with gancyclovir and/or foscarnet. Because these agents are virostatic, therapy in HIV-infected patients must be continued for life. Although 80% of patients initially demonstrate clinical regression or stabilization of disease, reactivation of the disease may occur in up to 50% of patients despite aggressive maintenance therapy with antivirals.

Acute retinal necrosis (ARN) is a necrotizing retinitis caused by members of the herpes virus family including herpes simplex, zoster, and CMV.[60] Bilateral involvement occurs in one third of cases (BARN). Although initially described in otherwise healthy patients, ARN has subsequently been commonly identified in immunocompromised hosts. The diagnosis is made on the basis of history and physical findings. Clinically, the anterior segment may demonstrate a mild to severe inflammatory reaction. The posterior segment findings include a retinal vasculitis primarily involving arteries, a mild to severe vitritis, and multifocal yellowish white patches of retinitis usually located between the midperiphery and ora serrata that eventually coalesce. Acute optic nerve edema and macula edema may also be seen during the acute stage of the disease. In contrast to CMV, retinal hemorrhage is not a prominent finding.

Treatment of ARN involves intravenous administration of acyclovir for 10 days followed by oral acyclovir for 4 to 6 weeks. Although of unproven efficacy, aspirin may be used to help prevent the vaso-obstructive complications. Topical and orally administered steroids may be used to suppress anterior segment and vitreous inflammation, respectively. As lesions regress and if visualization permits, laser photocoagulation may be performed posterior to necrotic retina to help prevent development of a retinal detachment. Due to full-thickness retinal necrosis and vitreous fibrosis, 75% of patients develop rhegmatogenous detachments with varying degrees of proliferative vitreoretinopathy. Scleral buckling and/or pars plana vitrectomy techniques should be used to repair ARN-related retinal detachments.

REFERENCES

1. Smith RE, Nozik RA. *Uveitis: A Clinical Approach to Diagnosis and Management*, 2nd ed. Baltimore: Williams & Wilkins; 1989:8–13.
2. Nussenblatt RB, Whitcup SM, Palestine AG. *Uveitis: Fundamentals and Clinical Practice*, 2nd ed. Chicago: Mosby Year Book; 1996:51–90.
3. Tabbara F, Nussenblatt RB. *Posterior Uveitis: Diagnosis and Management*. Newton, MA: Butterworth-Heinemann; 1994: 153–159.

4. Weiss MJ, Krause D. Uveitis. In: Vrabec MP, Florakis GF, eds. *Ophthalmic Essentials.* Cambridge, Mass: Blackwell Scientific; 1992:184–190.

5. Nussenblatt RB, Palestine AG, Chan CC, Roberge F. Standardization of vitreal inflammatory activity in intermediate and posterior uveitis. *Ophthalmology.* 1985; 92:467–471.

6. Kanski JJ. Juvenile arthritis and uveitis. *Surv Ophthalmol.* 1990;34(4):253–267.

7. Kanski JJ, Shun-Shin GA. Systemic uveitis syndromes in childhood: an analysis of 340 cases. *Ophthalmology.* 1984;91(10):1247–1252.

8. Giles CL. Uveitis in Childhood. 1. Anterior. *Ann Ophthalmol.* 1989;21:13–28.

9. Kanski JJ. Screening for uveitis in juvenile chronic arthritis. *Br J Ophthalmol* 1989;73:225–228.

10. Hemadt RK, Baer JC, Foster CS. Immunosuppressive drugs in the management of progressive corticosteroid resistant uveitis associated with juvenile rheumatoid arthritis. *Int Ophthalmol Clin.* 1992;32:241–252.

11. Schaller, JG. Ankylosing spondylitis of childhood onset. *Arthritis Rheum.* 1977;20:398–401.

12. Southwood TR, et al. Psoriatic arthritis in children. *Arthritis Rheum.* 1989;32(8):1007–1013.

13. Ostler HB, Dawson CR, Schachter J, Englemen EP. Reiters syndrome. *Am J Ophthalmol.* 1971; 71(5):986–991.

14. Lindsley CB, Schaller JG. Arthritis associated with inflammatory bowel disease in children. *J Pediatr.* 1974;84:16–20.

15. Salmon JF, Wright JP, Murray AD. Ocular inflammation in Crohns disease. *Ophthalmol* 1991;98:480–484.

16. Hoover DL, Khan JA, Giangiacomo J. Pediatric ocular sarcoidosis. *Surv Ophthalmol.* 1986;30(4):215–228.

17. Liesegang TJ. Clinical features and prognosis in Fuchs uveitis syndrome. *Arch. Ophthalmol.* 1982; 102:1153–1155.

18. Ohno S, et al. Ocular manifestations of Kawasakis disease. *Am J Ophthalmol.* 1982;93:713–717.

19. Burns JC, Joffe L, Sargent RA, et al. Anterior uveitis associated with Kawasaki syndrome. *Pediatr Infect Dis.* 1985;4:258–261.

20. Brockhurst RJ, Schepens CL, Okamura ID. Peripheral uveitis: description, complications and differential diagnosis. *Am J Ophthalmol.* 1960;49:1257–1266.

21. Hogan MJ, Kimura SJ, O'Connor GR. Peripheral retinitis and chronic cyclitis in children. *Trans Ophthalmol Soc UK.* 1965;85:39–52.

22. Althaus C, Sundmacher R. Intermediate uveitis: epidemiology, age, and sex distribution. *Dev Ophthalmol.* 1992;23:9–14.

23. Dining WJ. Intermediate uveitis: history terminology definition pars plantis: systemic disease associations. *Dev Ophthalmol.* 1992;23:3–8.

24. Kaplan HJ. Intermediate uveitis—a four step approach to treatment. In: Saari KM, ed. *Uveitis Update.* Amsterdam: Excerpta Medica; 1984:169–172.

25. Schlagel TF, Weber JC. Treatment of pars planitis. *Surv Ophthalmol.* 1977;22:120–130.

26. Moorthy RS, Inomata H, Rao NA. Vogt-Koyanagi-Harada syndrome. *Surv Ophthalmol.* 1995;39(4):265–292.

27. Michelson JB, Chisari FV. Bechets disease. *Surv Ophthalmol.* 1982;26(4):190–203.

28. Colvard DM, Robertson DM, O'Duffy JD. The ocular manifestations of Bechets disease. *Arch Ophthalmol.* 1977;95:1813–1817.

29. Whitcup SM, Salvo EC, Nussenblatt RB. Combined cyclosporin and corticosteroid treatment for sight threatening uveitis in Bechets disease. *Am J Ophthalmol.* 1994;118:39–45.

30. Margo CE, Hamed LM. Ocular syphilis. *Surv. Ophthalmol.* 1992;37(3):203–220.

31. Yoser SL, Forster, DJ, Rao NA. Systemic viral infections and their retinal and choroidal manifestations. *Surv Ophthalmol.* 1993;37(5):313–352.

32. Hennis HL, Scott AA, Apple DJ. Cytomegalovirus retinitis. *Surv Ophthalmol.* 1989;34(3):193–203.

33. Wolff SM. The ocular manifestations of congenital rubella. *Trans Am Ophthalmol Soc.* 1972;LXX:577–598.

34. Riffenburgh RS. Ocular manifestations of mumps. *Am J Ophthalmol.* 1961;66:739–743.

35. Robb RM, Watters GV. Ophthalmic manifestations of subacute sclerosing panencephalitis. *Arch Ophthalmol.* 1970;83:426–435.

36. Helm CJ, Holland GN. Ocular tuberculosis. *Surv Ophthalmol.* 1993;38(3):229–256.

37. Sen DK. Endogenous uveitis in Indian children: analysis of 94 cases. *J Pediatr Ophthalmol.* 1977;14:25–32.

38. Donahue HC. Ophthalmologic experience in a tuberculosis sanatorium. *Am J Ophthalmol.* 1967; 64(4): 742–748.

39. Rosen PH, Spalton DJ, Graham EM. Intraocular tuberculosis. *Eye.* 1990;4:486–492.

40. Ni C, Papale JJ, Robinson NL, Wu BF. Uveal tuberculosis. *Int Ophthalmol Clin.* 1982;22(3):103–124.

41. Winward KE, Smith JL, Culbertson WW, Hamelin AP. Ocular Lyme borreliosis. *Am J Ophthalmol.* 1989; 108: 651–657.

42. Karma A, et al. Diagnosis and clinical characteristics of ocular Lyme borreliosis. *Am J Ophthalmol.* 1994; 119: 127–135.

43. Winterkorn JKS. Lyme disease: neurologic and ophthalmic manifestations. *Surv Ophthalmol.* 1990; 35: 191–204.

44. Copeland RA Jr, Nozik RA, Shimokaji G. Uveitis in Lyme disease. *Ophthalmology.* 1989;107:127.

45. Dawson CR, Togni B. Herpes simplex eye infections: clinical manifestations, pathogenesis and management. *Surv Ophthalmol.* 1976;21(2):121–135.

46. Witmer R, Iwamoto T. Electron microscope observation of herpes-like particles in the iris. *Arch Ophthalmol.* 1968;79:331–337.

47. O'Connor GR. Recurrent herpes simplex in humans. *Surv Ophthalmol.* 1976;21:165–170.

48. Karbassi M, Raizman MB, Schuman JS. Herpes zoster ophthalmicus. *Surv Ophthalmol.* 1992;36(6):395–410.

49. Ostler HB, Thygeson P. The ocular manifestations of herpes zoster, varicella infectious mononucleosis and cytomegalovirus disease. *Surv Ophthalmol.* 1976; 21(2): 148–159.

50. Womack LW, Liesegang TJ. Complications of herpes zoster ophthalmicus. *Arch Ophthalmol.* 1983;101:42–45.

51. Perkins ES. Ocular toxoplasmosis. *Br J Ophthalmol.* 1973;57:1–15.

52. Giles CL. Uveitis in childhood. III. Posterior. *Ann Ophthalmol.* 1989;21:23–28.

53. Matthews JD, Weiter JJ. Outer retinal toxoplasmosis. *Ophthalmology.* 1988;95:941–946.

54. Weiss MJ, Velazquez N, Hofeldt AJ. Serologic tests in the diagnosis of toxoplasmic retinochoroiditis. *Am J Ophthalmol.* 1990;109:407–411.

55. O'Connor GR. Chemotherapy of toxoplasmosis and toxocariasis. In: Srinivasan BD, ed. *Ocular Therapeutics.* New York: Masson Publishing;1980;chap. 5:51–58.

56. Shields JA. Ocular toxocariasis: a review. *Surv Ophthalmol.* 1984;28(5):361–379.

57. Searl SS, Moazed K, Albert DM, Marcus LC. Ocular toxocariasis presenting as leukocoria in a patient with low ELISA titers to *Toxocara canis. Ophthalmology.* 1981; 88: 1302–1306.

58. de Smet MD. Ocular consequences of human immunodeficiency virus infection. *Ophthalmol Clin North Am.* 1993;6(1):117–126.

59. Dennehy PJ, Warman R, Flynn JT, Scott GB, Mastrucci MT. Ocular manifestations in pediatric patients with acquired immunodeficiency syndrome. *Arch Ophthalmol.* 1989;107:978–982.

60. Duker JS, Blumenkranz MS. Diagnosis and management of the acute retinal necrosis syndrome. *Surv Ophthalmol.* 1991;35(5):327–343.

61. Hennis HL, Scott AA, Apple DJ. Cytomegalovirus retinitis. *Surv Ophthalmol.* 1989;34(3):193–203.

18
■ ■ ■

Glaucomas

DAVID S. WALTON

Glaucoma in children is unusual; however, when intraocular disease is suspected in childhood the possibility of a primary or secondary elevation (or depression) of intraocular pressure must always be considered. Previously recognized causes of glaucoma in childhood are listed in Table 18–1. The diversity among these conditions should be noted.

■ Signs and Symptoms

The symptoms of childhood glaucoma are highly variable. Although some children are asymptomatic, others develop intense light sensitivity associated with corneal opacification, epiphora, and loss of vision. There may be a gradual occurrence of these problems, or alternatively a child may be asymptomatic for months and then develop these signs and symptoms acutely. Rapid elevation of eye pressure causes pain. Abnormal enlargement of the cornea and eye occurs in children under 3 years of age secondary to an elevated intraocular pressure. Review of past facial photographs often confirms the presence of this defect many months prior to its recognition by the child's parents. A cloudy cornea is the most common first sign of childhood glaucoma seen by parents or physicians in children with

unsuspected glaucoma (Fig. 18–1). When bilateral and slow in onset, it may be accepted as normal for many months. The loss of corneal transparency is caused by edema of the corneal epithelium and stroma. **Careful inspection of the cornea may reveal breaks in Descemet's membrane (Haab's striae), which is evidence for a raised intraocular pressure in early childhood** (Fig. 18–2).

Signs and Symptoms of Glaucoma

Signs and Symptoms of Glaucoma
Light sensitivity
Pain
Epiphora
Irritability
Vomiting
Cloudy cornea
Corneal enlargement
Elevated pressure

In addition to ocular signs and symptoms of glaucoma, secondary systemic abnormalities may occur and are especially common with acute glaucoma. Irritability, loss of appetite, and vomiting are seen and may be misunderstood before the ocular abnormality is recognized. Other systemic abnormalities may also provide information to help explain the cause of the pediatric glaucoma (Table 18–1).

TABLE 18–1. Table of Primary and Secondary Childhood Glaucomas

I. Primary glaucomas
  A. Congenital open-angle glaucoma
    1. Congenital
    2. Infantile
    3. Late recognized
  B. Autosomal dominant juvenile glaucoma
  C. Primary angle-closure glaucoma
  D. Associated with systemic abnormalities
    1. Sturge-Weber syndrome
    2. Neurofibromatosis (NF-1)
    3. Stickler's syndrome
    4. Oculocerebrorenal (Lowe's) syndrome
    5. Rieger's syndrome
    6. Hepatocerebrorenal syndrome
    7. Marfan syndrome
    8. Rubinstein-Taybi syndrome
    9. Infantile glaucoma associated with mental retardation and paralysis
    10. Oculodentodigital dysplasia
    11. Open-angle glaucoma associated with microcornea and absence of frontal sinuses
    12. Mucopolysaccharidosis
    13. Trisomy 13
    14. Cutis marmorata telangiectasia congenita
    15. Warburg syndrome
    16. Kniest syndrome (skeletal dysplasia)
    17. Michel's syndrome
    18. Nonprogressive hemiatrophy
  E. Associated with ocular abnormalities
    1. Congenital glaucoma with iris and pupillary abnormalities
    2. Aniridia
      a. Congenital glaucoma
      b. Acquired glaucoma
    3. Congenital ocular melanosis
    4. Sclerocornea
    5. Iridotrabecular dysgenesis
    6. Peters' syndrome
    7. Iridotrabecular dysgenesis and ectropion uveae
    8. Posterior polymorphous dystrophy
    9. Idiopathic or familial elevated episcleral venous pressure
    10. Anterior corneal staphylom
    11. Congenital microcoria with myopia
    12. Congenital hereditary endothelial dystrophy
    13. Congenital hereditary iris stromal hypoplasia

II. Secondary glaucomas
  A. Traumatic glaucoma
    1. Acute glaucoma
      a. Angle concussion
      b. Hyphema
      c. Ghost cell glaucoma
    2. Late-onset glaucoma with angle recession
    3. Arteriovenous fistula
  B. Secondary to intraocular neoplasm
    1. Retinoblastoma
    2. Juvenile xanthogranuloma
    3. Leukemia
    4. Melanoma
    5. Melanocytoma
    6. Iris rhabdomyosarcoma
    7. Aggressive nevi of the iris
  C. Secondary to uveitis
    1. Open-angle glaucoma
    2. Angle-blockage glaucoma
      a. Synechial angle closure
      b. Iris bombe with pupillary block
  D. Lens-induced glaucoma
    1. Subluxation-dislocation and pupillary block
      a. Marfan syndrome
      b. Homocystinuria
    2. Spherophakia and pupillary block
    3. Phacolytic glaucoma
  E. Secondary to surgery for congenital cataract
    1. Lens material blockage of the trabecular meshwork (acute or subacute)
    2. Pupillary block
    3. Chronic open-angle glaucoma associated with angle defects
  F. Steroid-induced glaucoma
  G. Secondary to rubeosis
    1. Retinoblastoma
    2. Coats' disease
    3. Medulloepithelioma
    4. Familial exudative vitreoretinopathy
  H. Secondary angle-closure glaucoma
    1. Retinopathy of prematurity
    2. Microphthalmos
    3. Nanophthalmos
    4. Retinoblastoma
    5. Persistent hyperplastic primary vitreous
    6. Congenital pupillary iris–lens membrane
  I. Glaucoma associated with increased venous pressure
    1. Carotid or dural-venous fistula
    2. Orbital disease
  J. Secondary to maternal rubella
  K. Secondary to intraocular infection
    1. Acute recurrent toxoplasmosis
    2. Acute herpetic iritis
  L. Ciliary block (malignant) glaucoma

■ Examination

Examination of children for glaucoma utilizes skills exercised in a complete pediatric eye examination. Prior to performing the ocular examination, it is necessary to obtain a detailed medical history. To perform the ocular exami- nation, the examiner must have appropriate instruments and skill to perform the necessary assessments quickly and successfully. The exam- ination of the young glaucoma patient will often be performed in both an office and an operating room setting under anesthesia (examination under anesthesia [EUA]).

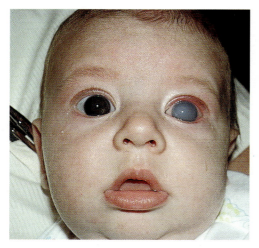

FIGURE 18–1. This 4-month-old developed sudden opacification of the left cornea, which was his first sign of congenital glaucoma. Bilateral corneal enlargement was also present.

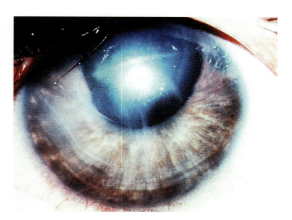

FIGURE 18–2. The cornea of this child with infantile glaucoma shows a central vertical break in Descemet's membrane associated with curvilinear peripheral corneal breaks.

Examination Instruments for Glaucoma

Focused flashlight
Hand-held slit lamp
Hand-held tonometer
Indirect ophthalmoscope
10 and 14D indirect lenses
Binocular loupe
Direct ophthalmoscope
Scleral transilluminator
Koeppe lens
Barkan viewing scope

The examination should begin with an estimate of vision (see Chapter 2). Is nystagmus present? Is there unusual avoidance of light? Strabismus? Pupillary reactivity should be noted. (This may be difficult if the corneas are cloudy or if the pupils are formed abnormally.) When possible, older children should have formal visual field testing.

Pediatric Glaucoma Examination

History
Observation for light sensitivity
Vision assessment
Anterior segment examination
   Cornea
   Anterior chamber
   Iris
   Pupil
Lens assessment
Fundoscopy
Gonioscopy
Tonometry
Ultrasonography

Inspection of the Anterior Segment

Ideally, young children are examined using a loupe and hand-held instruments. A formal slit lamp examination is usually possible in children 3 years of age and older. The corneal size is estimated, and any asymmetrical enlargement is noted. Measurement with a ruler is difficult in a young child. Asymmetric enlargement is more evident by inspection than by formal measurement.

The corneal clarity or presence of opacities should be noted. Corneal opacification related to increased pressure may be diffuse and/or localized. When diffuse, corneal edema is likely and may be associated with diffuse stromal opacification as well. Corneal edema causes a loss of corneal luster, reflections from the corneal surface are irregular, and an associated opacity at the level of Bowman's membrane may be present. A localized stromal opacity is usually associated with a break in Descemet's membrane. The opacity may be quite large, involving as much as half of the cornea. Localized stromal opacities associated with breaks in Descemet's membrane seen in newborn children are often very dense. The inspection of the cornea should include a careful inspection of Descemet's membrane. In older children, a break in Descemet's membrane is often associated with a clear cornea and may be the most certain evidence that a congenital glaucoma was present. Breaks in Descemet's membrane, appear as curvilinear parallel lines. During the inspection of Descemet's membrane, abnormal peripheral or central iridocorneal attachments should be identified. Diffuse irregular opacities associated with polymorphous corneal dystrophy should be ruled out.

Depth of the Anterior Chamber

Early glaucoma causes abnormal deepening of the anterior chamber associated with ocular enlargement.

Irides

Careful inspection of the irides is mandatory. The size, character, and reactivity of the pupils should be noted. Abnormally large pupils are seen with severe congenital glaucoma, whereas abnormally small pupils would be expected with Lowe syndrome. An ectropion uveae may be an isolated congenital iris defect with congenital glaucoma and be unilateral or bilateral or be associated with infantile glaucoma and neurofibromatosis (NF-1). The iris leaf should be carefully assessed. A normal iris is found with hereditary primary infantile glaucoma, whereas a quite abnormal stroma is expected with severe congenital glaucoma, hereditary iris hypoplasia and glaucoma, and certain secondary glaucomas. The abnormal convexity of the iris is an important sign of glaucoma secondary to pupillary blockage.

Lens

The lens is usually normal in most cases of pediatric glaucoma. Lowe syndrome is one cause of both cataracts and infantile glaucoma. Evidence of lens dislocation also should be assessed.

Additional Studies

Fundoscopy by direct or indirect ophthalmoscopy is important to assess the condition of the optic nerve head and to identify optic pallor or cupping. Opacification of the cornea may limit the reliability of this examination when a child is initially evaluated.

Tonometry is the most important component of the ocular examination of the child for glaucoma. Goldmann applanation tonometry for an older child is done as with an adult patient. The evaluation of the younger and less cooperative child takes more time and may be done with less confidence. With the assistance of the child's parent to encourage cooperation, it is usually possible to reliably measure a child's eye pressure (Fig. 18–3). To accomplish this a Schiotz, hand-held applanation or Tono-pen tonometer may be used. I prefer a hand-held applanation tonometer. This instrument allows accurate pressure measurements with the child in an upright position. Readings at moments of maximum cooperation can be easily selected and done repetitively.

Gonioscopy is a very important part of any examination for glaucoma. This exam may be difficult to perform in the office but if possible should be attempted. Koeppe gonioscopy or slit lamp gonioscopy can be attempted. I prefer the Koeppe technique for children. Careful qualitative assessment of the trabecular meshwork, scleral spur, and ciliary body band should be carried out.

Ultrasonography can add important information to the examination of a young child with glaucoma, which often may be accompanied by limited ability to view the posterior segment. Glaucoma is commonly present in eyes with advanced retinoblastoma and may also complicate Coats' disease, a ciliary body tumor, and a small percent of patients with a retinal detachment. In infancy, glaucoma commonly is seen with the progressive posterior segment defects of Norrie's disease.

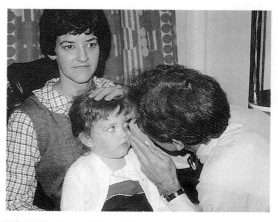

FIGURE 18–3. The office examination of a child with glaucoma often can include reliable tonometry. A hand-held applanation instrument is useful for this purpose.

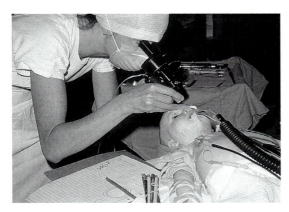

FIGURE 18–4. Kreppe gonioscopy is an important component of the operating room assessment of a child with glaucoma.

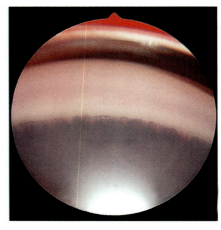

FIGURE 18–5. Gonioscopy at higher magnification (6× or 9×) utilizing a hand-held magnification unit can provide detailed information pertaining to the developmental status of the filtration angle.

Operating Room

EUA is an important component of the full assessment of any child with glaucoma.

Information to Be Obtained under EUA

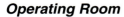

Intraocular pressure
Corneal height and width
Assessment of cornea
Assessment of anterior chamber
Assessment of irides gonioscopy
Assessment of lens
Assessment of vitreous
Dilated retinoscopy
Retinal status
Optic nerve

Careful assessment to determine the presence of uncontrolled glaucoma and its cause and the presence of associated abnormalities should not be postponed until the EUA.

General anesthesia agents directly alter the intraocular pressure. Ketamine anesthesia falsely elevates eye pressure readings. Many inhalation agents depress the pressure. The pressure must be obtained early in the induction with use of inhalation agents.

Gonioscopy is most effective and reliable under general anesthesia. Many types of gonioscopic lenses are now available and allow viewing of the angle by various techniques. For instance, a mirrored lens allows viewing with an operating room microscope. I prefer the direct view obtained using a Koeppe lens and hand-held microscope and viewing light (Figs. 18–4 and 18–5). This same viewing system can also be used in the office setting utilizing a loupe for magnification with less cooperative young patients (Fig. 18–6). Goniosurgery requires previous detailed gonioscopy to determine the specific type of glaucoma.

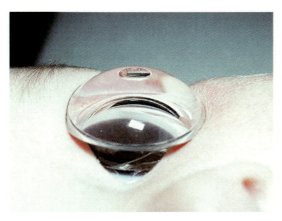

FIGURE 18–6. The direct view of the filtration angle obtained during an office examination and gonioscopy employing a loupe for additional magnification provides important information.

■ Differential Diagnosis

Only the confirmation of a persistent elevation of eye pressure establishes the diagnosis of glaucoma in a child. Most anterior segment defects seen in patients with glaucoma can occur without glaucoma or can be caused by other disease mechanisms.

Epiphora is seen with punctal or naso-lacrimal ductal obstruction or with miscellaneous causes of corneal irritation. Cloudiness of the cornea may be seen with storage diseases causing epithelial and/or stromal opacification; mucolipidosis type IV, for example, strongly suggests glaucoma because the clinical opacification is confined to the epithelium. Breaks in Descemet's membrane may also be seen with birth trauma caused by forceps. Extreme central positioning of Schwalbe's line may suggest a break in Descemet's membrane on initial inspection. Enlargement of the cornea may be seen with hereditary megalo-cornea and in Marfan syndrome. In some families larger corneas are characteristic; enlargement over 13 mm in the first year of life is exceptional for normal corneas.

A child may present with all the physical signs of infantile glaucoma, including residual stromal opacification, corneal enlargement, breaks in Descemet's membrane, deepening of the anterior chamber, abnormal gonioscopic findings, and disc cupping, but possess normal eye pressures. These findings may be present in one eye, with similar findings and glaucoma in the fellow eye. Such a clinical enigma is consistent with a spontaneous cure of intraocular pressure. A recurrence of glaucoma would not be expected. Eye pressures may also be normal for several weeks after birth in a child with obvious signs of congenital glaucoma. In this setting a return of elevated pressures would be expected.

After glaucoma is diagnosed it is important and helpful to use all the information now available from the history and physical examination to determine the type of pediatric glaucoma present (Table 18–1).

Response to treatment is not uniform between patients and in different types of pediatric glaucoma. The specific type of glaucoma present and the severity of the angle anomaly must be considered in the management of childhood glaucoma. The risk for either a primary or secondary glaucoma must be considered in the interpretation of the patient's glaucoma.

■ Primary Childhood Glaucoma

Congenital Open Angle Glaucoma

Congenital open angle glaucoma is the most common primary glaucoma seen in early childhood. Some patients are recognized shortly after birth, but diagnosis more often occurs between 3 and 9 months of age (Fig. 18–7). Cases are usually sporadic, and inheritance is thought to be consistent with polygenic or multifactorial inheritance. The gene defect has been linked to a gene defect on chromosome 1 p.[1]

The inherited defect seems confined to the filtration angle with other anterior segment abnormalities caused by the resultant eye pressure. Gonioscopy reveals an anterior positioning of the peripheral iris in many patients associated with opacification of tissues covering the ciliary body band area and scleral spur. This primary glaucoma typically responds well to goniosurgery.

Juvenile Open Angle Glaucoma

Juvenile open angle glaucoma is rare, bilateral, and acquired with significant pressure elevations, often beginning late in the first decade of life. Its inheritance is consistent with autosomal dominant inheritance, and the genetic defect has been linked to the chromosome 1 q.[2] Affected children are most often myopic. Gonioscopy is essentially normal; however,

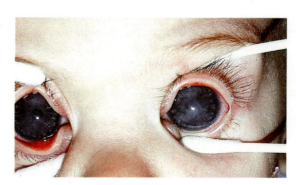

FIGURE 18–7. This child's infantile glaucoma was recognized at 10 months of age. Enlargement of each cornea is advanced, and diffuse corneal opacification is present, which is associated with multiple breaks in Descemet's membrane.

some patients possess an unusual number of fine iris processes. Some patients respond well to goniosurgery, whereas others will prove unresponsive and require filtration glaucoma surgery.

Primary Glaucoma Associated with Systemic Abnormalities

Sturge-Weber Syndrome

The Sturge-Weber syndrome is associated with an upper facial nevus flammeus and variable abnormal vascularity of the leptomeninges. Glaucoma may be congenital or acquired and is typically unilateral on the affected side of the face, but involvement may also be bilateral. Gonioscopy reveals a varied abnormality with decreased visibility of the scleral spur and level of insertion of the iris. Abnormal episcleral and conjunctival vessels are constant, and melanosis of the iris is common. Goniosurgery is usually not successful in controlling the eye pressure. Medical glaucoma treatment and filtration surgery are both often helpful.

Glaucoma is also seen with other systemic syndromes including neurofibromatosis, Lowe syndrome, Rieger's syndrome, and others (Table 18–1).

Primary Glaucoma Associated with Ocular Anomalies

Aniridia

Aniridia is an important eye disease frequently complicated by glaucoma. Congenital anomalies are present consisting of near complete absence of the iris, macular hypoplasia, small corneas, and filtration angle defects (Fig. 18–8). After birth, slowly progressive angle defects occur leading to obstruction of the trabecular meshwork. Cataract formation and progressive corneal opacification also complicate this condition. Aniridia is bilateral and demonstrates autosomal dominant transmission. Its gene has been cloned and is in the PAX6 region of chromosome 11 p.[3] Aniridia may occur secondary to a molecular genetic defect or be caused by a larger chromosomal deletion. Because of the proximity of the Wilms' tumor gene to the aniridia gene, chromosomal deletions put patients at risk for the development of this tumor and other systemic defects.

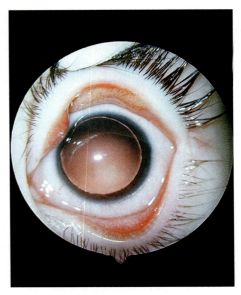

FIGURE 18–8. The ocular signs of aniridia, including near absence of the irides, are demonstrated in this young child. Note the clarity of both the cornea and the lens.

Early in life serial gonioscopy of aniridia patients may reveal a progressive forward shift of the peripheral iris stump over the trabecular meshwork. Goniosurgery to interrupt this development may be helpful.[4] Treatment of established aniridic glaucoma is difficult. Medical treatment and filtration surgery have been successful for some patients.

Peters' Anomaly

Peters' anomaly consists of a congenital central leukoma associated with absence of Descemet's membrane associated with attachments from its periphery to the iris stroma posteriorly. Corneolenticular attachments may also be present and may be associated with a central cataract. Glaucoma complicates a minority of patients with this anomaly. Peters' anomaly may be unilateral or bilateral and is most often sporadic, although autosomal dominant transmission may occur. This condition has also been associated with a defect in the PAX6 region of chromosome 11 p.[5]

Glaucoma may complicate other conditions expressing ocular anterior segment defects, including familial hypoplasia of the iris, posterior polymorphous dystrophy, and anterior iridotrabecular dysgenesis conditions.

■ Secondary Childhood Glaucoma

Glaucoma may complicate many childhood eye diseases and conditions (Table 18–1), which collectively represent the most common cause of childhood glaucoma. Management of a secondary glaucoma often requires control of the complicating eye pressure and treatment of the primary eye condition.

Trauma

Trauma to the anterior segment may cause immediate and secondary (delayed) hemorrhage. Glaucoma frequently complicates a secondary hemorrhage and may complicate the long term residual effects of injury to the trabecular meshwork. Glaucoma complicating a secondary hemorrhage may be initially treated medically, but paracentesis followed by anterior chamber washout is necessary if the pressure cannot be adequately controlled.

Neoplasia

The most frequent cause of glaucoma secondary to ocular tumor in childhood is retinoblastoma associated with rubeosis irides. Other causes include leukemia, lymphoma, and medulloepithelioma.

Chronic Anterior Uveitis

Chronic iridocyclitis is a relatively common cause of childhood glaucoma and complicates approximately one third of patients with this condition. Because patients are usually receiving topical steroids, their adverse effect on the eye pressure is often considered. Unlike a steroid induced glaucoma, gonioscopy usually reveals increased opacification of the trabecular meshwork inferiorly with fine synechiae to the ciliary body band and posterior trabecular meshwork. Medical glaucoma treatment is often helpful, but some cases will require surgical intervention. Goniosurgery can be of lasting benefit and should be considered.

Glaucoma Following Pediatric Cataract Surgery

Glaucoma following congenital cataract surgery may occur in the interval immediately after surgery secondary to pupillary block. More commonly, it occurs anytime thereafter, more insidiously, secondary to postoperative injury to the trabecular meshwork of undetermined cause. Typically, such glaucoma is recognized 1 to 3 years following lens surgery. Gonioscopy in such cases reveals abnormal forward insertion of the iris on the posterior trabecular meshwork. Medical treatment with a beta blocker or carbonic anhydrase inhibitor may be helpful, but surgery is usually required.

Other causes of secondary glaucoma in childhood include steroid glaucoma, lens induced glaucoma associated with lens subluxation, and pupillary block glaucoma associated with retinopathy of prematurity or microphthalmia.

■ Treatment of Childhood Glaucoma

Both medical and surgical treatment of glaucoma are employed for children. Systemic effects of drugs, even given topically, must be considered and parents carefully instructed in their administration and potential for complications.

Medical Treatment

Miotics are rarely indicated for children with glaucoma except to induce miosis when this is desired. Beta blocking agents are effective and usually can be given daily. **The most effective drug for childhood glaucoma is the carbonic anhydrase inhibitor acetazolamide.** A dose of 15 mg/kg/d may be administered. In children under 1 year of age a supplementary base seems helpful to lessen the metabolic acidosis. Sodium bicarbonate 1 mEq/kg/d or Bicitra 1 cc/kg/d may be administered to accomplish this goal. Topical dorzolamide may have a favorable effect on the eye pressure, but its beneficial effect usually is of short duration.

Surgical Management

Goniosurgery, filtration surgery, glaucoma implants procedures, iridotomy, cycloablation, and enucleation are types of procedures performed for childhood glaucoma. Of these techniques, only goniosurgery is now unique to childhood glaucoma surgery.

Goniotomy was first performed for children with congenital glaucoma by Barkan.[6] Approximately 80% of children with primary congenital open angle glaucoma can be cured with this procedure. External trabeculotomy is a procedure in which the trabeculum is excised as with a goniotomy but by way of an external approach.

Filtration surgery is often necessary for pediatric glaucomas unresponsive to goniotomy. Trabeculectomy is now the preferred procedure. Adjunctive use of an antimetabolite is often considered.

Placement of a glaucoma implant is an additional and important procedure for some resistant childhood glaucomas. It is especially useful in childhood aphakic glaucoma. In this procedure a small silicone tube is positioned in the anterior or posterior chamber and permanently attached to an external plate, which creates a reservoir from which aqueous humor is absorbed.

Cycloablative procedures utilizing laser energy or localized freezing produce permanent ciliary body injury and are done to decrease aqueous humor production to lessen eye pressure. Complications are frequent, and repeat procedures are often required.

Enucleation is indicated for deformed eyes that are painful, unsightly, and blind. Decision for enucleation is often delayed but represents an important treatment to benefit some children.

REFERENCES

1. Akarsu AN, Turacli ME, Altan SG, Barsoum-Homsy M, Cheverette L, Sayle BS, Sarfarazi M. A second locus (GLC3B) for primary congenital glaucoma (buphthalmos) maps to the 1p36 region. *Hum Mol Genet.* 1996; 5:1199–1203.

2. Sheffield VC, Stone EM, Alward WL, Drack AV, Johnson AT, Streb LN, Nichols BE. Genetic linkage of familial open angle glaucoma to chromosome 1 q21-q31. *Nature Genet.* 1993;4:47–50.

3. Ton CCT, et al. Positional cloning and characterization of a paired box- and homeobox-containing gene from the aniridia region. *Cell.* 1991;67:1059–1074.

4. Walton DS. Aniridic glaucoma: The results of goniosurgery to prevent and treat this problem. *Trans Am Ophthal Soc.* 1986;84:59–70.

5. Hanson IM, et al. Mutations at the PAX6 locus are found in heterogeneous anterior segment malformations including Peters' anomaly. *Nature Genet.* 1994; 6:168–173.

6. Barkan O. Techniques of goniotomy for congenital glaucoma. *Arch Ophthalmol.* 1949;41:65–82.

Pediatric Ophthalmology
Edited by P. F. Gallin
Thieme Medical Publishers, Inc.
New York © 2000

19

Leukocoria

STELLA DOUROS, SAN DEEP JAIN, B. DAVID GORMAN, AND ARTHUR M. COTLIAR

When white light enters the eye, it passes through the transparent ocular media (i.e., cornea, aqueous, lens, and vitreous) until it reaches the retina and choroid. The highly vascular choroid is responsible for the normal red fundus glow. The red reflex is the blurred illuminated image of the patient's retina that is formed in the pupillary plane.

Under normal circumstances, the pupil of a patient will appear black when examined with a penlight. The red reflex can be observed only when the observing eye and the illuminating point are coaxial. This alignment can be easily achieved by using a direct ophthalmoscope. The red reflex should be evaluated in a darkened room using a bright direct ophthalmoscope light. Normally the red reflex from both pupils should be symmetrical. Slight luminosity of the pupil may be seen with a penlight examination in highly hyperopic eyes and in pathological conditions where the retina is displaced

forward as in retinal detachment or an intraocular tumor. The emergent rays under these circumstances are divergent; therefore, it is not necessary for the observing eye to be coaxial, and the pupil will appear feebly illuminated even with a penlight examination (Figs. 19–1 and 19–2).

Leukocoria literally means "white pupil." It is a gross sign of intraocular pathology. Ocular conditions that interrupt the path of the light rays as they strike the vascular choroid may cause a whitish reflex to be produced at the pupil instead of the normal red reflex (Table 19–1). Because enucleation, chemotherapy, and radiation are favored treatments for malignant lesions such as retinoblastoma, the problem of differentiating nonmalignant lesions is more than academic.[1] Table 19–2 lists important differentiating features of common conditions that cause leukocoria. Leukocoria is an important clinical sign that should prompt an urgent

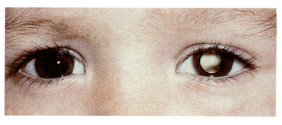

FIGURE 19–1. Unilateral leukocoria (left eye).

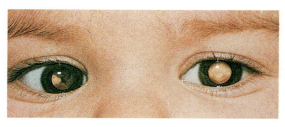

FIGURE 19–2. Bilateral leukocoria.

TABLE 19–1. Differential Diagnosis of Leukocoria

Congenital
    Cataracts
    Persistent hyperplastic primary vitreous
    Retinopathy of prematurity
    Familial exudative vitreoretinopathy
    Coats' disease (retinal telengectasia)
    Fundus colobomas
    Medullated nerve fibers
Tumors
    Retinoblastoma
    Astrocytoma
    Diktyoma
Infections
    Endophthalmitis
    Toxocariasis
    Toxoplasmosis

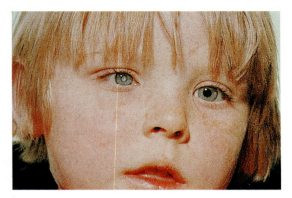

FIGURE 19–3. Congenital cataract prominently visible in the pupil of the right eye.

detailed general physical and ophthalmologic examination to identify the underlying pathology. Table 19–3 lists some of the signs that may help to identify the underlying pathology.

■ Congenital Cataracts

Cataracts are the most common cause of childhood leukocoria (Fig. 19–3). Visually disabling, bilateral, congenital cataracts often present with early nystagmus (by 3 months), which is indicative of a poor prognosis for visual recovery. Early surgical removal of congenital cataracts is associated with the best visual prognosis. Congenital cataracts are reported to occur in 1 out of 250 newborns.[2,3] It is significant that approximately one third of cataracts in children are hereditary, another third are associated with various syndromes or other diseases, and the final third are idiopathic.[4] Genetic and metabolic disease syndromes (e.g., Down syndrome, Lowe's syndrome, galactosemia) and intrauterine maternal infections with TORCH (*t*oxoplasmosis, *o*ther infections, *r*ubella, *c*ytomegalovirus, *h*erpes simplex) organisms are known specific causes of congenital cataracts.

Congenital cataracts can be polar (anterior or posterior), sutural, nuclear (pearly white nuclear cataract of rubella), capsular, or lamellar (most common). Of the various morphologic types of cataracts, anterior polar, posterior lentiglobus, and unilateral persistent hyperplastic primary vitreous (PHPV) are not usually related to systemic disorders. Many of the metabolic diseases can be treated, or further deterioration can be prevented with appropriate

TABLE 19–2. Typical Features of Common Conditions Causing Leukocoria

Common Conditions	Heredity	Usual Age at Diagnosis	Laterality	Typical Features
Congenital cataracts	Inherited (AD) (commonly)	Congenital (at birth)	Bilateral	Amblyopia Associated disease syndromes
Retinoblastoma	$\frac{2}{3}$ sporadic $\frac{1}{3}$ inherited (AD)	1–3 y <1 y	Bilateral Unilateral	Exophytic or endophytic growth Calcification on CT scan
PHPV	Sporadic	Congenital (at birth)	Unilateral	Visible ciliary processes Retrolental fibrovascular plaque Intraocular hemorrhage, ACG
Coats' disease	Sporadic	8–10 y	Unilateral	Massive subretinal exudation Retinal telengectasia
Retinopathy of prematurity	Sporadic	4–6 wk	Bilateral	Prematurity or low birth weight Incomplete retinal vascularization Neovascularization

AD, autosomal dominant; ACG, angle closure glaucoma; PHPV, persistent hyperplastic primary vitreous.

TABLE 19–3. Ocular Signs in Leukocoria and Associated Clinical Condition

Vision	Fixation Preference Amblyopia	All Conditions May Cause
Slit Lamp Exam		
Lids/lashes	Colobomas	Associated with fundus colobomas
Cornea	Corneal diameter	Microcornea in PHPV (persistant hyperplastic primary vitreous)
Anterior chamber	Shallow	PHPV
	Pseudohypopyon	Masquerade syndrome, retinoblastoma
Iris	Colobomas	Associated with fundus colobomas
	Visible ciliary processes	PHPV
	Hyperchromic heterochromia	Extensive rubeosis, ROP
Lens	Cataracts	Hereditary cataracts, PHPV, Stage V ROP, evidence against retinoblastoma
	Mittendorf's dots	PHPV
Eye movements	Nystagmus	All conditions may cause
	Pseudoexotropia	Macular dragging—ROP
Intraocular Pressure and Gonioscopy		
	Angle closure glaucoma	PHPV, stage V ROP
	Cataract and glaucoma	Congenital rubella, Lowe's syndrome
Fundus (dilate with cyclomydril eye drops × 3 q 5 min in infants, avoid phenylephrine)		
Vitreous	Hemorrhage	Fibrovascular membrane as in ROP, PHPV
	Seeding/opacification	Retinoblastoma
Retina	Exudative detachment	Coats' disease
	Tractional detachment	ROP, PHPV
	Elevated lesion	Toxocariasis, retinoblastoma
	Fibrovascular proliferation	ROP, FEVR (familial exudative vitreoretinopathy)
Ultrasound (A or B Scan)		
	Microphthalmos	PHPV, evidence against retinoblastoma
	Calcification	Retinoblastoma
CT Scan	Calcification	Retinoblastoma
Laboratory Investigations		
	CBC with differential	Eosinophilia in toxocariasis
	ELISA	Toxocariasis
	TORCH titers, VDRL	Bilateral cataracts
	Urine for amino acids	Bilateral cataracts

treatment.[5] Modern diagnostic techniques such as ultrasonography or magnetic resonance imaging can help identify posterior segment lesions behind the lens and opacified lens.[6]

Early surgical intervention (as soon as possible) and visual rehabilitation are the mainstays of management for visually significant congenital cataracts. A lensectomy (limbal or pars plana approach) is usually performed. Posterior capsulectomy and anterior vitrectomy are usually performed to prevent posterior capsular opacification. Visual rehabilitation is obtained with an intraocular lens (preferred, depending on age),

contact lens, or aphakic glasses. Postoperative amblyopia therapy may require eye patching.

■ Retinoblastoma

Retinoblastoma is the most common malignant intraocular tumor of childhood.[7,8] It is a neuroblastic tumor that is caused by a mutation in the long arm of chromosome 13. It is familial in one third of cases (bilateral tumors) and sporadic in two thirds of cases (unilateral tumors) and typically is diagnosed at approximately

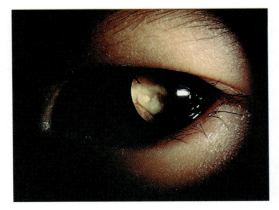

FIGURE 19–4. Leukocoria secondary to retino-blastoma.

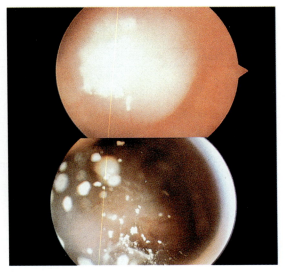

FIGURE 19–5. Fundus photograph of retino-blastoma, endophytic type.

1 year of age. The most common initial sign is leukocoria (Fig. 19–4) followed by strabismus. Two growth patterns have been identified: endo-phytic, which occurs when tumor breaks through the internal limiting membrane and is visible in the vitreous cavity as a whitish mass (Fig. 19–5), and exophytic, which occurs when tumor grows in the subretinal space producing a yellowish mass with overlying dilated and tortu-ous retinal vessels (Fig. 19–6). Radiographic or ultrasonographic demonstration of intraocular calcification aids in the diagnosis. Treatments include enucleation external-beam radiother-apy, radioactive plaque treatment, cryotherapy, and photocoagulation. Radiotherapy or chemotherapy may be used in an attempt to pre-serve at least one globe in bilateral cases.

■ Persistent Hyperplastic Primary Vitreous

Present at birth, persistent hyperplastic pri-mary vitreous (PHPV) is unilateral in over 90% of cases. When it presents bilaterally, chromo-somal defects may be present. Pathophysiolog-ically, PHPV develops when the fibrovascular component of the primary vitreous fails to involute by the seventh month of gestation when the secondary or mature vitreous devel-ops. PHPV presents as a white fibrovascular mass behind or extending to the lens. Leuko-

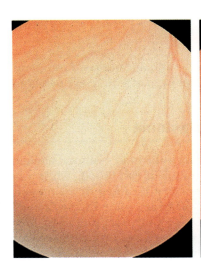
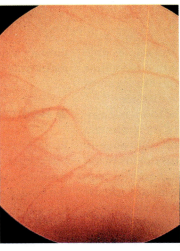

FIGURE 19–6. Fundus photograph of retinoblastoma, exophytic type.

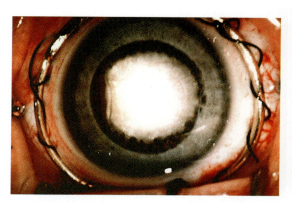

FIGURE 19–7. Persistent hyperplastic primary vitreous.

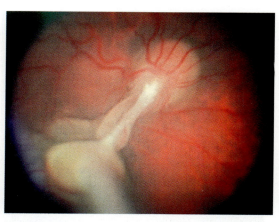

FIGURE 19–8. Toxocara granuloma attached to the optic nerve by a stalk (courtesy of Dr. William Freeman).

coria may result from the PHPV material itself or from the secondary cataract that frequently is present (Fig. 19–7). The eye is slightly microphthalmic and on dilation of the pupil may show elongated ciliary processes, which are particularly diagnostic of this disorder. Various degrees of severity may occur, ranging from mild persistent stalks that do not interfere with visual function and development to massive retinal tractional detachments and intraocular hemorrhage. Some time later, the eye also may lose all useful vision from secondary angle closure glaucoma as the lens swells. Modern surgical techniques have salvaged many eyes; however, the risk of glaucoma remains.[9]

■ Toxocariasis

When ingested by the human host, the lifecycle of *Toxocara canis* is abbreviated compared with that in its primary hosts.[10] In humans, the larvae hatch and bore through the intestine into the portal circulation but do not regain entry into the gastrointestinal tract to become mature worms. Therefore, the infection cannot be detected by stool samples. Migrating larvae gain entry to the eye through the short ciliary arteries and thus produce the most common presentation of a submacular granuloma. On the other hand, it is believed that, if the central reti-

nal artery is the portal of entry, a peripheral granuloma may present.

Ellsworth identified Toxocara granuloma as one of the few lesions that, when well visualized, can still be confused with retinoblastoma[11] (although retinal astrocytoma and tuberous sclerosis are the only other lesions mentioned). At times a dark central area can be seen perhaps representing remains of larvae.[10] A fibrotic tract leading to the disc also may be seen and is of diagnostic usefulness (Fig. 19–8). Toxocara may present with severe inflammation (perhaps when the worm or worms die[12]). This diffuse endophthalmitis with leukocoria can be confused with advanced and diffuse intraocular retinoblastoma. Other causes of uveitis that present in children can cause a white reflex and be confused with advanced retinoblastoma.[13] Vitritis, as occurs in toxoplasmosis, can obscure the retinal view, requiring the aid of imaging techniques such as ultrasound, computed tomography, or nuclear magnetic resonance. Intermediate uveitis with pars plana snowballs and vitreous "seeding" may be confusing as well. Response to steroids does not rule out malignant disease.

■ Coats' Disease

Although the early presentation of Coats' disease is fairly typical and easily recognized (Fig. 19–9),

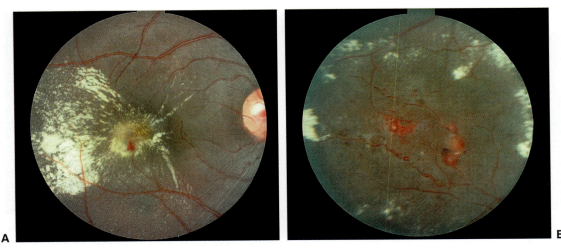

FIGURE 19–9. Coats' disease. **(A)** Exudative response in posterior pole in patient with Coats' disease. **(B)** Peripheral vascular anomaly in same patient (courtesy of Dr. Alfred Nadel and Dr. Barbara Phillips).

more advanced cases with massive subretinal exudation and detachment may be among the most difficult differential diagnoses. Advanced cases of Coats' disease are difficult to distinguish from retinoblastoma.[14] Coats' disease appears predominantly in young males (80%) and is usually unilateral (90%). It is not known whether family history or heredity predisposes certain individuals to Coats' disease. Although the average age of onset is in childhood (age 8 years), presentation in infancy is not uncommon.[15] In the early stages, characteristic findings include "light-bulb" telangiectatic vessels, miliary aneurysms, arteriovenous anastomoses, and capillary nonperfusion.[16] As a result of the vascular incompetence, collections of exudate may develop. The presence of apparently isolated macular exudate in a young child requires careful scrutiny of the retinal periphery to detect the responsible vascular anomalies. More extensive subretinal exudation may lead to retinal detachment and an apparent retrolental mass that causes prominent leukocoria. Diagnosis may be aided ultrasonographically by the finding of typical echoes from cholesterol crystals in subretinal fluid.[17] Treatment in the early stages consists of cryotherapy to the telangiectatic areas, laser photocoagulation to the abnormal blood vessels and surrounding retina, and drainage of subretinal fluid with or without buckling.

■ Retinopathy of Prematurity

Retinopathy of prematurity (ROP) is a vasoproliferative retinopathy of premature and low birth weight infants.[18] The process of retinal vascularization begins from the optic disc in the 16th week of gestation and proceeds toward the retinal periphery, reaching the nasal ora serrata at approximately 36 weeks' gestation and the temporal ora serrata at 40 weeks. Therefore, in premature infants vascularization of the anterior retina is incomplete at birth. Exposure to excessive concentrations of oxygen during this period can result in capillary endothelial cell toxicity and cessation of the normal vascularization process, and abnormal neovascularzation may occur. Eventually, fibroglial proliferation may extend into the vitreous, causing retinal traction and detachment. The end stage of ROP may present as a retrolental white mass (hence the term *retrolental fibroplasia*).

The American Academy of Pediatrics recommends that all high-risk infants (less than 36 weeks' gestation or birth weights of 2000 g who have received oxygen therapy) should be examined at the time of discharge from the nursery and subsequently at certain intervals, depending on the presence or absence of ROP and the grade of ROP. The pupil is dilated, and indirect ophthalmoscopy is performed, usually in the neonatal unit. An examination schedule is recommended for infants weighing less than

1500 g. The first exam is commonly performed 6 weeks postpartum and repeated every 1 to 2 weeks until retinal vascularization is complete or regression of prethreshold ROP occurs. The risk of developing ROP is high in infants with birth weights of less than 1250 g or with gestation ages of less than 28 weeks. Signs of ROP can be seen in 66% of infants with birth weights of less than 1251 g and 82% of those with birth weights of less than 1000 g.

An international classification has been developed to accurately stage acute ROP.[19] The International Classification of Retinopathy of Prematurity begins by defining three zones in which to identify the pathology (Fig. 19–10). Zone I consists of a circle posteriorly with the optic nerve as its center and the radius equal to twice the distance from the optic nerve to the foveola. Zone II is a band that stretches from the periphery of zone I to the outside edge of a circle whose center is again the disc but whose radius extends to the nasal ora serrata. Zone III consists of everything else, the periphery of the retina in all areas except the nasal periphery.

The classification system also identifies five stages of disease. Stage I consists of the appearance of a narrow white line present at the junction of vascular and avascular retina. Stage II consists of a thickening of this line or ridge of activity. In Stage III vessels are seen growing from the retina in this region into the vitreous cavity. Stage IV consists of retinal detachment, with macula attached (stage IV-a) or macula detached (stage IV-b). Stage V consists of a total retinal detachment. In addition, two more descriptive terms are used: *plus* disease describes the finding of dilated, tortuous vessels in the posterior pole commonly with dilated iris vessels, and *rush* disease is used to identify Zone I involvement with extensive *plus* disease.

The role of the ophthalmologist in the management of ROP is first to identify and stage the disease according to the international classification and then to follow the eye for progression to threshold disease, which is the indication for treatment. Threshold disease is defined as Stage III, Zone I or II ROP with *plus* disease, with 5 confluent or 8 cumulative hours

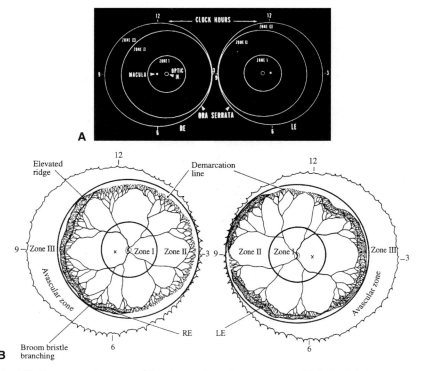

FIGURE 19–10. (A) Zones and stages of retinopathy of prematurity (ROP). **(B)** Example of threshold disease ROP.

of extraretinal neovascularization. The Cryo-ROP study has shown that cryotherapy to the avascular anterior retina reduces the incidence of an unfavorable outcome by approximately 50%.[20] Photocoagulation instead of cryotherapy is now feasible with portable laser using indirect ophthalmoscopy delivery systems and is preferable. More advanced disease may require retinal detachment surgery, lensectomy, and vitrectomy.

■ Coloboma of the Retina and Choroid

White sclera that is visible through an abnormal retina in the absence of the retinal pigment epithelium and the choroid can yield a prominent leukocoria effect (Fig. 19–11). Coloboma results from the failure of the embryonic fissure to fuse normally. The effect can be manifest in the optic nerve (Fig. 19–12), the choroid, and the retina, and anteriorly in the ciliary body and the iris. The various structures can be included either individually or collectively; the more serious anomalies may present with microphthalmia or orbital cyst. The visual potential of these eyes depends on the extent of normal macular development and the avoidance of anisometropic amblyopia.[21] Retinal detachments may develop later from breaks of the abnormal retinal tissue within the coloboma.[22]

■ Retinal Dysplasia

Retinal dysplasia appears prominently in all lists of lesions mistaken for retinoblastoma.[23] More a descriptive term rather than one delineating a particular entity, *retinal dysplasia* is associated with a multitude of cerebral and systemic anomalies as well as chromosomal aberrations. The diagnostic triad of Norrie's disease is congenital, bilateral blindness from retinal dysplasia, mental retardation, and deafness. The gene has been identified on the X chromosome, and its normal product, Norrin, is believed to affect endothelial cell migration and proliferation. Abnormal alleles of this gene are responsible for Norrie disease, X-linked exudative vitreoretinopathy, and exudative vitreoretinopathy. The finding of abnormal peripheral retinal findings similar to regressed ROP in genetically uninvolved children of female carriers suggests that abnormal Norrin can have an adverse transplacental effect.[24]

■ Angiomatosis Retinae (von Hippel-Lindau Disease)

The clinical appearance of angiomatosis retinae can be confused with retinoblastoma when it is clearly visible as a distinct retinal tumor or tumors, unilateral or bilateral, with feeder ves-

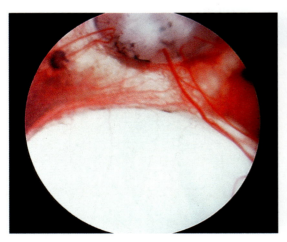

FIGURE 19–11. Inferior coloboma.

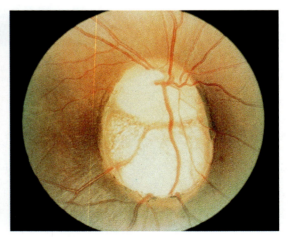

FIGURE 19–12. Optic disc coloboma presenting as leukocoria.

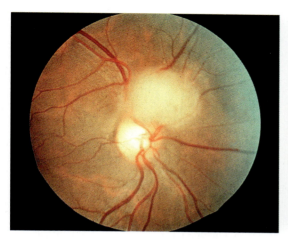

FIGURE 19–13. Astrocytic hamartoma in tuberous sclerosis.

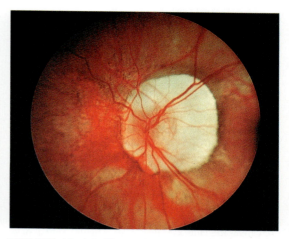

FIGURE 19–14. Extensive myopic chorioretinal degeneration presenting as leukocoria.

sels. Likewise, it is a diagnostic problem in a later stage when an overlying retinal detachment and secondary gliotic changes mimic one presentation of retinoblastoma. The association of retinal angiomas with cerebellar meningioblastoma is termed von Hippel-Lindau disease, which may be accompanied by pheochromocytoma or renal cell carcinoma.[25] The von Hippel-Lindau gene has been localized and cloned, and its role as a tumor suppressor gene is better understood.[26,27]

■ Tuberous Sclerosis

Tuberous sclerosis, or Bourneville's disease, presents with astrocytic hamartomas of the retina associated with mental retardation, epilepsy, and adenoma sebaceum of the skin. The retina shows a gray-white, raised astrocytic hamartoma classically described as "mulberry-like" (Fig. 19–13). Seeding of the lesion to other parts of the eye is possible, further confusing the differential diagnosis with retinoblastoma. However, the skin changes of tuberous sclerosis are characteristic and include the angiofibromas of adenoma sebaceum, frequently in a butterfly distribution on the face, shagreen patches of raised peau-de-orange surfaced skin, and hypomelanotic, oval "ash leaf" lesions more readily visualized with a Wood lamp. Tuberous

sclerosis has yielded to the probing research of molecular geneticists, who have located a gene and its product, tuberin, which is being studied to determine its physiological effects.[28]

■ Other Conditions

High myopia with chorioretinal degeneration can produce leukocoria if reflection from the exposed white of the sclera is extensive enough or appropriately located (Fig. 19–14). Other benign conditions such as extensive myelination of the nerve fibers can give rise to a white reflex (Fig. 19–15). Both conditions should be readily recognized during routine examination.

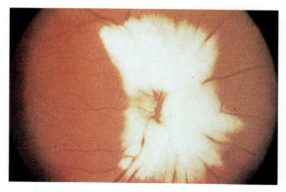

FIGURE 19–15. Myelinated nerve fibers presenting as leukocoria.

Less frequently reported etiologies that may be confused with retinoblastoma include endophthalmitis, juvenile xanthogranuloma, incontinentia pigmenti, and diktyoma.

REFERENCES

1. Howard GM, Ellsworth RM. Differential diagnosis in retinoblastoma: a statistical survey of 500 children. I. Relative frequency of lesions which simulate retinoblastoma. *Am J Ophthalmol.* 1965; 60:610–618.
2. Nelson LB, Ullman S. Congenital and developmental cataracts. In: Duane TJ, ed. *Clinical Ophthalmology.* Philadelphia, PA: JB Lippincott; 1994; 1:1–9.
3. Francois J. *Congenital Cataracts.* Springfield, IL: Charles C Thomas; 1963.
4. Cheng KP, Hiles DA, Biglan AV. The differential diagnosis of leukocoria. *Pediatric Ann.* 1990; 19:376–386.
5. Gitzelman R. Deficiency of erythrocyte galactokinase in a patient with galactose diabetes. *Lancet.* 1965;2:670.
6. De Potter P, Shields CL, Shields JA, et al. The role of magnetic resonance imaging in children with intraocular tumors and simulating lesions. *Ophthalmology.* 1996; 103:1774–1783.
7. Abramson DH, Servodidio CA. Retinoblastoma. *Optom Clin.* 1993; 3:49–61.
8. Abramson DH, Frank CM, Susman M, et al. Presenting signs of retinoblastoma. *J Pediatr.* 1998; 132:505–508.
9. Johnson CP, Keech RV. Prevalence of glaucoma after surgery for PHPV and infantile cataracts. *J Pediatr Ophthalmol Strabismus.* 1996; 33:14–17.
10. Shields JA. Ocular toxocariasis: a review. *Surv Ophthalmol.* 1984; 28:361–381.
11. Ellsworth RM. Retinoblastoma. In: Duane TJ, ed. *Clinical Ophthalmology.* Philadelphia, PA: JB Lippincott; 1994;3:ch.35.
12. Byers B, Kimura SJ. Uveitis after death of a larva in the vitreous cavity. *Am J Ophthalmol.* 1974; 77:63–66.
13. Stafford WR, Yanoff M, Parnell BL. Retinoblastomas initially misdiagnosed as primary ocular inflammations. *Arch Ophthal.* 1962; 82:771–773.
14. Steidl SM, Hirose T, Sang D, Hartnett DE. Difficulties in excluding the diagnosis of retinoblastoma in cases of advanced Coats' disease: a clinicopathologic report. *Ophthalmologica.* 1996; 210:336–340.
15. Duke-Elder S, Dobree JH. Diseases of the retina. In: Duke-Elder S, ed. *System of Ophthalmology.* London: Henry Kimpton; 1978; 10:164–178.
16. Francois J. Differential diagnosis of leukocoria in children. *Ann Ophthalmol.* 1978; 10:1375–1382.
17. Green RL, Byrne SF. Diagnostic ophthalmic ultrasound. In: Ryan SJ, ed. *Retina.* St. Louis, MO: CV Mosby; 1989; 255.
18. Flynn JT, Boncalari E, Bachynski BN, et al. Retinopathy of prematurity: diagnosis, severity and natural history. *Ophthalmology.* 1987; 94:620.
19. The Committee for Classification of Retinopathy of Prematurity: an international classification of retinopathy of prematurity. *Arch Ophthalmol.* 1984; 102:1130–1134.
20. Multicenter Trial of Cryotherapy for Retinopathy of Prematurity: preliminary results. *Arch Ophthalmol.* 1988; 106:471–479.
21. Olsen TW, Summers CG, Knobloch WH. Predicting visual acuity in children with colobomas involving the optic nerve. *J Pediatr Ophthalmol Strabismus.* 1996; 33: 47–51.
22. Gopal L, Badrinath SS, Sharma T, et al. Pattern of retinal breaks and retinal detachments in eyes with choroidal coloboma. *Ophthalmology.* 1995; 102:1212–1217.
23. Gunalp I, Gunduz K, Arslan Y. Retinoblastoma in Turkey: diagnosis and clinical characteristics. *Ophthalmic Genet.* 1996; 17:21–27.
24. Mintz-Hittner HA, Ferrell RE, Sims KB, et al. Peripheral retinopathy in offspring of carriers of Norrie disease gene mutations. Possible transplacental effect of abnormal Norrin. *Ophthalmology.* 1996; 103:2128–2134.
25. Duker JS, Brown GC. Vascular anomalies of the fundus. In: Duane TA, ed. *Clinical Ophthalmology.* Philadelphia, PA: JB Lippincott; 1994;3:ch.22.
26. Decker HJ, Weidt EJ, Brieger J. The von Hippel-Lindau tumor suppressor gene: a rare and intriguing disease opening new insight into basic mechanisms of carcinogenesis. *Cancer Genet Cytogenet.* 1997; 93:74–83.
27. Wizigmann-Voos S, Plate KH. Pathology, genetics and cell biology of hemangioblastomas. *Histol Histopathol.* 1996; 11:1049–1061.
28. Xiao GH, Shoarinjad F, Jin F, et al. The tuberous sclerosis 2 gene product, tuberin, functions as a Rab% GTPase activating protein (APG) in modulating endocytosis. *J Biol Chem.* 1997; 272:6097–6100.

Pediatric Ophthalmology
Edited by P. F. Gallin
Thieme Medical Publishers, Inc.
New York © 2000

20
###

Pediatric Cataracts

RICHARD E. BRAUNSTEIN AND ARTHUR M. COTLIAR

Evaluating children with cataracts is very difficult because children with cataracts are not just small adults with cataracts. They present numerous problems and challenges that involve medical, social, and surgical issues.

The care of children with cataracts begins with the first ophthalmologic examination and extends until at least 9 years of age due to the window of amblyopia. Often they develop additional ophthalmologic problems later in life. The ability to examine an infant and determine whether a lens opacity is visually significant, requiring urgent surgery, or inconsequential is an acquired skill with little room for error. Often, care of the pediatric cataract patient involves the coordination of a number of different specialists, including geneticists, pediatricians, social workers, and ophthalmologists.

■ Signs and Symptoms

Pediatric cataracts are often an incidental finding, especially when they are monocular. The management of pediatric cataracts varies greatly with patient age, extent of amblyopia, and significance of lens opacity. The presence of an opacity and the difficulty in diagnosis become two separate entities. Newborns are screened at birth, and any abnormality in the red reflex usu-

ally is brought to the attention of an ophthalmologist. Because newborns are examined with direct ophthalmoscopes, which constrict reactive pupils, partial and visually significant lens opacities are difficult to diagnose. Routine well baby pediatrician visits may detect a lens opacity in the red reflex. However, it is the appearance of a "funny looking eye" or different red reflexes on family photographs that can bring this to medical attention. Children with dense bilateral cataracts may present with nystagmus. Other findings that may prompt examination include strabismus and complaints of glare/photophobia. Failure to perform visually oriented tasks may not be noted, especially if the opacity is in one eye and the child functions normally with the other. Children with signs of developmental delay (i.e., failure to reach normal milestones), or features of clinical syndromes associated with ocular involvement should be routinely referred for comprehensive ophthalmologic evaluation.

Clinical Presentation of Congenital Cataracts

Leukocoria
Opacity in red reflex
Nystagmus
Strabismus
Photophobia/glare
Known systemic disorder associated with cataracts
Decreased visual interest
Developmental delay

■ Examination

Work-up of pediatric cataracts includes a thorough review of the maternal history, including illness during pregnancy, drug use (therapeutic or illicit), and birth history. Historically, congenital rubella accounted for up to 20% of all congenital lens opacities, but this has been significantly reduced through immunization programs. Other infections reportedly associated with congenital cataract include toxoplasmosis, herpes, measles, mumps, and vaccinia. Exposure to radiation during pregnancy and maternal use of corticosteroids and sulfa drugs may result in lens opacities. A history of low birth weight or maternal malnutrition during pregnancy is reportedly associated with congenital cataracts.

Systemic Disorders

There are many systemic syndromes, both metabolic and/or genetic, whose features include lens disorders. All children with unknown genetic syndromes and syndromes with ocular involvement should have eye examinations as soon as possible. Often, the presence and specific type of opacity can lead to a systemic diagnosis. Although a comprehensive discussion of each of these syndromes is not appropriate here, a comprehensive list is provided (Table 20–1). The medical evaluation of children with cataracts can be quite extensive and costly, but associated abnormalities usually allow the pediatrician and geneticist to direct the work-up appropriately. The one disorder that must not be overlooked is galactokinase deficiency, which may cause a cataract in otherwise healthy children. Unlike galactosemia, in which the enzyme galactose-1-phosphate uridyl transferase is absent, resulting in numerous systemic findings, the absence of galactokinase may result in cataract only, and dietary intervention may reverse or halt disease progression.

Genetics

A family history of cataract may be elicited during the medical work-up. The various forms of inheritance, of which autosomal dominant is the most frequent, have been described elsewhere. Up to one third of congenital cataracts in healthy children are idiopathic, often representing new genetic mutations.[1]

Ophthalmic Examination

In infants and very young children it is not possible to measure formal visual acuity. However, findings such as searching nystagmus with bilateral cataracts or strabismus with cataract suggest extremely poor vision that requires rapid intervention.

Evaluating Congenital Cataracts

Direct ophthalmoscopy or retinoscopy
Central opacity and/or surrounding distortion **greater than 3 mm** is significant
Slit lamp exam when possible
Rule out associated abnormalities of cornea, iris, or pupil
Hand held slit lamp or EUA
Rule out glaucoma (congenital rubella and Lowe's syndrome)
Fundus exam or B scan

In very young patients, multiple techniques are useful for evaluating the lens. The two basic techniques involve either direct slit lamp style viewing, or assessment of the lens opacity with respect to the red reflex. A portable slit lamp can be very helpful in evaluating the size, density, and location within the lens (anterior, posterior, central, etc.) of the opacity. The use of retinoscopy in a dilated eye allows the opacity to be visualized against the red reflex (back illuminated) and is extremely useful (Figs. 20–1 and 20–2). **If the opacity is central, greater than 3 mm, and/or impeding retinoscopy or funduscopy, it is usually visually significant**. A comparison of bilateral lens opacities may be important to plan for timing and necessity of surgery on one or both eyes. If an adequate examination cannot be performed in the office, an examination under anesthesia is usually performed, with surgery immediately following the exam if appropriate. An attempt should be made to identify any associated ocular abnormalities either preoperatively or at the time of surgery because they may affect the prognosis and management. This includes strabismus, corneal size, corneal opacities, iris structure, glaucoma, microphthalmos, persistent hyperplastic primary vitreous, and retinal abnormalities. Particular attention should be directed to the lens in terms of size, shape, and position.

TABLE 20–1. Cataracts Associated with Systemic Syndromes

Syndrome	Systemic Manifestations
Cataracts Associated with Skeletal Disease	
Albright's hereditary	Short stature, subcutaneous calcification, osteodystrophy brachydactyly
Chondrodysplasia punctata	Dysplastic skeletal changes, dermatosis of the skin, saddlenose deformity, pathognomonic radiologic findings in epiphysis
Majewski's syndrome	Neonatal dwarfism, polydactyly, narrow thorax, cleft lip and palate, visceral deformities
Myotonic dystrophy	Muscle wasting, hypogonadism, cardiac changes, baldness
Osteogenesis imperfecta	Bone fractures, deafness, skull anomalies, ligament hypercongenital flexibility, discoloration of dentition
Cataracts Associated with Dermatological Disorders	
Atopic dermatitis	Red, thickened, crusty skin, allergic history
Cockayne syndrome	Dwarfism, precocious senile appearance, deafness, retardation
Congenital ichthyosis	Fish-scale skin, hyperkeratosis, lack of hair
Incontinentia pigmenti	Skin pigmentation, hypodontia, skeletal defects, mental deficiency, microcephaly
Rothmund syndrome	Telangiectasia, hypogonadism, vascular skin lesions, saddlenose deformity, congenital bone defects
Cataracts Associated with Central Nervous System Syndromes	
Laurence-Moon-Bardet-Biedl	Retinitis pigmentosa, nystagmus, strabismus, polydactyly, mental retardation
Marinesco-Sjogren	Oligophrenia, spinocerebellar ataxia, nystagmus, mental retardation
Sjogren-Larson syndrome	Ichthyosis, spasticity, short stature, mental retardation, oligophrenia
Cataracts Associated with Craniofacial Syndromes	
Hallerman-Streiff syndrome	Over 90% have congenital cataracts, small stature, malar hypoplasia, micrognathia, abnormal dentition, bird-like facies
Pierre Robin syndrome	Cataracts uncommon, micrognathia, cleft palate, glossoptosis
Alport's syndrome	Cataracts uncommon, oxycephalic skull, normal intelligence, finger-fusion, congenital heart defects, polycystic kidneys
Crouzon's syndrome	Cataracts uncommon, brachycephaly, broadened nasal root, irregular dentition, mental retardation
Smith-Lemli-Opitz	Cataracts common, microcephaly, mental deficiency, syndactyly, hypospadias, cryptorchidism
Cataracts Associated with Multisystem Syndromes	
Noonan syndrome	Webbed neck, low-set ears, typical facies, pulmonary stenosis
Werner syndrome	Arrested growth, premature graying, scleroderma-like changes, arteriosclerosis, diabetes mellitus, hypogonadism, osteoporosis, premature senility

From KW Wright, *Pediatric Ophthalmology and Strabismus;* St. Louis, MO: Mosby Year Book; 1995, p. 379. Reprinted by permission.

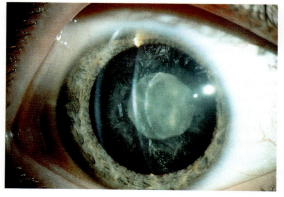

FIGURE 20–1. Visually significant cataract seen with direct illumination through dilated pupil.

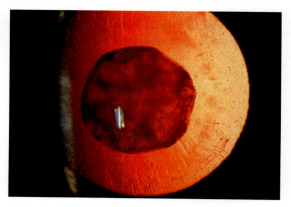

FIGURE 20–2. Visually significant cataract seen with retro-illumination (back-illuminated) against the red reflex.

Social Concerns

The importance of understanding a child's social situation cannot be over-emphasized because family support, commitment, and understanding are critical in the management of pediatric cataracts. Without adequate post-operative care, uncontrolled intraocular inflammation or glaucoma may result in permanent visual loss or complete blindness. Surgical success with dense amblyopia because of a family's inability to understand and provide appropriate amblyopia treatment (e.g., patching) or aphakic correction (e.g., contact lenses) is unacceptable. An attempt to address these issues preoperatively is medically appropriate and critical to successful pediatric cataract management.

Ectopia Lentis

Dislocated lenses in children are difficult to manage and have many systemic and genetic associations. A discussion of these syndromes is not appropriate here. As in the evaluation of children with cataracts, genetic, medical, and social evaluations are important, combined with skillful ophthalmologic assessments. An understanding of lens position and stability within the visual axis plays an important part in the management of induced refractive errors and the necessity of surgical intervention.

Treatment

After the diagnosis of cataract is made and the appropriate medical and genetic evaluations are initiated, treatment of the lens opacity must be addressed. Lenticular abnormalities may be associated with significant refractive errors and anisometropia. When possible, a careful cycloplegic retinoscopic examination should be performed and, if appropriate, glasses prescribed. In unilateral or asymmetric cataracts, occlusion therapy for amblyopia management should be initiated. Pharmacological dilatation of the pupil may be beneficial for central lens opacities allowing the child to view through the clear peripheral lens. This is usually not tolerated for very long, but it can be used as a temporary measure if surgery needs to be delayed for medical reasons.

In newborns, a significant unilateral cataract should be removed as soon as possible. This is a medical emergency. If the child is medically unstable and cannot tolerate general anesthesia, surgery will be necessarily delayed. All reasonable attempts should be made to operate and begin visual rehabilitation as soon as possible within the first 6 weeks of life because the prognosis for good vision is dramatically reduced thereafter due to dense, irreversible amblyopia. With bilateral cataracts, there is less urgency although surgery should be performed as soon as possible, no later than 4 months. Removal of the lens opacity is the first step, but treatment of the resultant aphakia with spectacles or contact lenses may prove to be a greater challenge. The management of infants with unilateral aphakia and contact lenses will not be discussed here but suffice it to say that this is a formidable task for physician and family. The use of intraocular lenses in this age group is still controversial. Most surgeons will leave newborns aphakic and address visual rehabilitation with appropriate optical correction. In unilateral aphakia, contact lenses are essential to allow for any chance of binocular vision. With bilateral cataract surgery, vision can be corrected with either contact lenses (preferably) or aphakic spectacles.

Although controversial in newborns, improved techniques and experience have made intraocular lenses acceptable in children 2 years of age and older. Although reports in the literature document successful lens implantation in children as young as 4 months of age, most pediatric ophthalmic surgeons would not implant lenses in children less than 2 years old. Factors that make intraocular lens implantation difficult in this group include changing axial length, corneal curvature, increased tissue reactivity, decreased scleral rigidity, smaller size, and long life span after surgery.[2]

In children with cataracts who initially had good vision or small lens opacities, there is less urgency to surgical intervention. Within the amblyopic period, surgery should be performed when vision deteriorates. This is often a clinical judgment. If the child is 9 years or older, surgery may be delayed with a good long-term prognosis. Treatment of these patients is similar to surgery in adults because the eye is larger, allowing for an adult surgical technique with placement of an intraocular lens.

Surgical Technique

Incision

Cataract extraction in children is similar to that in adults, beginning with proper wound construction. A scleral pocket-type incision with a limbal-based conjunctival flap is utilized for either the phacoemulsification handpiece or the vitrector, depending on the type of cataract and age of the patient. In cases utilizing a vitrector for lens removal, we prefer a separate clear corneal incision for placement of a chamber maintaining cannula providing irrigation separate from the vitrectomy handpiece. Additional sideport incisions are made to accommodate a second instrument if desired.

Anterior Capsulectomy

The anterior chamber is filled with a high molecular weight viscoelastic to facilitate the anterior capsulectomy. A continuous tear capsulorhexis is preferred because this facilitates secure in-the-bag intraocular lens placement. The increased elasticity of the anterior capsule in children combined with increased vitreous pressure makes performing a continuous curvilinear capsulorhexis more difficult in a pediatric than in an adult eye. The initial tear should be smaller than normal because it tends to spiral outward in the pediatric eye. If the tear cannot be completed in a circular fashion, the vitrector can be used to perform a mechanized can-opener style capsulectomy.[3]

Lensectomy

Because the lens of the pediatric eye is usually soft, the removal of lens material in pediatric cases can be accomplished with a number of different techniques. These include the irrigation/aspiration handpiece, a vitrectomy unit, or the phacoemulsification handpiece. Although no ultrasound may actually be required for lens removal, the phacoemulsification handpiece provides the most efficient method of lens removal. In smaller eyes, the vitrectomy handpiece is helpful because of its reduced size. Hydrodissection and hydrodelineation can be utilized to facilitate lens removal. The irrigation/aspiration handpiece is normally required to strip the cortical material from the capsule.

Posterior Capsulectomy and Anterior Vitrectomy

Posterior capsule opacification following cataract surgery in children occurs with a higher frequency than adults, with rates approaching 90% 3 years after surgery.[4] Postoperative management of an opacified posterior capsule in a child is difficult because Nd:YAG capsulotomy is often impossible due to the child's inability to cooperate with the treatment. This often necessitates a return to the operating room for surgical posterior capsulectomy.

Recognition of this problem has led to the use of posterior capsulectomy at the time of cataract surgery in any patient who will not be able to cooperate for a laser capsulotomy postoperatively. After filling the capsular bag with a high molecular weight viscoelastic agent, a continuous tear posterior capsulorhexis can be performed. The diameter of the capsulectomy should be slightly smaller than the optic diameter of the intraocular lens. Alternatively, an automated vitrector can be used to create the posterior capsulectomy.

The decision to perform an anterior vitrectomy at the time of cataract surgery is still controversial. We believe this is mandatory. Many surgeons believe that the anterior vitreous provides a scaffold on which cells proliferate, resulting in opacification in the visual axis. An anterior vitrectomy is performed after the posterior capsulectomy to prevent development of a secondary cataract. More recently, posterior optic capture of an intraocular lens implanted within the capsular bag has been introduced as a method of reducing secondary cataract, without the need for vitrectomy. Following intraocular lens placement and posterior capsulorhexis, the optic is pushed posteriorly through the posterior capsulorhexis without tearing the edges of the capsular opening. This allows for apposition of the anterior and posterior capsule leaflets for nearly 360 degrees, which theoretically blocks proliferations into the visual axis.[5]

Intraocular Lenses

Implanting lenses in pediatric eyes requires an understanding of the growth of the pediatric eye and the expected refractive change of that eye over the child's lifetime. Based on postmortem data, 90% of crystalline lens growth occurs during the first 2 years of life.[6] After the age of 2 years, standard size capsular bag style intraocular lenses with a diameter of 12.0 to 12.5 mm can be safely implanted in children. In children younger than 2 years, a downsized intraocular lens with a diameter of 10.0 mm may be necessary to prevent extensive stretching and distortion of the capsular bag. Considerable controversy exists over the optimal refractive goal in pediatric intraocular implantation. Assuming a shift toward myopia through childhood, it is reasonable to aim for a small hyperopic refractive error postoperatively. This is modified according to patient age and status of the fellow eye.[4]

Finally, a brief mention should be made of the use of foldable intraocular lenses in children. Theoretic benefits to the use of foldable intraocular lenses relate to the reduced incision size with greater wound stability for postoperative security and less induced astigmatism, improving the refractive predictability. Little information is available regarding the long-term safety of these lenses in young children, although we have experience utilizing foldable acrylic lenses in older children with excellent results.

Follow-Up

The postoperative management of the pediatric cataract patient is quite different from that of the adult patient. In general, there is much more intraocular inflammation, and aggressive corticosteroid use is often necessary. The correction of aphakia with contact lenses or spectacles requires careful retinoscopy and tremendous effort from physician, staff, and families. Regular examinations are essential to monitor vision, refraction, clarity of the visual axis, intraocular inflammation, and intraocular pressure. In small children, office examinations are often inadequate, and examinations under anesthesia are required.

Amblyopia therapy involves aphakic correction if necessary and patching. We generally patch monocular cataract patients every day for a half day at a time. Bilateral cataract patients are monitored for amblyopia development and treated accordingly. Amblyopia is often the limiting factor in vision following cataract surgery in children.

The postoperative period involves continued family education. A successful outcome can only be achieved through the hard work and persistence of physician and family working together. Pediatric contact lens wear requires careful lens fitting, parental teaching, and close follow-up. Often, the parents become frustrated from the tremendous demands of caring for these children, and the physician is required to help support the family in any way possible. With all of our surgical advances, it is still the tremendous dedication from families, physician, and staff that are the essential ingredients in successful pediatric cataract surgery.

REFERENCES

1. Merin S, Crawford JS. The etiology of congenital cataract: a survey. *Can J Ophthalmol.* 1971;6:178–182.
2. Wilson ME, et al. Current trends in the use of intraocular lenses in children. *J Cataract Refract Surg.* 1994;20:579–583.
3. Wilson ME, et al. Mechanized anterior capsulectomy as an alternative to manual capsulorhexis in children undergoing intraocular lens implantation. *J Peditar Ophthalmol Strabismus.* 1996;33:237–240.
4. Plager DA, et al. Capsular management and refractive error in pediatric intraocular lenses. *Ophthalmology.* 1997;104:600–607.
5. Gimbel HV. Posterior capsulorhexis with optic capture in pediatric cataract and intraocular lens surgery. *Ophthalmology.* 1996;103:1871–1875.
6. Wilson ME, et al. Intraocular lenses for pediatric implantation: biomaterial, designs, and sizing. *J Cataract Refract Surg.* 1994;20:584–591.
7. Wright KW. *Pediatric Ophthalmology and Strabismus.* St. Louis, MO: Mosby Year Book; 1995.

Pediatric Ophthalmology
Edited by P. F. Gallin
Thieme Medical Publishers, Inc.
New York © 2000

21
■■■

Pediatric Retinal Examination and Diseases

THOMAS E. FLYNN, JOHN T. FLYNN, AND STANLEY CHANG

The safe and informative retinal examination of children under 18 years of age is one of the most difficult challenges facing both the pediatric ophthalmologist and the general ophthalmologist caring for children. This chapter will focus on the indications and techniques for such examinations and will briefly cover important entities that need to be considered any time a child complains of a decrease or change in vision or unusual visual behaviors are noted. An exhaustive treatise on all pediatric retinal diseases is beyond the scope of this work, and can be found elsewhere.[1-3]

■ Retinal Examinations in Children

When Should Children Have Dilated Fundus Examinations?

The indications, frequencies, and techniques of general pediatric examinations are covered elsewhere.[1-3] Some clues to the need for an especially careful and detailed retinal examination include a family history of progressive visual loss or blindness, night blindness, nystagmus or strabismus, or enucleation. Consanguinity, maternal drug or alcohol use, prenatal exposure to viruses (including HIV if known) and other serious infections, or therapeutic medication use during pregnancy indicate a high risk of retinal problems. Low birth weight, difficult labor and delivery with asphyxia, and a prolonged stay in the hospital after birth indicate serious medical problems. A history of a lack of early visual behaviors or peculiar eye position or movements is also important. Children in the foster care system may be seen without a complete or accurate medical or social history of either mother or child; these children should be considered high risk and examined promptly and thoroughly.

The indications for retinal examination vary considerably by the age of the child. An infant who has clear media, an abnormal Bruckner test (see below), and nystagmus requires urgent evaluation. A toddler manifesting a change in visual behavior, inattention to formerly attractive objects, or loss of previously attained developmental milestones needs a retinal evaluation. A school-aged child with falling grades, difficulty with reading or seeing the blackboard, and poor attention should be thoroughly examined for retinal pathology. At least one dilated fundus examination along with a retinoscopic manifest in all children prior to starting school has been advocated by many specialists and is certainly the ideal protocol to recommend. Fewer than 5% of children in the United States ever receive such an evaluation.

How Do I Examine a Child's Retina When He Won't Sit Still?

Although adults recognize the advantages in putting up with the inconvenience of a retinal examination, the benefits are often lost on children. A few strategies can be tried before arranging for an examination under anesthesia (EUA). First, do not rush into putting drops in the eye and beginning scleral depression immediately after entering the office. Spend a few moments speaking to the child and parents in a normal tone about nonthreatening subjects. Allow the family a few moments to become comfortable with you. If necessary, let the child play in the exam room or waiting room to calm down and become bored.

Second, plan a strategy appropriate for the child's age. Infants may be wrapped in blankets like a papoose for quick peeks in the eye. Alternatively, a mother's lap with the child's legs under her elbows and the child's elbows pinned to his ears works as well as a papoose board. Infants will tolerate a great deal if they are fed during the examination. Teenagers can frequently be persuaded to go along with an examination to get away from your office. Children between these two age groups can be nearly impossible to examine. Attractive loud toys or interesting videos can be helpful. Keeping the examiner's head out of the line of sight of the unexamined eye is important if you are trying to distract the child. If necessary, employ fathers, grandparents, or other accompanying adults if strong-arm tactics are used—your office personnel should be reserved for other tasks such as drops, vision testing, and assistance with later exams. Use a 28- or 30-diopter lens and low light intensity to scan the retina quickly and determine whether further evaluation is needed. Unfortunately, bribery, threats, or distractions are often attempted with limited success. Some pediatricians may try sedation with benzodiazepines, intramuscular DPT (Demerol, Phenergan, Thorazine), or chloral hydrate for younger children with some success; this strategy should be used with caution as sedatives may have dangerous side effects.

Third, plan an examination at quiet times when the office is empty; examining a retina in a minimally cooperative child is time consuming at best. The added stimulation of a crowded office, ringing telephones, and your impatience to move on to another patient will affect any child. If you have tried your best and cannot see the retina well enough to accurately localize and draw a lesion in the retina, perform the EUA.

What Dilating Drops Do I Use?

In infants use Cyclogyl 0.5%, one drop twice in the eye; see the infant 30 to 40 minutes later. In toddlers, apply Cyclogyl 0.5% (light iris) or Cyclogyl 1% (dark iris) combined with Neosynephrine 2.5%, one drop of each twice in each eye; see the child 30 to 40 minutes later. Older children and teenagers may be dilated in the same manner as adults. Dilation may be difficult in premature infants with pulmonary disease in the hospital; the doses mentioned for infants may be doubled, but the child needs to be watched closely for increased body warmth and irritability.

How Do I Do an Exam under Anesthesia?

The risks of EUA when done by an experienced anesthesiologist familiar with pediatric patients and techniques are low.[4] In many large hospitals, anesthesiologists boarded in both disciplines are available for this purpose. The examination is performed under general anesthesia given by mask without prior sedation and without an in-dwelling intravenous line.

When Do I Do a Fluorescein Angiogram?

Fluorescein angiography[5] is performed when one of three concerns exists: (1) when retinal or choroidal ischemia is suspected, (2) when abnormal blood vessel growth or anatomy is noted, and (3) when abnormal vascular permeability exists, such as with macular edema. In children, diseases that lead to ischemia in the retina are uncommon but include important disorders such as familial exudative vitreoretinopathy, incontinentia pigmenti, sickle cell disease, and retinopathy of prematurity (ROP). Abnormal blood vessel growth may occur in the setting of retinal ischemia or in retinoblastoma or other tumors, or they may exist in hamartomatous lesions occurring in the phakomatoses or Coats' disease. Usually these conditions are confirmed with ophthalmoscopy alone. However, angiography may help to differentiate one type of lesion from another based on filling pattern and presence of leakage in late phase images. Third, permeable retinal vasculature may occur in any condition causing an abnormality of vessels. This is most critical when it causes macular edema, commonly in patients with intermediate uveitis or long-standing juvenile onset diabetes mellitus. Characteristic angiographic appearance also helps in the diagnosis of conditions such as Stargardt's or Best's diseases.

Intravenous bolus injections of fluorescein sodium are required to accurately assess the arteriovenous transit in an eye as well as imaging lesions such as microaneurysms, which are best seen in early phase pictures before leakage obscures them. In school-aged and adolescent children, minimal dose adjustment may be made on adult dosing schedules. In younger children and those unable to tolerate or cooperate with intravenous injections, several studies suggest protocols for oral administration of dye. With computerized imaging systems and software, image enhancement allows accurate visualization of abnormal vessels, ischemic retina, and macular edema with reasonable accuracy. The transit of dye is, however, gradual and delayed.

When Should I Obtain Electrophysiologic Studies?

Useful clues to the need for electrophysiologic studies include family histories of visual loss with a normal retinal exam and obvious decreased vision, attenuation of the retinal vasculature in any child with unexplained visual problems, or a suspected storage disease with a retinal component (e.g., Batten-Vogt-Spielmayer family). Two other types of pediatric patients are also referred for electrophysiologic testing. The first group is children suspected of having an inherited retinal dystrophy such as retinitis pigmentosa (RP) or a vitreoretinopathy and related systemic syndromes. The second broad category is children with apparent subnormal vision with strabismus or nystagmus without obvious retinal abnormalities on examination.

In any patient with congenital nystagmus, after ruling out a sensory etiology such as cataract, a thorough battery of tests must be done to diagnose the cause. More than 90% of patients with congenital nystagmus have been found to have one of a group of diagnoses affecting retinal function: albinism, Leber's congenital amaurosis and related RP, achromatopsia, or congenital stationary night blindness (CSNB). In each case, early fundus examination may be normal, and in all cases visual behaviors and responses are minimal or absent. The use of electrophysiologic testing may differentiate these entities from each other and from delayed visual maturation in which physiologically normal eyes fail to maintain fixation. Serial use of electrophysiologic testing may also show improvement in retinal function from infancy to early childhood, as expected in albinism, achromatopsia, and CSNB.

Electroretinography (ERG) measures the responses of rods and cones to light stimuli (Fig. 21–1). Standardized protocols allow selective evaluation of each photoreceptor; cone dystrophies can be distinguished from early RP with appropriate ERG testing. ERG testing is performed serially to distinguish progressive loss of photoreceptor function, usually hereditary, from nonprogressive pigmentary retinopathies. The ERG measured in response to pattern stimuli can provide one measure of visual acuity and function in young children. A good ERG requires a well-sedated child; an excellent technician may be able to talk a cooperative child through a single eye ERG without sedation.

Leber's congenital amaurosis (LCA, Fig. 21–2) early-onset RP, and related systemic syndromes show normal or nearly normal fundus appearances early in life with an extinguished ERG. Although other diseases such as achromatopsia or CSNB may have barely recordable ERGs, these typically improve with age. The deficit in LCA and RP will not improve. Delayed visual maturation will also show normal fundi and poor or absent fixation responses, with normal ERG on testing. Distinguishing rod and cone responses will assist in diagnosis; the absence of rods is consistent with early-onset

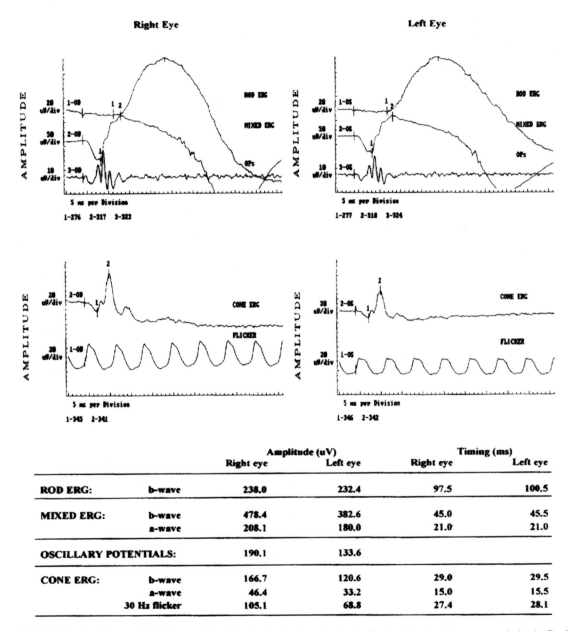

FIGURE 21–1. Normal ERG in a child with single flash rod, single flash mixed rod–cone, and single flash cone and flicker response labeled.

		Amplitude (uV)		Timing (ms)	
		Right eye	Left eye	Right eye	Left eye
ROD ERG:	b-wave	238.0	232.4	97.5	100.5
MIXED ERG:	b-wave	478.4	382.6	45.0	45.5
	a-wave	208.1	180.0	21.0	21.0
OSCILLARY POTENTIALS:		190.1	133.6		
CONE ERG:	b-wave	166.7	120.6	29.0	29.5
	a-wave	46.4	33.2	15.0	15.5
	30 Hz flicker	105.1	68.8	27.4	28.1

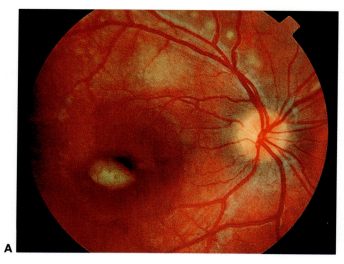

A

FIGURE 21–2. Extinguished ERG, both rod and cone responses in Leber's congenital amaurosis.

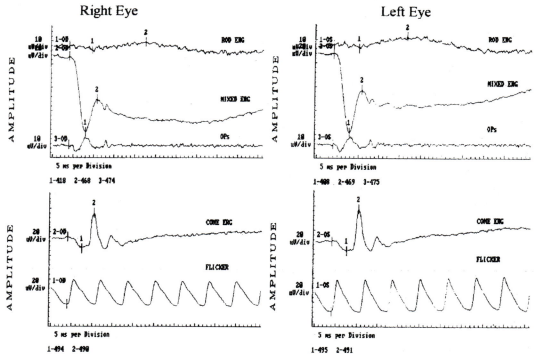

		Amplitude (uV)		Timing (ms)	
		right eye	left eye	right eye	left eye
ROD ERG:	b-wave	18.9	27.0	92.5	88.0
MIXED ERG:	b-wave	139.4	178.4	34.0	34.0
	a-wave	326.6	334.6	20.0	19.0
OSCILLARY POTENTIALS:		52.6	47.1		
CONE ERG:	b-wave	153.8	174.0	32.0	31.0
	a-wave	44.2	38.8	17.0	17.5
	30 Hz flicker	98.0	127.6	31.8	31.0

B

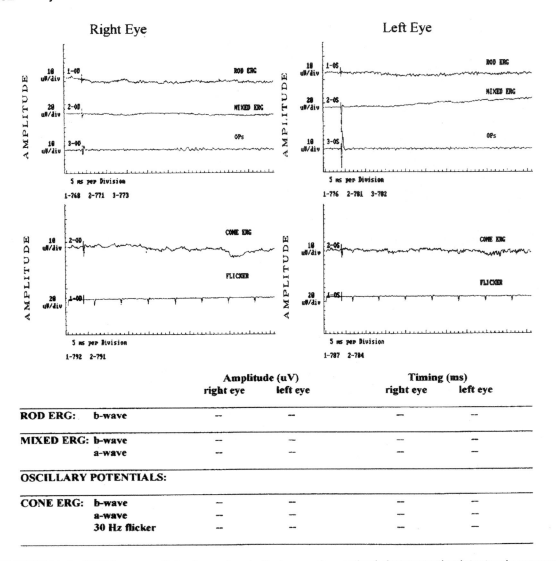

FIGURE 21–3. ERG in congenital achromatopsia (rod monochromatism) demonstrating intact rod response and absent cone response.

RP, and the absence of cones is consistent with achromatopsia and variants (Fig. 21–3). Thus, ERGs and other electrophysiologic tests are crucial in diagnosing the cause of poor visual development in young children.

The visual evoked potential (VEP) measures the electroencephalogram during repetitive visual stimulation; a tracing averaging many VEPs, the visual evoked response, will detect posterior visual pathway diseases, even in the presence of normal ERG results. The latency of the wave form indicates the state of conduction along the optic nerve; the amplitude of the wave indicates visual acuity. Along with the ERG, the VER can provide useful information about visual function in infants and preverbal children as well as diagnose neurologic causes of poor visual function.

Electrooculography (EOG) measures an electrical potential existing between retinal pigment epithelium (RPE) cells and photoreceptors; the difference between the voltage measured in light- and dark-adapted conditions is expressed as a ratio. A subnormal ratio is observed in 100%

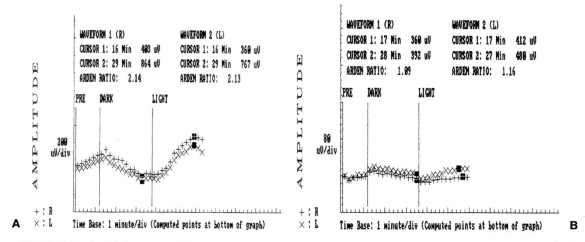

FIGURE 21–4. EOG tracing **(A)** showing abnormal (>2) light–dark ratio in a case of Best's Disease **(B)**.

of patients with visual loss due to Best's disease (Fig. 21–4). The EOG, even with normal vision and ERG studies, is the best test for this disease.

In no instance is electrophysiologic testing[6] ordered in isolation. Along with a thorough history and a good ophthalmic examination and genetic and laboratory testing where appropriate, this methodology is combined with visual field, color testing, and dark adaptometry to diagnose the causes of poor vision in children.

When Should I Get an Ultrasound?

A B-scan ultrasound is appropriate to evaluate all eyes in which the posterior pole and retina cannot be directly viewed due to media opacity. In children, corneal opacity and cataract limiting the view of the posterior pole are the most common reasons for ultrasonographic imaging. Often the exam done through closed lids in a drowsy child or hungry infant provides all the information needed without general anesthesia. In most cases, the retina is imaged to rule out retinal detachment in the presence of trauma, hyphema, or vitreous hemorrhage. Thickening of the choroid or choroidal effusions can be evaluated in children with chronic uveitis and hypotony. With extreme care an ultrasound probe can be used in a cooperative child to rule out an intraocular foreign body, although this technique is dangerous with any suspected ruptured globe and is not generally recommended. In addition, details of orbital and intraconal

anatomy, such as the echo-free "T-sign" of fluid behind the globe in posterior scleritis or orbital pseudotumor, or the presence of enlarged rectus muscles in various diseases may be imaged. In each case, an ultrasound is obtained relatively rapidly in situations in which computed tomography (CT) scanning or magnetic resonance imaging (not for metallic foreign bodies) can also provide valuable information.

In certain diseases, most typically in retinoblastoma causing leukocoria (Fig. 21–5) or in choroidal osteoma, the ultrasound characteristics of the lesion may provide a clue as to its identity. The presence of echoes typical of calcification assist in diagnosing each of these tumors.

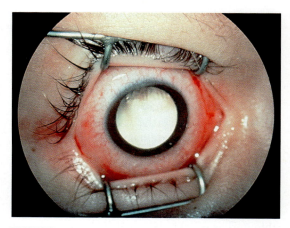

FIGURE 21–5. Leukocoria from a massive intraocular retinoblastoma.

What Abnormalities Should be Referred to Specialists?

If you are confident of your diagnosis and the suspected condition has no specialized treatment, there is no real need for a specialist referral. If you are in doubt about the diagnosis or if your diagnosis carries genetic, social, or familial implications (e.g., Tay-Sach's or congenital syphilis), it is wise to refer to a specialist for a confirmatory opinion. Retinoblastoma and ROP are two conditions for which specific treatments exist, which occur at sufficiently low frequency that an individual general ophthalmologist may see few cases in a clinical lifetime. Because of the complexity of management these diseases are best left to specialists. Given the significant risks of legal liability to those caring for children with ROP, retinoblastoma, or similar diseases, referral to specialists may be regarded as self-preservation.

What Abnormalities Must I Report to Child Protective Services?

The best advice is *better to overcall than undercall*, to avoid learning belatedly of the death of an infant whom you had seen. A nonverbal or pre-verbal child with little or no history, an eccentric pupil, a cataract, retinal or subhyaloid hemorrhages, and retinal tears or dialyses are usual subjects for referrals. The "blood and thunder" fundus or Terson's pattern of bleeding signifies a mortal injury and is the result of a gradual buildup of violence by the perpetrator; such findings are rare. It is important to keep unexpected settings in mind, such as a consult for "fever of unknown origin," which may be the result of a beating administered by a clever caregiver who leaves no obvious bruises. Older children may not tell the examiner about ongoing child abuse, even under direct questioning. Thus, the art lies in having a heightened sense of awareness before the violence reaches the stage of irreversible damage and death.

How Do I Tell Parents about Abnormal Findings?

Telling the truth, as simply and honestly as possible and as quickly as possible, is the only policy. More harm and misery are caused by failing to confront reality than by facing it explicitly. A clinician can note an abnormality and if uncertain about its significance simply say, "I don't know, but I know where to send you to find out." Misinformation, false hopes, and deliberate equivocation will rebound to your ultimate discredit.

■ Specific Conditions

Retinopathy of Prematurity

ROP is a disease that affects preterm and low-birth-weight infants receiving supplemental oxygen administration after birth.[7] The Multicenter Trial of Cryotherapy for Retinopathy of Prematurity defines high-risk infants as those with birth weights of 1250 g or less. The study concluded that, the lower the birth weight, the higher the risk of developing ROP; a 90% risk of ROP was noted for infants weighing less than 750 g. The pathology of ROP reaches its peak at 1 to 3 months after birth, with retinal detachment and other blinding complications following thereafter. Because treatment has been found effective in preventing the blinding effects of ROP, examination of all low-birth-weight infants and infants receiving supplemental oxygen at birth is mandatory.

The vessels of the retina grow from the optic nerve to the periphery, reaching the ora on the temporal retina after birth. To find and stage the pathology in infants with ROP, an examiner must see the retina beyond the equator for 360 degrees. The committee of ophthalmologists developing the International Classification of Retinopathy of Prematurity found three parameters significant: location of the process (zone), extent in clock hours of pathology, and the severity or appearance of the abnormal vessels. The CRYO-ROP study defined threshold disease requiring cryotherapy as more than five contiguous or eight cumulative (total) clock hours of (stage 3) neovascular proliferation extending from a ridge of issue at the demarcation of vascularized and nonvascular retina in zone I or II with plus disease. Zone I is a circle centered on the disc with radius of twice the distance from the optic disc to the macula. Zone II is a circle extending from zone I to the nasal ora, leaving a small residual temporal crescent (zone III). Plus disease is defined as dilatation and tortuosity of vessels in the posterior pole as well as adjacent to the ridge of developing blood vessels. Retinal lesions are categorized by the highest stage of disease observed in each clock hour. Treatment of threshold disease with cryopexy or laser via indirect ophthalmoscopy significantly decreases progression to more advanced disease.

Regression of most nonthreshold disease without serious vascular or retinal sequelae is the most common outcome in eyes with ROP. Advanced ROP, if untreated or unsuccessfully treated, leads to retinal detachment on the basis of traction originating at the line of vascularizing tissue. This is defined as stage 4 disease if a partial detachment, with or without extension to the macula (A and B, respectively), exists. Stage 5 disease includes funnel detachments, staged further depending on the anatomy of the funnel. Because the visual outcomes of detachment surgery for stage 4B and stage 5 disease are often poor, prevention of progression is key.[8] Surgery of complicated retinal detachments involves vitrectomy with adjunctive instrumentation and techniques and is best left to vitreoretinal surgeons specializing in this field. Visual rehabilitation, particularly after lensectomy, is a critical determinant of final visual function and is best handled by pediatric ophthalmologists working with a motivated family. Thus, the consequences of missed or delayed diagnosis of ROP for long-term visual recovery are grave.

Initial screening examinations of low birthweight infants always begin (often occur) in the neonatal intensive care unit. Although controversy exists about the indications and timing of initial examination, a screening examination at 4 to 6 weeks of age or 32 to 34 weeks after conception in infants weighing 1500 g or less at birth is reasonable. Eyes with zone II disease, which is less than stage 2, can be seen every 2 weeks. Any zone I or zone II disease that is more advanced than stage 2 but not yet threshold (prethreshold) should be examined weekly or more often. Examinations should occur on schedule until either threshold is reached or the retina vascularizes through zone III.

Infants are dilated with drops containing 0.5% cyclopentolate, 0.5% tropicamide, and 2.5% phenylephrine (see above) in dilute form. Drops are given two times, 5 to 10 minutes apart. Although systemic hypertension is a consideration with mydriatics, adequate pupillary dilation is critical to allow visualization beyond the equator. Alternatively, new technology has been developed that allows photographic visualization and computer storage of images through undilated pupils with a wide angle contact hand-held camera probe (Fig. 21–6). Indirect ophthalmoscopy is performed 30 to 60 minutes after drops are instilled, using a 28- or 30-diopter lens. A lid speculum is inserted after instillation of topical anesthetic; a lens loupe or small culture swab is used for scleral depression. Depression is used to rotate the peripheral retina into view while avoiding excessive pressure on the eye (causing pulsation of the cranial retinal artery or blanching of the optic nerve) or causing bradycardia (the oculocardiac reflex). A retinal drawing showing the extent and tabulating the severity of vascular changes is advisable even if the disease appears mild, both for your benefit and for other examiners who might be consulted in the future. Updated drawings should be made on each serial examination until all pathologic changes have stabilized or resolved. You should advise both the neonatal intensive care unit team and the family of your findings.

In the event that prethreshold or threshold disease is found, you must arrange for prompt referral and follow-up with a pediatric ophthalmologist specializing in treatment of ROP if you

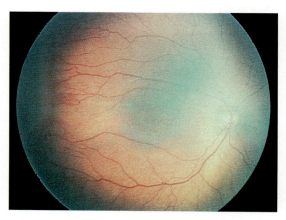

FIGURE 21–6. Digitized image of ROP taken with the wide-angle RET CAM 120®.

choose not to treat this yourself. It is prudent to call the family at home to insure that the follow-up recommendations are being complied with.

Regressed ROP has a number of permanent sequelae that may be noted on examination of healthy children and adults. These include most commonly myopia, astigmatism, anisometropia, and strabismus. Less common are glaucoma, traction-rhegmatogenous retinal detachment, peripheral retinal folds, avascularity of the peripheral retina, lattice degeneration, macular ectopia, vascular tortuosity or straightening, and myopia, among others.

Specific methods for treating the vascular lesions of ROP are beyond the scope of this chapter. Both cryopexy and laser applied to nonvascularized retina arrest the progression of ROP to retinal detachment and other blinding sequelae. Only prompt examination and appropriate recognition of the staging of ROP, as well as indications for therapy, will allow either treatment to benefit your patient.

Retinal Detachment

Retinal detachments in children[9] are uncommon and usually due to underlying disease such as ROP or retinoblastoma, a syndrome such as Stickler's syndrome, or trauma (Fig. 21–7). Retinal detachments may be serous, rhegmatogenous, or tractional. In each case, diagnosis of the underlying cause of the detachment is important to the child's health and long-term visual function. Detailed reviews of the causes of retinal detachments in children can be found elsewhere.[1–3]

Detachment of the retina often occurs in the setting of obvious abnormality of the structure of the eye and body. Abnormalities of vitreous and retinal development will be reviewed briefly in the next section. Other abnormalities, typical of adults such as lattice degeneration or high myopia are correlated with an increased frequency of retinal detachments in children. Conditions may be inherited or occur sporadically and often occur together in the same eye; each may be signs of familial degenerative disorders.

Three hereditary systemic disorders have increased risk of retinal detachment. Marfan's syndrome combines tall stature, long and hyperextensible joints, aortic dilatation and dissection, and other heart valve abnormalities with ocular abnormalities. These include myopia, bilateral ectopia lentis (dislocated superior and temporal, Fig. 21–8), iris changes, and retinal detachments in 10 to 20% of eyes. These usually occur with lens dislocation or cataract surgery. Although axial myopia is correlated with the frequency of retinal detachment, lattice degeneration and vitreous abnormalities are incidental findings.

Homocystinuria is an autosomal recessive condition combining tall stature, long limbs with restricted mobility, malar flush, hypertensive and occlusive cardiovascular disease, and mental retardation in 50% of affected patients with ocular abnormalities. These include bilateral lens dislocation in 90% of patients (displaced downward), myopia in some patients, and retinal detachment as a consequence of lens dislocation or surgery in up to 10% of affected eyes. Other retinal or vitreous findings

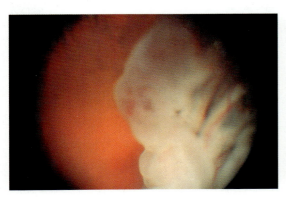

FIGURE 21–7. Giant retinal tear, which may occur in cases of trauma.

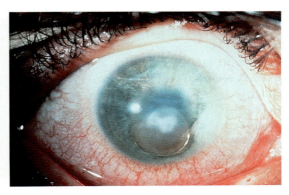

FIGURE 21–8. Ectopia lentis in Marfan's syndrome.

do not affect the risk of developing retinal detachment. One form of homocystinuria, the Hermansky-Pudlak syndrome, features platelet abnormalities, with increased risk of thrombotic vascular occlusions and death after general anesthesia. This may be associated with albinism.

Ehlers-Danlos syndrome is a group of hereditary disorders of which type VI is autosomal recessive, combining elastic and fragile skin, hyperextensible joints, and tendency toward hemorrhagic diathesis with ocular abnormalities. These include blue and fragile sclera, keratoconus, angioid streaks, lattice and other pigmentary degenerations of the peripheral retina, and a low risk of retinal detachment related to the presence of myopia. The scleral thinning and bleeding abnormalities may make retinal reattachment surgery hazardous.

Five entities may cause congenital retinal detachments. Persistent hyperplastic primary vitreous (PHPV) may exhibit vitreous membranes with retinal folds or detachments in one or both eyes, with or without the typical microphthalmos or anterior changes associated with PHPV. Retinal dysplasia refers to a spectrum of severe abnormalities of retinal development due to various causes, including Trisomy 13, inherited syndromes, and intrauterine infection. Falciform retinal folds typically occur in the inferotemporal quadrant, extending anteriorly from the optic nerve head; these often occur in structurally normal eyes and may represent a milder form of abnormal retinal development than the other disorders in this group. Norrie's disease is an X-linked hereditary disorder combining bilateral leukocoria and retinal dysplasia with mental retardation (25% of affected boys) or deafness. Incontinentia pigmenti (Fig. 21–9) is a hereditary disorder almost always lethal for males displaying abnormalities of skin pigmentation with dental and neurologic disorders, along with various changes in the retina including avascular retina, pigmentary disturbances of RPE, and retinal detachment. Although some remedy may be attempted in milder forms of ocular abnormalities to improve or preserve vision, the role of the ophthalmologist is frequently to assist in the diagnosis of these disorders.

Leukocoria is sometimes encountered in one or both eyes. The occurrence of retinal detachment on ultrasound in any eye with leukocoria should immediately raise the suspicion of retinoblastoma and other tumors of the posterior segment, ROP, PHPV, toxocara, and the various causes of retinal dysplasia.

Several isolated abnormalities of ocular development or structure may be associated with complicated retinal detachments. The morning glory disc and congenital optic pits are anomalies of optic nerve head formation. Both show abnormalities of vessel anatomy, at the optic nerve head. The morning glory disc (Fig. 21–10) is more often unilateral and may be associated with systemic abnormalities, including basal encephalocele. Optic pits are not associated with systemic abnormalities. Both are

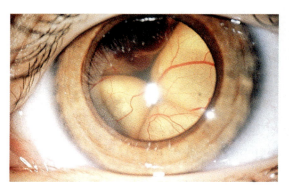

FIGURE 21–9. Retinal detachment in incontinentia pigmenti.

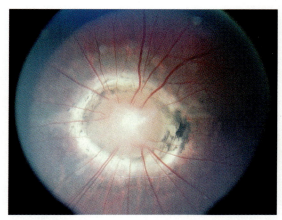

FIGURE 21–10. Morning glory disk, which is associated with an increased risk of localized retinal detachment.

associated with an increased risk of localized retinal detachment in 25 to 37% of affected eyes. Morning glory discs often cause serous and rhegmatogenous retinal detachments with holes located in the anomalous disc, whereas optic pits may produce detachment related to macular retinoschisis. In both cases, anomalous production or circulation of sub- or intraretinal fluid is proposed as the pathogenesis of the retinal detachment. Therapy of the retinal detachments is controversial with various authors advocating laser, intravitreal gas injection, or vitrectomy, internal drainage of subretinal fluid, laser, and some form of long-acting retinal tamponade such as gas or silicone oil.

Coloboma of the optic nerve and coloboma of the retina and choroid (Fig. 21–11) represent anomalous development of the optic nerve papilla and incomplete closure of the fetal fissure; the involved portion of the optic nerve or retina is often inferior and nasal. Both are associated with systemic abnormalities, including basal encephalocele in the former and the CHARGE association in the latter. Some cases of each are hereditary and bilateral. Both are associated with the development of complicated rhegmatogenous retinal detachments with the causative breaks originating in the area of abnormal tissue. Vitrectomy, internal drainage, laser or cryopexy, and long-acting tamponade are now advocated as effective management of the associated retinal detachment.

Giant retinal tears may be associated with colobomas of the lens.

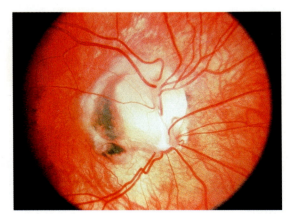

FIGURE 21–11. Coloboma of the optic nerve and choroid.

Bilateral nontraumatic inferotemporal retinal dialyses may be associated with chronic slowly progressive retinal detachment, often with extensive demarcation lines.

Ocular trauma, often as a result of blunt trauma inflicted by parents or other caregivers, is an important cause of retinal abnormalities in children. It has been estimated that 40% of battered children show some form of ocular damage. The abuse is frequently manifest in the first 4 years of life. Infants with head injuries may present with retinal hemorrhages, cotton wool spots, subhyaloid and vitreous hemorrhages, disc swelling, or peripapillary hemorrhage ("blood and thunder," Terson's or Purtscher's retinopathy due to violent thoracic compression). Imaging of the central nervous system may show associated intracranial or subdural hemorrhage, cerebral edema, and midline shifts. Retinal dialyses may be found in the superonasal and inferotemporal pars plana, often with associated avulsion of the vitreous base. Irregular and large retinal breaks, sometimes with underlying RPE changes and choroidal atrophy, represent a later response to severe blunt trauma. The inferotemporal quadrant is vulnerable because it is least protected from direct trauma by the orbit. Retinoschisis, macular scarring or hole, vitreous traction in the periphery, choroidal rupture scars concentric to the disc, posterior and peripapillary retinal tears or avulsion, and optic atrophy may be permanent sequelae of blunt trauma. A number of conditions can lead to retinal hemorrhages in infants found unresponsive, but none of the other etiologies, including CPR, show both hemorrhages and other signs of retinal or vitreous base trauma. Thus, a thorough and exacting retinal examination in all children with loss of consciousness, seizures, or cardiac arrest can assist in the correct diagnosis of battered child syndrome.

Vitreoretinopathies

A number of disorders of vitreous formation combined with abnormalities of retinal anatomy can predispose to complicated retinal detachments.[1–3,9] Several of these syndromes are associated with these entities as well.

Stickler's syndrome, also termed hereditary progressive arthroophthalmopathy, combines significant ocular pathology with orthopedic and midfacial anomalies in an autosomal dominant inheritance pattern. Ocular abnormalities include high myopia, a clear vitreous space with membranes and strands (the "optically empty" vitreous), perivascular pigmentary disturbances, and glaucoma. Cataract formation is the rule in the fourth and fifth decades; complicated retinal detachments occur in nearly 50% of affected eyes.

Systemic abnormalities include growth disturbances at the epiphyseal plates of weight-bearing joints. Facial anomalies such as cleft palate, bifid uvula, and the Pierre-Robin anomaly may lead the child's parents to seek pediatric attention before the ocular pathology is noted. Hearing loss may occur in later childhood. Cardiac abnormalities, such as mitral valve prolapse, occur in up to 46% of affected children.

Definitive management of children with Stickler's syndrome should be undertaken by a team of specialists, with an orientation toward evaluating the entire family. Genetic counseling, orthopedic intervention, ear, nose, and throat, and plastic surgical evaluation as well as cardiologic consultation may all be required. Because pedigrees show heterogeneous genetic alterations, with variable penetrance, the presence of this syndrome may be missed in less affected family members.

Ophthalmologic management includes serial retinoscopic or manifest refractions and follow-up with special attention to early lens changes to prevent the development of amblyopia. Retinal examinations must be thorough to recognize the presence of retinal breaks and tears. Complicated retinal detachments, giant tears, and multiple posterior breaks associated with retinal detachment are all features of this syndrome. These require specialized vitreoretinal surgery.

Wagner's disease is autosomal dominantly inherited and includes some of the ocular features of Stickler's syndrome, including moderate myopia, cataract formation, an optically empty vitreous with strands, and perivascular pigmentation and sheathing. Progressive atrophy of the retina and choroid, nyctalopia, and peripheral visual field loss will all come to an ophthalmologist's attention in early adulthood.

ERG testing shows loss of B-wave amplitude, which may progress to extinguished electrical activity in the retina (Fig. 21–12). Early cataract formation is also noted in Wagner's disease. No association with systemic anomalies or retinal detachment has been noted. Management of ocular abnormalities is conservative. Similar retinal findings without systemic anomalies, combined with a high risk of retinal detachment, may be termed Jansen's syndrome.

Goldmann-Favre syndrome is an autosomal recessive degeneration of the retina that leads to profound visual loss due to retinoschisis, progressive pigmentary degeneration reminiscent of retinitis pigmentosa (RP), and early cataract formation. Affected children present in the first and second decades complaining of poor vision and increasing difficulty with night vision. Retinal examination reveals peripheral retinoschisis that progresses centripetally, a macula with cystic changes and a "beaten metal" reflex, vitreous strands, disc pallor, and vascular sheathing. Fluorescein angiography distinguishes the maculopathy by its absence of leakage. ERG testing reveals loss of scotopic A-wave amplitude early, progressing to loss of ERG activity, and marked abnormal dark adaptation. Visual fields may show peripheral ring scotomas similar to those seen in RP. Loss of visual acuity in childhood is often severe with vision reduced to 20/200 in each eye.

Familial exudative vitreoretinopathy combines the salient retinal findings of ROP with an autosomal dominant inheritance pattern, without a history of prematurity or perinatal oxygen administration. Findings vary from vitreous abnormalities with an area of peripheral "white without pressure" to a ridge of retinal tissue with fibrovascular proliferation bordering an avascular area of retina. Dilated and tortuous retinal vessels with subretinal exudate, peripheral tractional retinal detachment, and dragging of the macula temporally may be noted. Visual loss may be due to amblyopia, cataract, band keratopathy, glaucoma, cystoid macular edema, massive subretinal exudates or extensive retinal detachment, or vitreous hemorrhage. Mild cases remain stable with little likelihood of visual loss after age 20, although retinal detachment may occur later in life near the ridge of fibrovascular tissue.

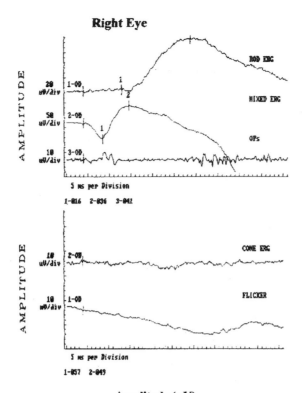

	Amplitude (uV) right eye	Timing (ms) right eye
ROD ERG: b-wave	202.1	123.5
MIXED ERG: b-wave	339.3	53.0
a-wave	164.1	22.5
OSCILLARY POTENTIALS:	54.3	
CONE ERG: b-wave	--	--
a-wave	--	--
30 Hz flicker	--	--

FIGURE 21–12. ERG in Wagner's syndrome showing loss of the scotopic (rod) a-wave.

Early examination and diagnosis may allow treatment of the avascular retina as well as prompt identification of retinal breaks, which may lead to retinal detachment in almost 30% of affected eyes. Tractional detachments in childhood are best managed with vitrectomy techniques, whereas rhegmatogenous detachments later in life may be managed with scleral buckling.

X-linked juvenile retinoschisis affects boys and presents with superficial cystic spaces in the retina, arranged in a stellate pattern around the fovea. These lesions do not manifest the pattern of leakage of fluorescein dye noted on angiography with other causes of macular edema. The cystic spaces may merge forming the characteristic foveal schisis with radial striae. Peripheral retinoschisis, originating in the inferotemporal quadrant, complicates half of the cases of foveal schisis. Narrowing and sheathing of retinal vessels, peripheral pigmentary changes similar to RP, vitreous hemorrhage, and, uncommonly, retinal detachments may all occur in the periphery. Vision is limited by both macular damage, which appears as an atrophic retina overlying RPE changes and extensive peripheral field loss (absolute scotomata) in areas of retinoschisis. Visions of 20/200 are common in the sixth and seventh decades. Serial loss of rod and cone function on ERG, dark adaptation, and color vision are often noted.

Although scleral buckle surgery can be employed to repair most retinal detachments, reserving vitrectomy for vitreous hemorrhage or complicated retinal detachments, the ultimate prognosis for good vision is poor. Some female carriers and female homozygotes may show a limited form of this disorder.

Inherited, Metabolic, and Storage Diseases

A large and bewildering array of hereditary, metabolic, and storage diseases shows characteristic retinal changes.[1–3,5,10] Fortunately, you will rarely be examining such children in complete isolation. A family history, a pediatric referral for suspicion of multisystem storage disease, or the presence of obvious abnormalities of the body, facies, or the anterior segment will alert the clinician to the presence of genetic diseases. A tertiary care institution can accept responsibility for characterizing the gene locus of the disorder, establishing the pedigree, and counseling the family once you have validated the suspicion of a hereditary disorder. The vast majority of these conditions are autosomal recessive or X-linked recessive.

The cherry red spot in the macula is one of the characteristic signs seen in retinal practice. Although the underlying cause in adults is often vascular occlusion, in children the lesion is due to accumulation of material in the retinal ganglion cells. The spot represents the thin foveolar retina showing the underlying RPE and choroid. This appearance may be seen in

- Sphingolipidoses: hexosaminidase deficiency, GM_2 gangliosidosis, type I (Tay-Sachs) and type II (Sandhoff's); sphingomyelinase deficiency, Niemann-Pick, types A, B, and C (Fig. 21–13); β-galactosidase deficiency (A, B, and C), Landing's disease; glucocerebrosidase deficiency, Gaucher's disease; galactocerebroside β-galactosidase (galactocerebrosidase) deficiency, Krabbe's disease.

- Lysosomal ceramidase deficiency, Farber's disease.

- Sulfatase A deficiency, metachromatic leukodystrophy.

- Mucolipidoses: lysosomal neuraminidase deficiency, sialidosis, type I (cherry red spot myoclonus syndrome) and type II; nephrosialidosis; with β-galactosidase deficiency, galactosialidosis (Goldberg-Cotlier syndrome).

These changes should not be confused with macular holes or hemorrhages, which may occur in the setting of traumatic retinopathy. The cherry red appearance may also occur in any disease causing retinal edema in the posterior pole; it has been noted in subacute

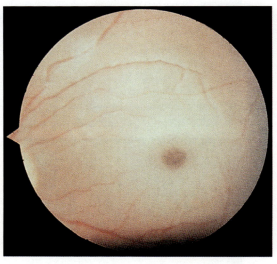

FIGURE 21–13. The cherry red spot of Niemann-Pick disease.

sclerosing panencephalitis (SSPE, rubeola) affecting the retina in this location.

Disturbances of macular pigmentation, typically in a bull's eye maculopathy pattern, may be a finding in

- Neuronal ceroid lipofuscinosis (Batten's disease); due to an uncharacterized defect, three types are described in children, based on age of onset: Haltia-Santavuori presents in infancy; Jansky-Bielschowsky, at 2 to 4 years of age; Spielmeyer-Vogt, at 6 to 7 years of age (Fig. 21–14).
- Hallervorden-Spatz disease, a neurodegenerative disorder of unknown cause.
- Primary hereditary hyperoxaluria, type I, a deficiency of hepatic peroxisomal alanine: glycolate aminotransferase.
- Bardet-Beidl syndrome and the related Laurence-Moon syndrome.
- Olivopontocerebellar atrophy, type III, a neurodegenerative disorder.
- Stargardt's disease, beginning with a beaten bronze appearance of the macula and blockage of background choroidal flourescence (Fig. 21–15); may have

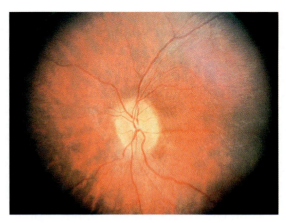

FIGURE 21–14. The fundus appearance in Speilmeyer-Vogt's disease.

peripheral fleck retinopathy. It progresses to geographic atrophy of the macula in later life.

- Bassen-Kornzweig syndrome, abetalipoproteinemia treated with vitamin A and E supplementation.
- Cone dystrophies and cone–rod dystrophies, inherited or sporadic, may change from a normal macular appearance to a bull's eye later.

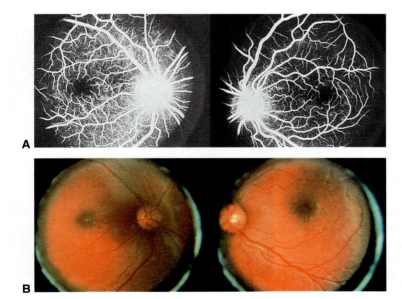

FIGURE 21–15. Blockage of background choroidal flourescence in early Stargardt's disease **(A)** and "beaten bronze" fundus appearance **(B)**.

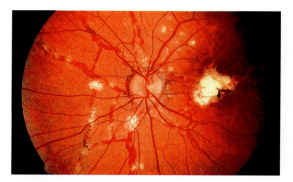

FIGURE 21–16. Angioid streaks in PXE.

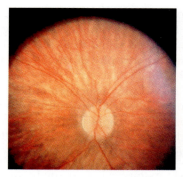

FIGURE 21–17. Fundus appearance in Leber's congenital amaurosis demonstrating attenuated retinal vasculature, "pepper and salt" PE changes.

Kearns-Sayre syndrome, a multisystem disorder of mitochondrial genes and function, is typically associated with a diffuse pigmentary disturbance; its early appearance in the macula may be confused with a bull's eye pattern. This can also be true of other inherited diseases not typically thought to cause maculopathy.

Half of children seen with angioid streaks (Fig. 21–16), which may appear red, gray, or yellow, have no associated systemic diseases; the other half may have

- Hemoglobinopathies: sickle cell disease, thalassemia, hereditary spherocytosis and heterozygous disorders.
- Pseudoxanthoma elasticum.
- Paget's disease of bone.
- Ehlers-Danlos syndrome.
- Bassen-Kornzweig syndrome (abetalipoproteinemia).
- Acromegaly.
- Calcinosis.

The streaks often do not develop until the end of the first or second decades of life. Angioid streaks carry a 50% risk of development of subretinal neovascular membranes affecting the macula, which carries a poor prognosis for vision.

Colobomas or large scars in the macula may be seen in several inherited disorders, in addition to idiopathic, inflammatory, or infectious diseases such as Toxoplasmosis, and in myopia. These include

- Late progressive cone dystrophy.
- Leber's congenital amaurosis (Fig. 21–17), with severe visual dysfunction in infancy and hyperopia.
- Aicardi's syndrome (Fig. 21–18), with large atrophic RPE lesions and agenesis of the *corpus callosum.*
- North Carolina macular dystrophy.

Large areas of atrophy of the choroid may occur in patients with myopia or in patients suffering prior trauma to the eye. Inherited causes include

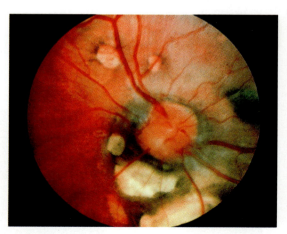

FIGURE 21–18. Lacunae defects in the PE in Aicardi's syndrome.

- Choroideremia, with night blindness in the first and second decades, progressing to extensive visual field loss with corresponding atrophy of the choroid, RPE, and retina.
- Gyrate atrophy, associated with deficiency of mitochondrial ornithine aminotransferase, with atrophy beginning in the midperiphery progressing centrally and anteriorly.

Similarly, extensive hypopigmentation of the fundus accompanies albinism, both ocular and oculocutaneous. Many patients show abnormalities such as iris transillumination defects, optic nerve and macular hypoplasia, myopia, strabismus, and nystagmus. Systemic problems may include susceptibility to infections, mental retardation, neurologic diseases (Chediak-Higashi disease), and coagulation defects (Hermansky Pudlak's disease).

Deposition of crystals, usually yellow or golden in color, may occur with medication use in adults or embolic particles, such as injected talc. Inherited causes include

- Bietti's crystalline tapetoretinal dystrophy, with crystals in the cornea, and extensive RPE atrophy.
- Cystinosis, with crystals in the cornea and renal disease.
- Hyperoxaluria, type I, with widespread deposition of oxalate crystals throughout the body and extensive RPE changes in the posterior pole.
- Gyrate atrophy, with small crystals in the RPE and unaffected choroid.

- Sjogren-Larsson syndrome, presenting with fine white crystals around the macula as well as skin abnormalities.

Various retinal disorders associated with flecks may also appear to be crystalline in nature. A diligent search for crystals elsewhere in the eye (cornea) and body as well as inborn errors of metabolism or multisystem dysfunction will distinguish crystalline disorders.

Chronic uveal effusions have been described in a patient with mucopolysaccharidosis type VI, Maroteaux-Lamy syndrome, which may be associated with abnormal thickening of the posterior sclera.

Inherited pigmentary retinopathies simulating retinitis pigmentosa will be discussed later.

Vascular Diseases of the Retina

Disorders of blood vessel formation in the eye may accompany systemic diseases or be isolated to the eye.[1–3,10]

Coats' disease (Fig. 21–19) is a noninherited disorder of unknown etiology that presents in the first and early second decades; it is unilateral 80% of the time and occurs in males more frequently than females (ratio 3:1). The significant retinal findings are areas of subretinal white or yellow exudate, hemorrhage, abnormal telangiectatic (light bulb shaped) vessels located near the subretinal exudates, and focal aneurysms of retinal vessels. The affected areas of retina may include the posterior pole, and the child may be referred for workup of leukocoria, strabismus, or poor vision in one eye. Flu-

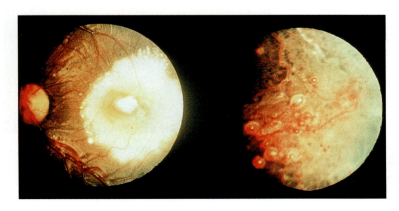

FIGURE 21–19. Coats' disease demonstrating subretinal cholesterol and telangectatic retinal vessels.

orescein angiography can be helpful in determining the location and extent of telangiectatic retinal vessels.

Because of the likelihood of enlargement of the areas of subretinal exudate and severely decreased vision, treatment to ablate the abnormal vessels with laser or cryopexy is undertaken. Vitrectomy may be required to drain massive areas of subretinal exudate or to clear away overlying hemorrhage to allow photocoagulation of the abnormal vessels.

Retinal findings characteristic of Coats' disease may be associated with another systemic or eye disease. This may occur in association with RP and related disorders, children with progressive facial hemiatrophy (Perry-Romberg syndrome), and young adults with fascioscapulohumeral muscular dystrophy, Alport's syndrome (nephritis, deafness, anterior lenticonus, and white retinal lesions), and tuberous sclerosis (see what follows).

Several hamartomatous tumors of the eye should be differentiated clearly. The choroidal hemangioma may occur as an isolated yellow choroidal lesion with an overlying serous detachment of the retina, often with lipid exudates. These usually become symptomatic only in adulthood but may be noted in children. On fluorescein angiogram large vascular channels in the choroid, diffuse leakage, and cystic degeneration of the overlying retina are noted. A more diffuse hemangioma found in Sturge-Weber syndrome can involve the entire choroid, imparting a red color to the affected fundus. The other elements are ipsilateral facial nevus flammeus, glaucoma, intracranial vascular malformations, and seizures in some cases. Retinal findings may include serous subretinal fluid and cystic changes in the retina and choroidal and retinal detachments after filtering procedures. The Sturge-Weber syndrome is one of a group of mainly dominantly inherited diseases called phacomatoses, which link hamartomas or other tumors of different organ systems. The other phakomatoses mentioned below are Westkamp-Cotlier syndrome, Von Hippel syndrome and variants, Wyburn-Mason syndrome, neurofibromatosis, and tuberous sclerosis (Bourneville's disease).

The cavernous hemangioma of the retina appears as a cluster of dark aneurysmal vessels surrounded by white or gray fibrous tissue; the lesion may appear as an elevated cluster of grapes. The lesions are found more often in females, usually in the second or third decade. The lesions are usually solitary but may be multifocal and bilateral. Fluorescein angiography reveals delayed and incomplete filling of the aneurysms and no leakage of dye. The retinal hemangiomas may be associated with angiomas occurring in the brain and skin, called Westkamp-Cotlier syndrome.

The capillary hemangioma of the retina usually appears as a large solitary pinkish or red globular lesion with large, anastomosing feeder vessels. They may be endophytic and easily visible on the retina or optic nerve or exophytic and buried under the retina or within the nerve. There is often leakage of subretinal fluid and retinal lipid exudates in the exophytic hemangiomas. The presence of abnormal anastomosing vessels within the lesion and leakage of fluid from the hemangioma are fluorescein angiographic hallmarks. The angiomas may show growth in size into adulthood and require treatment with laser, cryopexy, or diathermy if vision is affected. Vitrectomy may be necessary for a complication, such as vitreous hemorrhage or retinal traction. Syndromes include retinal findings alone in von Hippel's disease (Fig. 21–20). The combination of angiomas of the retina, central nervous system, and spine and hamartomas, tumors, or cysts of visceral organs (kidney, liver, pancreas, lung, and elsewhere) is termed von Hippel-Lindau disease. Diagnosing this dominantly inherited syndrome[11] is of critical

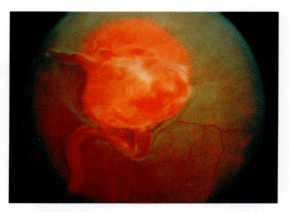

FIGURE 21–20. Retinal angioma typical of von Hippel's disease.

importance because of the high rate of occurrence of renal cell carcinoma, cerebellar angiomas, and pheochromocytoma.

Retinal vessels may take unusual forms in the child's eye. Among these is congenital retinal arterial tortuosity, idiopathic inherited retinal venous beading, and congenital prepapillary vascular loops. Although these phenomena are benign if they occur in isolation, other systemic disorders in children, such as leukemia, sickle cell, familial dysautonomia (Riley-Day syndrome), mucopolysaccharidosis type VI (Maroteaux-Lamy syndrome), and Fabry's disease, may cause tortuosity of retinal vessels in children. Venous beading may occur with diabetes, leukemia, and Alport's disease. Vascular loops of the optic disc may be identical in appearance to optociliary shunt vessels, which are seen in the setting of chronic disc edema in optic nerve meningiomas (part of neurofibromatosis type 2). These conditions, whether idiopathic or pathological, may be associated with visual loss if the circulation of the macula or optic nerve is affected. Fluorescein angiography can be valuable in distinguishing congenital from pathological vascular abnormalities, as can referral of the child for focused and careful pediatric examination.

Congenital enlargement of a large retinal vessel, termed a macrovessel, can involve a retinal vein or artery and may involve areas of nonperfusion of the retina or abnormal capillaries. The macrovessels may show a normal capillary bed between the arterial and venous sides or may constitute retinal arteriovenous or racemose aneurysms with extensive disturbances of retinal circulation and poor vision. Severe instances of racemose aneurysms may be associated with the nonhereditary Wyburn-Mason syndrome when arteriovenous malformations of the midbrain and periorbital area are found. Fluorescein angiography is indicated to stage the macrovessels and assess the surrounding retinal circulation. The clinical course of macrovessels is variable; treatment is only rarely indicated or helpful.

Retinal vascular abnormalities are common in childhood and may be associated with systemic diseases. The vascular changes due to diabetes, sickle cell and related hereditary hemoglobinopathies, and hypertension have the same pathogenesis as in adults. These tend to occur in adolescents in early stages of retinal disease. As noted above, trauma to the eye, head, and chest may present as a vascular lesion. Leukemia (Fig. 21–21) and related hyperviscosity syndromes may reveal themselves in children as visual loss due to diffuse retinal vascular disease. Retinal ischemia and abnormal vascular anatomy as a consequence of inflammatory and infectious diseases are covered elsewhere in this text. Attenuation of retinal vessels, often without neovascularization, occurs in diffuse pigmentary retinopathies, such as RP.

Retinitis Pigmentosa and Related Disorders

RP refers to a heterogeneous group of eye diseases that are classically marked by bilateral waxy pallor of the optic disc, vascular attenuation, progressive retinal pigmentary changes with retinal atrophy beginning in the periphery and traveling posteriorly, visual field defects,

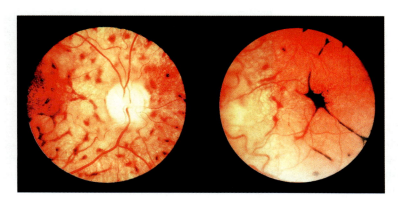

FIGURE 21–21. Fundus appearance "leopard spot" choroidopathy typical of the fundus appearance in acute lymphocytic leukemia in children.

loss of rod function greater than cone function on electrophysiologic testing, cataract, and relatively late preservation of central vision.[1-3,5,10] In young children this typical pattern is not the rule because most of these signs develop gradually over time. In addition, because RP is a heterogeneous assortment of gene mutations affecting different molecular entities, the inheritance of RP is sex linked, autosomal recessive, and dominant and occurs sporadically.[12] Finally, several nonclassical variants of RP exist, including some associated with extraocular organ system dysfunction.

The typical presentations of RP in children are of an asymptomatic child referred for examination because of a family history or a symptomatic child with night blindness, headaches, photopsias, and fluctuating vision during the day. As outlined above, a third presentation is that of an infant with absent visual responses and an extinguished ERG. A majority of older patients present with some abnormality of the macula, including cystoid macular edema, macular pucker, or pigment migration into the macula. A mild inflammatory component is often present on diagnosis.

The workup of any diffuse pigmentary disturbance in the retina includes a history oriented toward discovering evidence of any visual problem such as reduced vision, bumping into objects located beside the patient, or nyctalopia. A careful family history for similar visual disturbances and/or consanguinity must be obtained. A thorough eye exam including electrophysiologic studies should be performed. A Goldmann visual field (in a cooperative child), ERG, and dark adaptometry (difficult in children) are indicated for diagnosis of RP. The presence of large ring-shaped scotomas in the midperiphery leaving a small central island of vision and preserved areas of vision in the periphery are consistent with typical RP; symmetrical field loss is usual. A standard protocol for ERG testing distinguishes loss of rod function from cone dysfunction and allows serial measurements showing progressive loss of amplitude in RP. Abnormal dark adaptation testing reflects the loss of rod component of threshold sensitivity. Nonprogressive (pigmentary) night blinding disturbances of the retina such as CSNB (Fig. 21–22) can be distinguished from RP by these tests.

The primary mechanism leading to blindness in RP is a progressive loss of photoreceptors. Genetic analysis has implicated a wide variety of mutations in genes with abnormal gene products affecting photoreceptor viability and shown that RP is a heterogeneous series of related disorders. Differing patterns of inheritance occur in RP. Autosomal dominant RP constitutes 22% of cases; children will be referred for examination because of a family history. Nyctalopia begins late in the first or second decade, with slower progression and milder disease than other inherited forms of the disease. Autosomal recessive cases are estimated at 9 to 10% of cases; the absence of evidence of RP in either parent supports either this mode of inheritance or a sporadic or simplex case. Because of this confusion, recessive and simplex cases may be confused. Recessive cases are often more severe, and 40% are associated with some form of systemic disease or syndrome. X-linked RP is usually the most severe, leading to blindness in the third or fourth decade in most patients; female carriers often reveal some degree of abnormality on electrophysiologic testing or fundus examination.

RP may be associated with other disorders. A link with LCA has been proposed. Infants may be referred for lack of response to visual stimuli, strabismus, or nystagmus as well as presence of the oculodigital sign (the infant's poking his own eye). Associated disorders include deafness, polycystic kidneys, cardiomyopathy, and osteopetrosis. The ERG will be extinguished in both early-onset RP and LCA.

Usher syndrome combines deafness with RP; type I is more severe and includes vestibular dysfunction. Type II is milder and does not involve the vestibular system. Alstrom disease leads to atypical pigmentary retinopathy, early blindness, obesity, diabetes, and deafness. Bardet-Biedl syndrome combines obesity, hypogonadism, polydactyly, and mental retardation (Fig. 21–23). The neuronal ceroid lipofuscinoses (see above) present with neurological deterioration, which eventually leads to death, and pigmentary retinopathy. Renal failure and retinal degeneration occur in Senior-Loken syndrome. A large variety of other systemic syndromes is reviewed elsewhere.

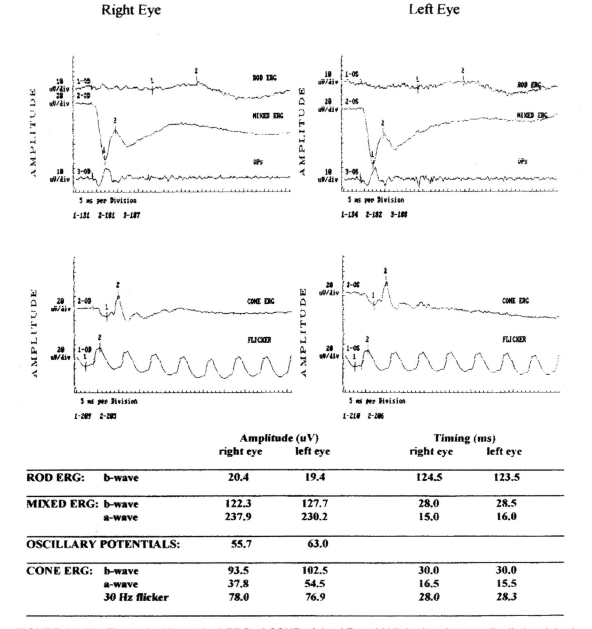

FIGURE 21–22. The typical "negative" ERG of CSNB of the AR and X-linked variety, easily distinguished from RP.

Retinitis punctata albescens shows numerous whitish spots in the retina, pigment migration sparing the macula, and other features typical of RP; this appearance may be seen with Alport's syndrome. Pigmentary disturbances are absent in RP sine pigmenti; unilateral, sectoral, and forms with preserved paraarterial RPE are unusual variants of this disease. These variants will often require electrophysiologic and field testing as well as examination of other family members to make the diagnosis.

The "salt and pepper" fundus may be confused with RP; the differential diagnosis differs, and the electrophysiologic and retinal features of RP are distinct from this entity. The most common cause of salt and pepper fundus

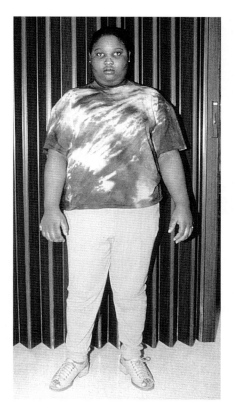

FIGURE 21–23. The typical body habitus of a Biedel Bardot patient with polydactyly.

changes is an intrauterine infection, such as rubella or syphilis. Syndromes associated with this appearance include Alstrom's, Cockayne's (cachexia, birdlike facies, and severe progressive neurologic deterioration), and carriers of X-linked choroideremia and ocular albinism. The mitochondrial encephalomyopathies (Kearns-Sayre but not MELAS, Leber's Hereditary Optic Neuropathy, or MERRF) can be associated with salt and pepper fundus changes. Fundus pulverulentis combines macular changes typical of a macular pattern dystrophy with mottled peripheral RPE changes.

Miscellaneous Dots and Spots

Retinoblastoma is the most common intraocular tumor occurring in children. Its pathogenesis and treament are covered elsewhere.[1–3,5,10] It appears in several important retinal differential diagnoses and will be discussed briefly here. Children may be diagnosed as having one of several common presentations.[1–3] First, any child with leukocoria or obvious heterochromia irides should be referred for examination; because a fundus examination is required for any child with strabismus, this is another common presentation. Retinoblastoma occurs sporadically in two thirds of cases and is dominantly inherited in the rest. Children with bilateral involvement will generally have a family history and be diagnosed earlier (mean age 13 months) than unilateral (24 months); "trilateral" involvement with pinealoma may occur in hereditary cases and is usually fatal. Retinoblastoma is diagnosed by age 5 in 90% of cases, although the disease may rarely present into the sixth decade of life. Overall mortality is 15% of patients, with extensive optic nerve invasion and age at diagnosis (2 to 7 years) closely associated with mortality. Additionally, recurrent or metastatic retinoblastoma may be fatal later in the course of the illness; in hereditary cases, secondary tumors may occur inside the field of therapeutic radiation (up to one third of patients) and outside (5 to 9%) over 30 years after treatment.

The appearance of retinoblastoma is variable. The tumor may present as a subretinal exophytic lesion with an overlying retinal detachment and telangiectatic vessels on the retinal surface. Tumors overlying the retina with white vitreous seeds may also be seen in endophytic lesions. Rarely, diffuse infiltrating disease may simulate uveitis and present with a pseudohypopyon. The presence of calcification and abnormally permeable vessels on fluorescein angiography ramifying into the tumor mass are features consistent with retinoblastoma. In addition, leukocoria may require ultrasound or CT scans to determine the presence of calcium inside the eye to diagnose retinoblastoma. This appearance must be differentiated from Coats' disease, *Toxocara*, PHPV, ROP, retinal dysplasia, FEVR, incontinentia pigmenti, and other causes of leukocoria and large retinal and subretinal masses.

The appearance of a single or multiple white retinal tumors represents another important differential diagnosis. Abnormal vessels and calcification support endophytic retinoblastoma; a related lesion that may also be calcified is the retinoma, which may have a white "fish flesh"

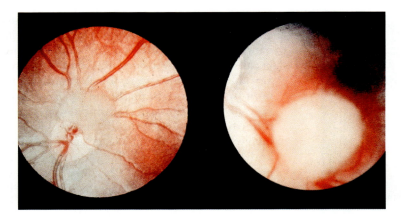

FIGURE 21–24. The typical mulberry-like lesion of Bourneville's disease.

appearance and surrounding RPE changes. This tumor occurs almost exclusively contralateral to an eye with retinoblastoma or in a family member of a patient with hereditary disease. It is felt to represent a regressed or incomplete form of retinoblastoma; malignant transformation of the benign retinoma is possible, and these lesions require close follow-up for this and for the development of secondary neoplastic tumors.

Astrocytic hamartomas (Fig. 21–24) may appear as white globular bodies arising from the surface of the retina and optic nerve, acquiring nodular calcified areas later in life (mulberry pattern). Single lesions may occur in normal chidren; the presence of multiple hamartomas supports the presence of tuberous sclerosis,[14] a phacomatosis combining calcified central nervous system hamartomas, multiple skin lesions, changes in the bones of the fingers and toes, hamartomas of the myocardium and kidneys, and lung disease. The clinical triad of seizures, mental retardation, and sebaceous adenomas of the skin may be seen. Any unknown white retinal lesion should occasion a careful pediatric and neurologic examination. Other elements in the differential diagnosis include granulomas such as *Toxocara* (Fig. 21–25) and benign lesions such as the combined RPE and retinal hamartoma.

The combined hamartoma may occur at the optic nerve head or elsewhere in the retina. Typically, the lesion is peripapillary, slightly elevated, and slate gray in color with surrounding RPE changes. Occurrence elsewhere in the retina is marked by slightly less pigmentation. Visual loss may result from serous exudation at the edge of the lesion, subretinal neovascular

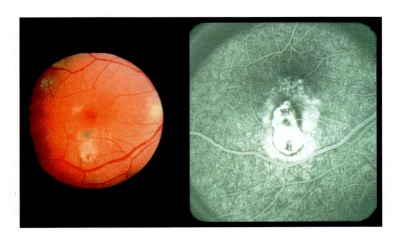

FIGURE 21–25. *Toxocara* granuloma in the macula resulting in vertical diplopia due to retinal traction (courtesy of Don Gass, my patient in his atlas).

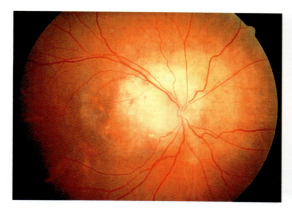

FIGURE 21–26. Fundus appearance of a choroidal osteoma.

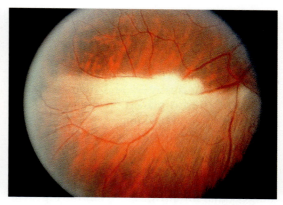

FIGURE 21–27. Myelinated nerve fibers.

membrane growth, and retinal traction. Fluorescein angiography reveals abnormally permeable capillary growth within the body of the tumor. These combined hamartomas may be associated with neurofibromatosis type 2.[15]

Choroidal osteoma (Fig. 21–26) is a subretinal tumor arising in the peripapillary and macular regions in young females; initially, the tumors may appear orange when deep to intact RPE. Later RPE changes may impart a white or mottled appearance to the tumor. Visual loss may occur because of serous retinal elevation or hemorrhagic complications of subretinal neovascularization. Fluorescein angiography may reveal sluggish blood flow in the tumor and late hyperfluorescence where the retina is elevated. Fine vascular spiders can be seen at the surface of the osteoma. Ultrasound and radiography can demonstrate calcification within the lesion. Osteomas may be bilateral in 20% of patients and multicentric and may show slow growth into adulthood.[16] The lesions may first present in adulthood where they may result from chronic inflammatory diseases of the posterior pole. The tumors consist of bone that lies in the choroid with abnormal blood vessels communicating with the choriocapillaris. The tumors are benign.

Myelinated nerve fibers (Fig. 21–27) usually arise from the optic nerve head and travel varying distances following arcuate nerve fiber bundles.[17] The lesions appear hard and white and lie in the inner retina without significant elevation. Because an absolute scotoma exists in the distribution of affected retina, a child with extensive myelinated nerve fibers may present with leukocoria or strabismus. No therapy or systemic associations are known for this abnormality.

■ Pediatric Retinal Surgery

Retinal detachments in pediatric patients are often delayed in diagnosis and become more complex compared to adults. In ROP, careful monitoring and the use of peripheral laser photocoagulation or cryotherapy for stage III retinopathy has reduced the number of patients progressing to tractional detachments requiring vitreoretinal surgery. In older children, most retinal detachments are associated with trauma or with hereditary conditions such as Stickler's syndrome, inferotemporal retinal dialysis, or retinoschisis. Often the diagnosis is delayed because young children do not alert parents of early symptoms and usually report symptoms after severe visual loss by macular involvement or by vitreous hemorrhage. Because of the delay in diagnosis, the retinal detachment is often associated with proliferative vitreoretinopathy. These changes are often seen as pigment dispersion in the vitreous, subretinal proliferation, and star or fixed folds.

Retinal surgery in the pediatric patient requires the close collaboration of a clinical team comprising the pediatric ophthalmologist, pediatrician, anesthesiologist, nurse, orthoptist, anesthesia should be considered relative to the overall medical status of the infant. The anesthetic risks are lower if the infant is greater than 44 to 50 weeks gestational age. Anesthetic complications in children include an increased risk of malignant hyperthermia in children undergoing strabismus surgery and increased vagal tone as traction is placed on the extraocular muscles for scleral buckling.

Laser photocoagulation in neonates with ROP is usually done in close proximity to the neonatal intensive care unit. The proximity allows continued surveillance of the patient by the neonatal intensive care team during treatment. A portable laser with indirect ophthalmoscopic laser delivery system is used. Green or infrared wavelengths are both effective in reducing the retinal neovascularization. Following dilation, topical anesthetics can be used with a scleral depressor to stabilize the eye during treatment. Cryotherapy can also be used to treat the peripheral ischemic retina. However, the advantages of laser photocoagulation are the ability to place more effective treatment in eyes with a posteriorly located ridge and a broad zone of avascular retina and, externally, less postoperative edema and inflammation.

Although careful monitoring and laser photocoagulation have greatly reduced the progression of stage III eyes with ROP, vitreoretinal surgery is still necessary in some eyes that develop stages IV or V. In stage IV-A and some stage IV-B eyes with tractional detachments, an encircling scleral buckle is sufficient. In more severe forms with more extraretinal fibrovascular proliferation, vitrectomy is necessary. A visual evoked potential (VEP) or electronic evoked response (EER) may be helpful in assessment of visual potential in these eyes. There have been various approaches in surgical management of ROP. An open-sky approach is used more routinely by some surgeons, whereas others reserve this for eyes with a clouded cornea. This approach offers a two-handed approach to membrane dissection. The closed vitrectomy approach is different from adult patients in that the small size of the eye and anterior vitreoretinal pathoanatomy requires more anterior entry sites through the pars plicata. In closed-funnel retinal detachments, often the lens must be aspirated. On open-funnel configurations, it may be possible to preserve the clear lens by placing the sclerotomy incisions slightly more posteriorly. The objective of the surgery is to release the traction, opening the funnel and flattening as much of the posterior retina as possible.

In children with complicated forms of retinal detachment such as giant retinal tears or traumatic retinal detachment with proliferative vitreoretinopathy, the surgical approach is similar to that used in adults. The differences are that often the posterior hyaloid is not separated, and this layer is more adherent to the retinal surface. There is also a generalized impression among retinal surgeons that children have a greater tendency to reproliferate compared with adults. Finally because of these factors and the difficulty with postoperative positioning and examination in the pediatric population, most vitreoretinal surgeons prefer the use of silicone oil as the primary agent for extended vitreoretinal tamponade.

Postoperatively it is important to work with the pediatric ophthalmologist in the visual rehabilitation and treatment of amblyopia. This may require fitting of a contact lens, working with parents in learning how to place the lens, and periods of occlusion therapy as necessary.

■ Conclusion

A broad overview of pediatric retinal disease has been presented along with a few practical suggestions on the techniques of pediatric retinal examination and therapy of some ocular conditions. The importance of performing thorough and accurate retinal examinations on children has been emphasized throughout this chapter in recognition of the difficulty of evaluating subtle findings in patients who are often uncooperative and even antagonistic. Surmounting these obstacles is critical because often a child's sight and sometimes life depends on your performing your task properly. It is strongly suggested that the reader read one or more of the encyclopedic texts of pediatric ophthalmology and follow the significant literature in this challenging field. Today's well-cared-for children will be tomorrow's loyal patients.

REFERENCES

1. Wright KW, ed. *Pediatric Ophthalmology and Strabismus.* St. Louis, MO: Mosby Year Book; 1997.
2. Taylor D, ed. *Paediatric Ophthalmology,* 2nd ed. Boston: Blackwell Science; 1997.
3. Nelson LB, Harley RD, eds. *Harley's Pediatric Ophthalmology* 4th ed. Philadelphia: WB Saunders; 1998.
4. Badgwell JM, ed. *Clinical Pediatric Anesthesia.* New York: Lippincott-Raven; 1998.
5. Gass JDM. *Stereoscopic Atlas of Macular Diseases,* 4th ed. St. Louis, MO: Mosby Year Book; 1997.
6. Fishman GA, Sokol S. *Electrophysiologic Testing in Disorders of the Retina, Optic Nerve, and Visual Pathway,* Ophthalmology Monographs, 2. San Francisco, CA: American Academy of Ophthalmology; 1990.
7. Flynn JT, Tasman. *Retinopathy of Prematurity: A Clinician's Guide.* New York: Springer-Verlag; 1992.
8. Cryotherapy for Retinopathy of Prematurity Cooperative Group. Multicenter trial of cryotherapy for retinopathy of prematurity: one year outcome—structure and function. *Arch Ophthalmol.* 1990;108:1408–1416.
9. Wilkinson CP, Rice TA, Michels RG, eds. *Michels Retinal Detachment,* 2nd ed. St. Louis, MO: Mosby Year Book; 1996.
10. Spencer WH, ed. *Ophthalmic Pathology: An Atlas and Textbook.* Philadelphia: WB Saunders; 1996.
11. Webster AR, Maher ER, Moore AT. Clinical characteristics of ocular angiomatosis in von Hippel-Lindau disease and correlation with germline mutation. *Arch Ophthalmol.* 1999;117:371–378.
12. Anderson RE, Lavail MM, eds. *Degenerative Diseases of the Retina.* New York: Plenum Publishing; 1995.
13. Shields JA, Shield CL, Parsons HM. Differential diagnosis of retinoblastoma. *Retina.* 1991;11:232–243.
14. McLean JM. Glial tumors of the retina in relation to tuberous sclerosis. *Am J Ophthalmol.* 1956;41:428–432.
15. Bouzas EA, Parry DM, Eldridge R, Kaiser-Kupfer MI. Familial occurrence of combined pigment epithelial and retinal hamartomas associated with neurofibromatosis. 2. *Retina.* 1992;12:103–107.
16. Gass JDM. New observations concerning choroidal osteomas. *Int Ophthalmol.* 1979;1:71–84.
17. Straatsma BR, Foos RY, Heckenlively JR, Taylor GN. Myelinated retinal nerve fibers. *Am J Ophthalmol.* 1981;91:25–38.

Pediatric Ophthalmology
Edited by P. F. Gallin
Thieme Medical Publishers, Inc.
New York © 2000

22
∎∎∎

Retinoblastoma

JERRY A. SHIELDS AND CAROL L. SHIELDS

Retinoblastoma is the most common and most important malignant intraocular tumor of childhood. It is important that the ophthalmologist makes a prompt and accurate diagnosis and refers the patient to an ocular oncologist for appropriate treatment. This chapter considers general aspects, clinical features, pathology, diagnostic approaches, and management of retinoblastoma. A more detailed discussion on these topics can be found in a reference devoted to intraocular tumors.[1–4]

∎ General Considerations

Retinoblastoma is the most common intraocular malignancy of childhood and is second to uveal melanoma as the most common primary intraocular malignancy in humans. Although estimates vary, it occurs with a frequency of approximately 1 in 15,000 live births. Approximately 6% of newly diagnosed retinoblastoma cases are familial and 94% are sporadic. All patients with familial retinoblastoma are at risk of passing the predisposition for tumor development to their offspring.[1] The details of the genetics and genetic counseling of patients with retinoblastoma are discussed in the literature[2] and are beyond the scope of this chapter.

There is no apparent predisposition for race or gender and no predilection for the right or left eye. The tumor occurs bilaterally in 25 to 35% of cases. In the multicentric or bilateral cases the average number of tumors per eye is five with a random distribution between the two eyes. The tumor is diagnosed at an average age of 18 months, with bilateral cases being recognized at an average age of 12 months and unilateral cases at 23 months. In rare instances, the tumor is first recognized at birth, in the teens, or even in adulthood.[1,5]

∎ Clinical Features

Most retinoblastomas present with leukocoria (a white pupillary reflex) (Fig. 22–1). When a retinoblastoma is small, it appears as a flat trans-

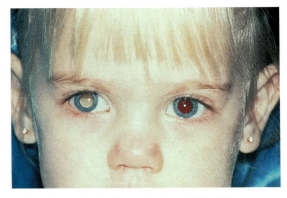

FIGURE 22–1. Leukocoria in a child with retinoblastoma.

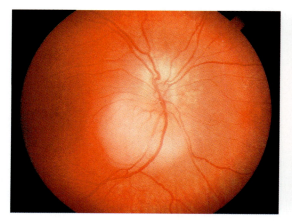

FIGURE 22–2. Small retinoblastoma inferior to optic disc.

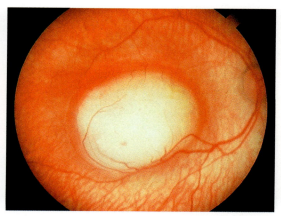

FIGURE 22–3. Slightly larger retinoblastoma showing white color.

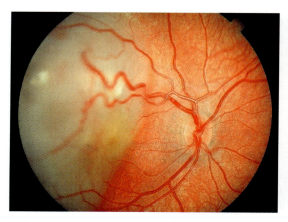

FIGURE 22–4. Retinoblastoma with dilated, tortuous retinal blood vessels.

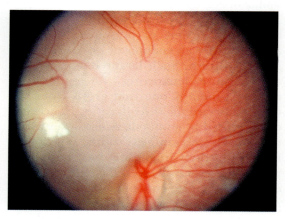

FIGURE 22–5. Retinoblastoma with vitreous seeding.

parent or slightly white lesion in the sensory retina (Fig. 22–2). Slightly larger tumors are less transparent and appear solid white (Fig. 22–3). As the tumor becomes larger, dilated tortuous retinal arteries and veins supply and drain the tumor (Fig. 22–4). Some retinoblastomas are associated with seeding of tumor cells into the overlying vitreous (Fig. 22–5). Some untreated retinoblastomas show foci of chalk-like calcification that has been likened to cottage cheese (Fig. 22–6). If a tumor is located in the foveal region, the child may develop either exotropia or esotropia. **Although most children with strabismus do not have retinoblastoma, it is important that every child with this finding have a**

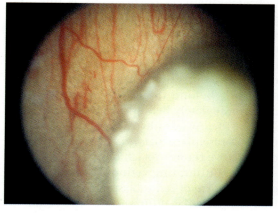

FIGURE 22–6. Retinoblastoma with foci of calcification.

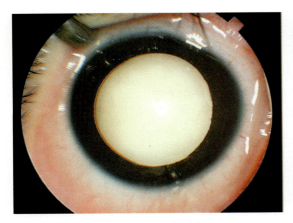

FIGURE 22–7. Endophytic retinoblastoma.

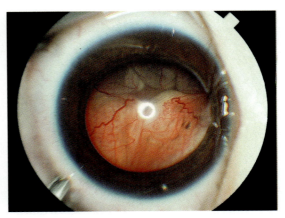

FIGURE 22–8. Exophytic retinoblastoma.

careful fundus examination to exclude the possibility of retinoblastoma.

More characteristically, retinoblastoma is larger at the time of presentation and it assumes either an endophytic or an exophytic growth pattern. Such larger tumors almost always cause leukocoria. An endophytic retinoblastoma is one that grows from the retina in toward the vitreous cavity. Hence, it is characterized by a white hazy mass over which no retinal vessels can be visualized (Fig. 22–7). Because of their friable nature, endophytic tumors can eventually seed the entire vitreous cavity and simulate endophthalmitis. An endophytic retinoblastoma can also seed into the anterior chamber and produce multiple nodules at the pupillary margin. With time, the cells may settle into the inferior portion of the angle and resemble a hypopyon.

An exophytic retinoblastoma is one that grows from the retina out into the subretinal space. In contrast to an endophytic tumor, the retinal vessels are apparent on the surface of the tumor. Such tumors produce a progressive retinal detachment, with the retina often displaced anteriorly behind the clear lens and a white mass immediately behind the detached retina (Fig. 22–8). An exophytic retinoblastoma can clinically resemble Coats' disease or other forms of exudative retinal detachment.

Diffuse infiltrating retinoblastoma is a less common form of retinoblastoma characterized by a relatively flat infiltration of the retina by tumor cells.[6,7] Because an obvious mass is not present, there is often a delay in diagnosis.

Therefore, diffuse retinoblastomas are usually recognized clinically at an older age than are typical cases of retinoblastoma. They frequently produce vitreous and anterior chamber seeding, which may be confused with intraocular inflammation. Fortunately, almost all reported cases of diffuse infiltrating retinoblastoma have been unilateral sporadic cases with a negative family history. Because of the extensive intraocular seeding in most instances, enucleation has been considered to be the best management.

Iris neovascularization (rubeosis iridis) occurs in 17% of all children with retinoblastoma and in about 50% of eyes with advanced retinoblastoma that require enucleation.[8] We believe that iris neovascularization usually accounts for the acquired heterochromia iridis that characterizes some cases of retinoblastoma. **Any infant with unexplained acquired heterochromia should be evaluated for possible retinoblastoma**. Spontaneous bleeding from these vessels may cause a hyphema.

Some necrotic retinoblastomas can produce severe secondary periocular inflammation, resulting in a clinical appearance of preseptal cellulitis or endophthalmitis.[9,10] In such cases computed tomography (CT) can reveal a large calcified intraocular mass with periocular soft tissue density suggesting extraocular extension of retinoblastoma. However, these advanced cases usually do not have evidence of extraocular extension after enucleation of the affected eye. The periocular inflammation seen with retinoblastoma appears to be secondary to necrosis within the tumor and not secondary to extraocular extension of the tumor. Tumors with true orbital extension are more likely to show extension to the brain and metastasis to regional lymph nodes.

Trilateral Retinoblastoma

In recent years it has been recognized that some children with the familial form of retinoblastoma can also develop a pinealoblastoma.[11,12] Because the pineal tumor has many similarities to retinoblastoma from embryological, pathologic, and immunologic standpoints, the pineal tumor can be detected with CT or magnetic resonance imaging (MRI). The prognosis for life is guarded. Most children who die from retinoblastoma have some degree of intracranial involvement, usually secondary to direct spread through the optic nerve or subarachnoid space. We believe that some earlier reported cases of presumed brain metastasis probably represented pinealoblastoma (trilateral retinoblastoma) that were misdiagnosed as metastatic retinoblastoma before the entity of trilateral retinoblastoma was recognized.

Retinocytoma

Recent evidence supports the existence of an uncommon benign variant of retinoblastoma that has been termed retinoma[13] or retinocytoma.[14] We believe that the term *retinoma* is too general because it could be interpreted to mean any tumor of the retina. Although no terminology is perfect, there is a stronger argument for using either the term *retinocytoma* or *spontaneously arrested retinoblastoma* to define this condition.[1] A retinocytoma carries the same genetic implications as an active retinoblastoma.[13,14]

Spontaneously Regressed Retinoblastoma

Complete spontaneous necrosis leading to regression and a "cure" is a well-known phenomenon that is said to occur more frequently in retinoblastoma than in any other malignant neoplasm.[1] It is characterized by a severe inflammatory reaction in an eye with retinoblastoma, sometimes followed by the development of phthisis bulbi. In cases of spontaneous regression of a smaller retinoblastoma, the eye may retain good vision (Fig. 22–9). It is not certain whether such tumor regression occurs secondary to vascular ischemia to the tumor or whether more complex immunopathologic mechanisms play a role. In any child with a phthisical eye of uncertain cause, the diagnosis of spontaneously regressed retinoblastoma should be considered. Spontaneously regressed retinoblastoma carries the same genetic implications as an active retinoblastoma.

■ Pathology

In most cases, retinoblastoma can be readily recognized in the sectioned eye by its typical appearance (Fig. 22–10). It is a chalky white, friable tumor with dense foci of calcification. An endophytic retinoblastoma usually produces

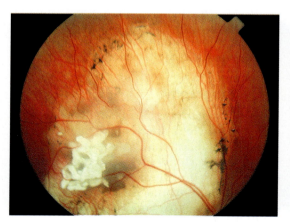

FIGURE 22–9. Spontaneously regressed retinoblastoma in an eye with good vision.

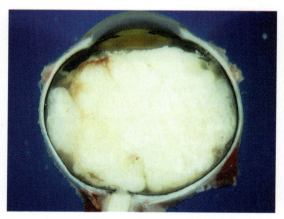

FIGURE 22–10. Grossly sectioned eye showing white retinoblastoma filling the interior of the eye.

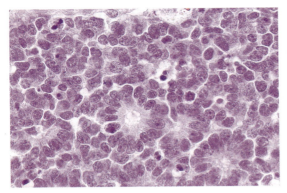

FIGURE 22–11. Photomicrograph of retinoblastoma showing Flexner-Wintersteiner rosettes (hematoxylin-eosin ×250). (Photomicrograph courtesy of Dr. Ralph C. Eagle, Jr.)

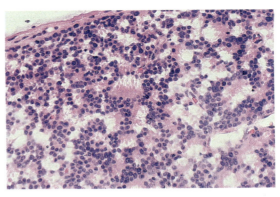

FIGURE 22–12. Photomicrograph of retinoblastoma showing fleurettes (hematoxylin-eosin ×250). (Photomicrograph courtesy of Dr. Ralph C. Eagle, Jr.)

seeding into the vitreous cavity. An exophytic tumor tends to push the retina anteriorly and to occupy the subretinal space. Some tumors have both endophytic and exophytic components, and others appear to be totally calcified as a result of marked necrosis.[1]

Cytologically, retinoblastomas make up a spectrum ranging from poorly differentiated to well differentiated tumors. The poorly differentiated tumor consists of small- to medium-sized round neuroblastic cells with large hyperchromatic nuclei and scanty cytoplasm. The well-differentiated retinoblastoma is characterized by the presence of rosettes and fleurettes. The Flexner-Wintersteiner rosette consists of columnar cells arranged around a clear central lumen (Fig. 22–11). The Flexner-Wintersteiner rosette is highly characteristic of retinoblastoma but is occasionally seen in other ophthalmic tumors such as medulloepithelioma. Some well-differentiated retinoblastomas and retinocytomas are also characterized by the presence of fleurettes. A fleurette is a lightly eosinophilic structure composed of groups of tumor cells that contain pear-shaped eosinophilic processes that project through the fenestrated membrane[1] (Fig. 22–12).

■ Diagnostic Approaches

In the patient with suspected retinoblastoma, a detailed history, general medical evaluation,

external ocular examination, slit lamp biomicroscopy, and indirect ophthalmoscopy should be obtained to substantiate the diagnosis.[3] In addition certain ancillary studies, such as fluorescein angiography, ultrasonography, CT, and MRI, can assist in the diagnosis.

Fluorescein Angiography

Fluorescein angiography can provide diagnostic and therapeutic information in selected children with discrete retinoblastoma.[3,15] Very small intraretinal tumors show only minimally dilated feeding vessels in the arterial phase, mild hypervascularity in the venous phase, and mild late staining of the mass (Fig. 22–13). Slightly larger intraretinal tumors show more intense hypervascularity and late staining. Moderate-sized tumors usually demonstrate markedly dilated feeding arteries and draining veins. Such tumors also show numerous fine capillary ramifications on the tumor surface.

Ultrasonography

Retinoblastomas have ultrasonographic features that usually help to differentiate them from the pseudoretinoblastomas.[3] A-scan ultrasonography typically shows constant high internal echoes within the tumor and rapid attenuation of the normal orbital pattern. There is frequently an anechoic area in the basal portion of the tumor nearest the sclera. B-scan ultra-

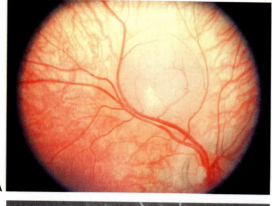

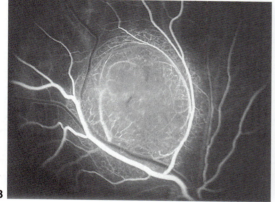

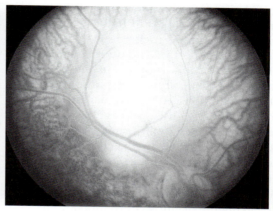

FIGURE 22–13. Fluorescein angiography of retinoblastoma. **(A)** Clinical appearance of tumor. **(B)** Arterial phase, showing two feeding arteries. **(C)** Late angiogram showing continued hyperfluorescence of the mass.

sonography characteristically shows a rounded or irregular intraocular mass with numerous highly reflective echoes within the lesion. A characteristic feature of B-scan is attenuation or absence of the normal soft tissue echoes in the orbit directly behind the tumor (Fig. 22–14). This occurs as a result of attenuation and reflection of the sound by the calcification within the mass. These reflective focal echoes within the tumor persist after the soft tissues echoes of

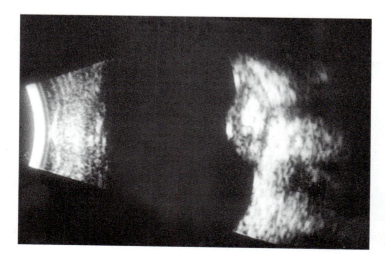

FIGURE 22–14. B-scan ultrasonography of retinoblastoma showing mass with calcification.

the eye have disappeared when the sensitivity of the ultrasound machine is lowered. Ultrasonography can be used to document tumor regression following radiotherapy.

Computed Tomography

Although both ultrasonography and CT can detect calcium in retinoblastoma, the advantage of CT over ultrasound is that it is better able to delineate extraocular extension of tumor and to detect the presence of an associated pinealoblastoma (trilateral retinoblastoma).

With CT, retinoblastoma typically appears as an intraocular mass with foci of calcification within the tumor in greater than 80% of tumors[3] (Fig. 22–15). The presence of intraocular calcification with CT is suggestive of retinoblastoma but is not pathognomonic. Other conditions, such as retinal astrocytoma, advanced Coats' disease, retinal angiomatosis, and nematode endophthalmitis, can occasionally produce intraocular calcification or even ossification that can lead to misdiagnosis with ultrasonography or CT. Therefore, all of the clinical findings should be taken into account in making the diagnosis of retinoblastoma.

Magnetic Resonance Imaging (MRI)

MRI may be of some diagnostic assistance in the evaluation of a child with suspected retinoblastoma.[16] A retinoblastoma is moderately hyperintense to vitreous on T1 weighted images and becomes hypointense on T2 weighted images.

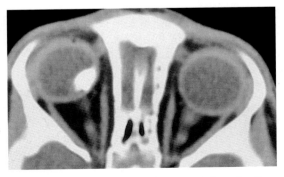

FIGURE 22–15. Computed tomography of retinoblastoma showing calcified intraocular mass.

Areas of calcification are often accentuated on T2 weighted images. Some authorities have reported that associated hemorrhage and exudation appear markedly different from retinoblastoma tissue on T2 weighted images. Thus, MRI has potential evaluating patients prior to treatment and in monitoring their response to therapy by helping to differentiate among active tumor, hemorrhage, and exudation. However, more studies will be necessary to determine the efficacy and limitations of MRI in the evaluation of children with suspected retinoblastoma.

■ Management

The management of retinoblastoma can be complex, and it is impossible to establish firm rules regarding treatment.[17,18] Each case must be individualized according to the entire clinical situation. Proper management necessitates the ability to use the various instruments, familiarity with the disease, and above all experience in dealing with such problems.[4] There are several options available for the treatment of retinoblastoma, and the method selected should depend on the size and extent of the tumor(s), whether there is unilateral or bilateral involvement, and the patient's systemic status. The methods that we currently advocate include enucleation, external beam irradiation, scleral plaque irradiation, photocoagulation, cryotherapy, chemotherapy, chemothermotherapy, and chemoreduction. In many cases, it may be necessary to employ various combinations of treatment to achieve a satisfactory result.[16]

Enucleation

Enucleation is probably indicated for all unilateral cases in which the tumor fills most of the globe and in which there is little hope of salvaging any viable retina or useful vision. In performing enucleation, it is important to obtain a long section of optic nerve because the main route of extension of the tumor is by way of the optic nerve to the central nervous system[19] (Fig. 22–16). A hydroxyapatite implant can be safely employed in children with retinoblastoma.[20] If

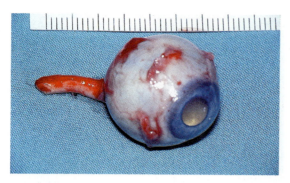

FIGURE 22–16. Eye enucleated for retinoblastoma showing long section of optic nerve.

half the retina is free from tumor, other methods of treatment can be considered as long as the parents have been fully informed as to the possibilities of metastasis and the complications of treatment. More details on indications and technique of enucleation are provided in the literature.[4] There has been a decreasing frequency of enucleation in recent years because of earlier diagnosis and more widespread use of conservative methods of management.[21]

External Beam Irradiation

In general, retinoblastoma is a very radiosensitive tumor, and irradiation can be an effective method of treatment[4,22] (Fig. 22–17). External

beam irradiation is most often used to treat the second eye after the eye with the more advanced tumor has been enucleated. The technique of external beam irradiation varies somewhat from center to center. The techniques, results, and complications of external beam irradiation are discussed in the literature.[4,22]

Perhaps the most important long-term complication of external beam irradiation is the development of radiation-induced tumors.[23,24] Radiation-induced orbital sarcomas, usually in the field of irradiation, are the most common, but other malignancies such as lymphoma and leukemias also have been recognized. The incidence of such tumors has greatly decreased because the total radiation doses were reduced from 8000 to 4000 cGy. More recently, new tumors distant from the site of irradiation are being detected. Furthermore many cases have been recognized in patients who had undergone no irradiation.[23,24]

Episcleral Plaque Brachytherapy

An increasingly employed alternative method of irradiation for retinoblastoma is the application of a radioactive plaque. The indications, techniques, complications, and results of plaque radiotherapy for retinoblastoma are discussed in the literature. Most tumors show dramatic regression after plaque treatment (Fig. 22–18). Plaque radiotherapy can be used

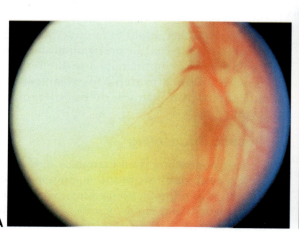
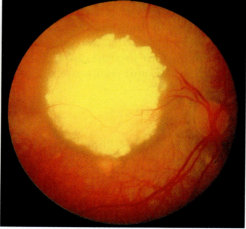

FIGURE 22–17. External beam irradiation for macular retinoblastoma. **(A)** Pretreatment appearance of tumor. **(B)** Appearance 3 months later showing calcified mass.

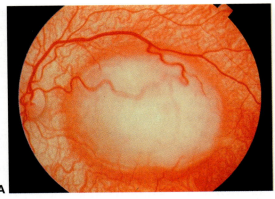
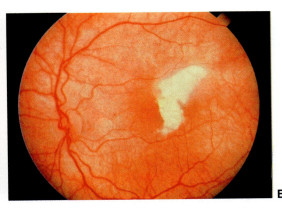

FIGURE 22–18. Plaque radiotherapy for macular retinoblastoma. **(A)** Pretreatment appearance of tumor. **(B)** Appearance 6 months later showing complete disappearance of the mass, with residual retinal pigment epithelial alterations.

successfully as a primary treatment of selected cases of unilateral or bilateral retinoblastoma or as a supplemental treatment after other treatment methods had failed.[25–27]

Cryotherapy

Cryotherapy is an effective method of eradicating selected small retinoblastomas.[4] It is generally used for small peripheral tumors that are confined to the sensory retina without vitreous seeding. The indications, techniques, and results are discussed n the literature.[4,28]

Laser Photocoagulation

Photocoagulation can be employed for selected small retinoblastomas. It may be used as primary treatment in some cases or as supplementary treatment in cases that were initially treated with irradiation or cryotherapy. The indications, techniques, and results are discussed in the literature.[4,29,30]

Chemotherapy

Chemotherapy has traditionally been used in cases of retinoblastoma that exhibit metastasis, orbital involvement, or invasion of the optic nerve detected after enucleation. The details of chemotherapy are discussed in the literature.[31]

Chemothermotherapy

In recent years there have been a number of important new developments in the management of children with retinoblastoma. These include chemothermotherapy and chemoreduction and combinations of these methods.[32]

Chemothermotherapy is a method of using chemotherapy (carboplatin) to sensitize a tumor to heat and then treat the tumor with heat by way of a diode laser delivery system.[32] This technique is currently gaining popularity in selected cases. It may be most applicable for small tumors near the optic disc (Fig. 22–19).

Chemoreduction

Chemoreduction is a method of decreasing a tumor size so that it can be treated with a more conservative method. This technique has recently gained popularity and is currently being employed more frequently[33–36] (Fig. 22–20). Eyes that would have undergone enucleation or external beam irradiation in the past are now being managed with chemoreduction followed by definitive management with radioactive plaques, thermotherapy, or cryotherapy.[33]

Genetic Counseling

Genetic counseling is an extremely important component of the overall management of patients with retinoblastoma. Karyotype studies of the patient and family members are helpful in this regard. Some patients with retinoblastoma have a deletion in the long arm of chromosome 13. This subject is discussed in more detail in the literature[2] and in Chapter 8.

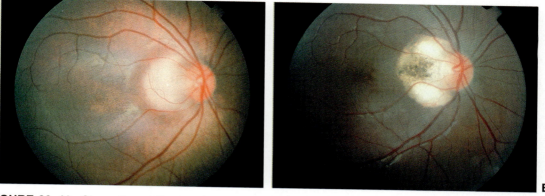

FIGURE 22–19. Chemothermotherapy for retinoblastoma. **(A)** Pretreatment appearance of small tumor. **(B)** Appearance 3 months later showing flat scar with pigment proliferation and no residual tumor.

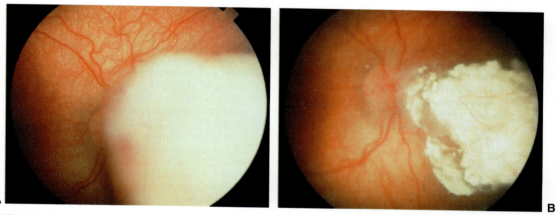

FIGURE 22–20. Chemoreduction for retinoblastoma. **(A)** Pretreatment appearance showing massive retinoblastoma behind the lens. **(B)** Appearance after chemotherapy showing marked decrease in size of the tumor. The residual tumor was subsequently treated with a radioactive plaque.

■ Summary

The treatment of retinoblastoma varies with the laterality and extent of the tumor. Most unilateral cases are managed by enucleation of the involved eye, except when the tumor is of small size when it is detected. In bilateral cases, an attempt to salvage the second eye is made by using irradiation, photocoagulation, or cryotherapy. In some cases a combination of these techniques is necessary. Chemothermotherapy and chemoreduction are more recently popularized methods of management that are currently gaining more advocates. Combinations of these newer techniques are being employed more often today. The prognosis for vision and life in patients with retinoblastoma has improved greatly during the last century. This has been largely due to earlier recognition and the use of modern therapeutic methods.

REFERENCES

1. Shields JA, Shields CL. Retinoblastoma: clinical and pathologic features. In: Shields JA, Shields CL, eds. *Intraocular Tumors: A Text and Atlas.* Philadelphia: WB Saunders; 1992:305–332.
2. Shields JA, Shields CL. Genetics of retinoblastoma. In: Shields JA, Shields CL, eds. *Intraocular Tumors: A Text and Atlas.* Philadelphia: WB Saunders; 1992:333–339.
3. Shields JA, Shields CL. Diagnostic approaches to retinoblastoma. In: Shields JA, Shields CL, eds. *Intraocular Tumors: A Text and Atlas.* Philadelphia: WB Saunders; 1992:363–376.

4. Shields JA, Shields CL. Management and prognosis of retinoblastoma. In: Shields JA, Shields CL, eds. *Intraocular Tumors: A Text and Atlas.* Philadelphia: WB Saunders; 1992:377–391.

5. Shields CL, Shields JA, Shah P. Retinoblastoma in older children. *Ophthalmology.* 1991;98:395–399.

6. Nicholson DH, Norton EW. Diffuse infiltrating retinoblastoma. *Trans Am Ophthalmol Soc.* 1980; 78:265–289.

7. Shields JA, Shields CL, Eagle RC, Blair CJ. Spontaneous pseudohypopyon secondary to diffuse infiltrating retinoblastoma. *Arch Ophthalmol.* 1988; 106:1301–1302.

8. Shields CL, et al. Prevalence and mechanisms of secondary intraocular pressure elevation in eyes with intraocular tumors. *Ophthalmology.* 1987; 94:839–846.

9. Shields JA, Shields CL, Suvarnamani C, Schroeder RP, DePotter P. Retinoblastoma manifesting as orbital cellulitis. *Am J Ophthalmol.* 1991;112:442–449.

10. Stafford WR, Yanoff M, Parnell B. Retinoblastoma initially misdiagnosed as primary ocular inflammation. *Arch Ophthalmol.* 1969; 82:771–773.

11. Zimmerman LE, et al. Trilateral retinoblastoma: ectopic intracranial retinoblastoma associated with bilateral retinoblastoma. *J Pediatr Ophthalmol Strabismus.* 1982; 19:310–315.

12. De Potter P, Shields CL, Shields JA. Clinical variations of trilateral retinoblastoma: a report of 13 cases. *J Pediatr Ophthalmol Strabismus.* 1994; 31:26–31.

13. Gallie BL, Ellsworth RM, Abramson DH, Phillips RA. Retinoma: spontaneous regression of retinoblastoma or benign manifestation of a mutation? *Br J Cancer.* 1982; 45:513–521.

14. Margo C, Hidayat A, Kopelman J, Zimmerman LE. Retinocytoma: a benign variant of retinoblastoma. *Arch Ophthalmol.* 1983; 101:1519–1531.

15. Shields JA, Sanborn GE, Augsburger JJ, Orlock D, Donoso LA. Fluorescein angiography of retinoblastoma. *Retina.* 1982; 2:206–214.

16. DePotter P, Shields JA, Shields CL. Tumors and pseudotumors of the retina. In: DePotter P, Shields JA, Shields CL, eds. *MRI of the Eye and Orbit.* Philadelphia: JB Lippincott, 1995:93–94.

17. Shields JA. Misconceptions and techniques in the management of retinoblastoma. The 1992 Paul Henkind Memorial Lecture. *Retina.* 1992; 12:320–330.

18. Shields JA, Shields CL, Donoso LA, Lieb WE. Changing concepts in the management of retinoblastoma. *Ophthalmic Surg.* 1990; 21:72–76.

19. Shields JA, Shields CL, De Potter P. Enucleation technique for children with retinoblastoma. *J Pediatr Ophthalmol Strabismus.* 1992; 29:213–215.

20. De Potter P, Shields CL, Shields JA, Singh AD. Use of the orbital hydroxyapatite implant in the pediatric population. *Arch Ophthalmol.* 1994; 112:208–212.

21. Shields JA, Shields CL, Sivalingam V. Decreasing frequency of enucleation in patients with retinoblastoma. *Am J Ophthalmol.* 1989; 108:185–188.

22. Abramson DH, et al. The management of unilateral retinoblastoma without primary enucleation. *Arch Ophthalmol.* 1982; 100:1249–1252.

23. Abramson DH, Ronner HJ, Ellsworth RM. Second tumors in nonirradiated bilateral retinoblastoma. *Am J Ophthalmol.* 1979; 87:624–627.

24. Roarty JD, McLean IW, Zimmerman LE. Incidence of second neoplasms in patients with bilateral retinoblastoma. *Ophthalmology.* 1988; 95:1583–1587.

25. Shields JA, et al. Episcleral plaque radiotherapy for retinoblastoma. *Ophthalmology.* 1989; 96:530–537.

26. Shields CL, Shields JA, Minelli S, DePotter P, Hernandez JC, Cater J, Brady LW. Regression of retinoblastoma after plaque radiotherapy. *Am J Ophthalmol.* 1993; 115:181–187.

27. Shields JA, Shields CL, De Potter P, Hernandez JC, Brady LW. Plaque radiotherapy for residual or recurrent retinoblastoma in 91 cases. *J Pediatr Ophthalmol Strabismus.* 1994; 31:242–245.

28. Shields JA, Parsons H, Shields CL, Giblin, ME. The role of cryotherapy in the management of retinoblastoma. *Am J Ophthalmol.* 1989;108:260–264.

29. Shields JA, Parsons H, Shields CL, Giblin, ME. The role of photocoagulation in the management of retinoblastoma. *Arch Ophthalmol.* 1990; 108:205–208.

30. Shields CL, Shields JA, Kiratli H, De Potter P. Treatment of retinoblastoma with indirect ophthalmoscope laser photocoagulation. *J Pediatr Ophthalmol Strabismus.* 1995; 32:317–322.

31. White L. Chemotherapy in retinoblastoma: current status and future directions. *Am J Pediatr Hemat Oncol.* 1991; 13:189–201.

32. Shields CL, Shields JA, De Potter P. New treatment modalities for retinoblastoma. *Curr Opin Ophthalmol.* 1996; 7:20–26.

33. Shields CL, De Potter P, Himmelstein B, Shields JA, Meadows AT, Maris J. Chemoreduction in the initial management of intraocular retinoblastoma. *Arch Ophthalmol.* 1996; 114:1330–1338.

34. Shields CL, Shields JA, De Potter P, Himmelstein B, Meadows AT. The effect of chemoreduction on retinoblastoma-induced retinal detachment. *J Pediatr Ophthalmol Strabismus.* 1997; 34:165–169.

35. Shields CL, Shields JA, Needle M, De Potter P, Kheterpal S, Hamada A, Meadows AT. Combined chemoreduction and adjuvant treatment for intraocular retinoblastoma. *Ophthalmology.* 1997; 104:2101–2111.

36. Shields JA, Shields CL, De Potter P, Needle M. Bilateral macular retinoblastoma managed by chemoreduction and chemothermotherapy. *Arch Ophthalmol.* 1996; 114:1426–1427.

Pediatric Ophthalmology
Edited by P. F. Gallin
Thieme Medical Publishers, Inc.
New York © 2000

23

∎∎∎

Orbital Diseases

MICHAEL KAZIM

The identification of an acute orbital process in a child produces an understandably high level of anxiety in the parents, referring pediatrician, and child. To maximize the amount of clinical information that is derived from the initial examination, it is important to begin the interaction by alleviating anxiety. In a relaxed setting, a great deal of information can be derived by simply observing a child from across the examination room. Important diagnostic clues include the discomfort of a child, the motility of the lids and globe, the presence of tearing or inflammation, or a focal mass effect in the lid and proptosis.

As the examination continues the history is derived from the child's caregiver. It should be detailed, containing a review of familial diseases, birth history, trauma, and medical history. The history of the current illness should be carefully taken as details of the pace of the disease will often provide insight into the disease.

Generally, diseases will evolve by one of three patterns. Rapidly evolving proptosis over the course of hours to days generally represents an infectious/inflammatory process or highly malignant lesion. Slowly evolving processes that grow over the course of months to years are generally benign. Proptosis with growth rates in between are a mixed array of lesions including fungal infections and low-grade malignancies. One of the more helpful examinations to determine the time course of the proptosis is a review of old full-face photographs.

The clinical examination should include an assessment of optic nerve function, including visual acuity, color vision, pupil response, and if the child is able a visual field examination. Proptosis can be estimated grossly by examining the child's globes from the submental view. More accurate measurements can be made with either a Leudde or a Hertel exophthalmometer. The presence of resistance to retropulsion and associated pain will provide information regarding the nature of the orbital disease. The displacement of the globe out of the axial plane gives an indication of the location of the lesion within the orbit.

Motility of the globe and the eyelids is measured as accurately as possible as is the sensory function in the trigeminal distribution. The localization of the lesion within the orbital apex, optic canal, and cavernous sinus is most easily made based on the performance of the sensory and motor nerves within these spaces.

The conjunctiva should be examined for chemosis (a sensitive measure of congestive ouflow obstruction), hemorrhage, and pigmented lesions. Iris nodules and pigment as well as cataract should be identified. The fundus should be examined for papilledema, venous or arterial dilation, and retinal or choroidal lesions.

The most common lesions to affect children are grouped by age in the following sections. The diseases are listed by incidence.

■ Birth

The disease entities that are apparent shortly after birth are virtually limited to congenital conditions. The lesions feature most commonly developmental anomalies and vascular hamartomas (Table 23–1).

TABLE 23–1. Tumors Present at Birth

Capillary hemangioma
Lipodermoid
Lacrimal mucocele
Hematic cyst
Encephalocele
Microphthalmos with cyst
Teratoma

Capillary Hemangioma

Capillary hemangiomas of childhood represent the most common benign orbital tumor in children. The lesions may be superficial to the orbital septum, deep within the orbit without apparent cutaneous involvement, or, in a minority, traverse both the intra- and extraorbital spaces (Fig. 23–1). The cutaneous tumors generally appear within the first month after birth. Typically a flat or only slightly elevated lesion is present at first. The lesions tend to grow rapidly in either a continuously progressive fashion or episodically in association with the child's growth pattern. Growth of the lesion can be anticipated for approximately 1 year, after which involution occurs for up to 4 or 5 years. Children should be monitored during the growth phase to assure that the growth of the tumor does not produce amblyopia (through obstruction of the visual axis or induced astigmatism) or severe cosmetic deformity.

Orbital hemangiomas can be more difficult to diagnose. Proptosis is the typical presenting feature and is generally identified by 1 month of age. There may be other cutaneous hemangiomas that suggest the orbital diagnosis. At Babies Hospital we have identified prematurity as a risk factor for the development of capillary hemangioma. Computed tomography (CT) or magnetic resonance imaging (MRI) will identify a noncircumscribed soft-tissue mass. Bone destruction, which is a typical feature of malignancy, is not identified in the case of capillary hemangioma. In some cases a biopsy is required to confirm the clinical suspicion and exclude the diagnosis of malignancy.

As in the case of the cutaneous lesions growth is anticipated during the first year, after which, involution occurs. Patients are monitored for the development of amblyopia and compressive optic neuropathy.

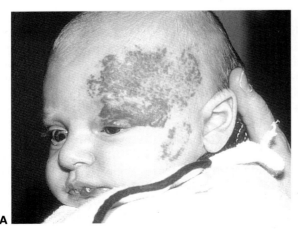
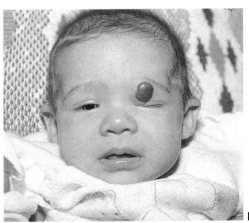

FIGURE 23–1. (A) Capillary hemangioma of the left brow and upper eyelid. **(B)** Capillary hemangioma of the left upper lid producing significant mechanical ptosis.

Lesions that extend from cutaneous to the deep orbit have radiographic and clinical features of both processes. The diagnosis is more apparent due to the cutaneous component; however, management may be difficult due to the diffuse involvement of the orbital and adnexal tissues.

Management of this group of lesions is guided by the development of ocular function and cosmetic deformity produced by the lesion. If the lesion is small and slow growing and does not retard visual development, conservative measures are indicated.

Observation at regular intervals will assure that the lesion continues to behave in a benign fashion. After maximal spontaneous resolution, surgical resection of the residual lesion can be considered.

Cutaneous lesions that obstruct the visual axis, producing amblyopia, astigmatism, or significant deformity are treated. Treatment varies with the patient; however, most patients receive corticosteroids by either local injection or systemic administration. Delivered locally, the dose is 40 to 80 mg of triamcinolone and 25 mg of methylprednisolone. If systemic therapy is chosen the dose of prednisone is 1.5 to 2.5 mg/kg daily with the dose and taper guided by the clinical response. The advantage of local therapy is the lower level of systemic absorption and adverse effect. Despite this patients require monitoring by a pediatrician for adrenal axis insufficiency and immunosupression during treatment. The risks of local therapy include atrophy of the overlying skin and the rare but catastrophic blindness resulting from ophthalmic artery occlusion due to propagation of the depo compound during the injection. To avoid injecting into the orbit, deep lesions are uniformly treated with systemic corticosteroids. Alternative therapy has included low-dose radiotherapy, which we presently do not routinely advocate because of the potential for long-term ill effects. Interferon has enjoyed some advocacy; however, it is routinely not indicated due to the need for long-term daily injections of the very costly compound.

When full spontaneous resolution of the orbital hemangiomas has occurred consideration of surgery is given in cases in which prop-

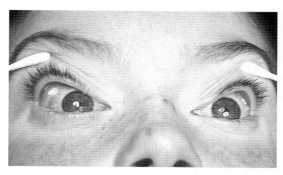

FIGURE 23–2. Lipodermoid of the right superior temporal cul-de-sac.

tosis persists. Preoperative noninvasive imaging provides the anatomic details required to plan an effective resection. Complete resection is not routinely possible or required.

Lipodermoid

Lipodermoids are relatively common tumors identified in the superotemporal quadrant of the anterior orbit consisting of fatty tissue (Fig. 23–2). The process is most commonly bilateral. The overlying conjunctiva routinely demonstrates hair follicles and aqueous and sebaceous glands. All three may produce ocular irritation and result in a clinical picture of conjunctivitis. The mass is mobile and does not impair ocular motility. The lateral canthal angle may be distorted due to associated maldevelopment. CT scan demonstrates a fat density lesion that may extend deeply into the orbit. The diagnosis of the lesion is made on clinical grounds. Excision of the lesion is contemplated to relieve ocular discomfort and for cosmesis. It should be remembered that no attempt should be made at complete resection as this risks damage to the lateral rectus muscle. Instead a conservative removal of the superficial component of the lesion will achieve the surgical goals.

Lacrimal Sac Mucocele

Lacrimal sac mucoceles result from congenital obstruction of both the valve of Hasner distally and the valve of Rosenmüller proximally. This results in a closed lacrimal sac that accumulates mucoid product, resulting in a firm bluish mass generally identified within the first week after

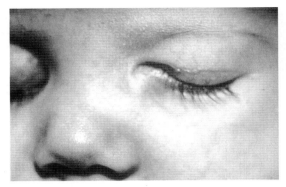

FIGURE 23–3. Mucocele of left nasolacrimal sac. Blue tinged discoloration of the skin is typical of this lesion.

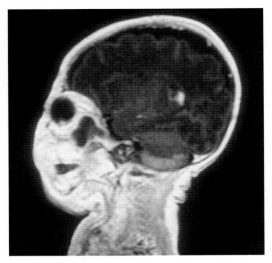

FIGURE 23–4. MRI hematic cyst of the posterior orbit.

birth (Fig. 23–3). These lesions are located beneath the medial canthal tendon and may displace the tendon and attached lower eyelid superiorly. The size of the mass is limited by the distensibility of the surrounding tissues, which is reached within 1 to 2 days. Lacrimal sac mucoceles must be distinguished from deep capillary hemangiomas that generally do not enlarge as rapidly in the first few days of life and encephaloceles that arise above the medial canthal tendon and are not bluish. Further evidence is provided by transillumination, which reveals the cystic nature of the mucocele. If there remains any uncertainty regarding the diagnosis, a CT scan is of value to exclude an encephalocele. Treatment of the mucocele by lacrimal probing is indicated at the earliest convenience to prevent progression to acute dacryocystitis, which often ensues within weeks after birth in these cases.

Hematic Cyst

Hematic cysts are an unusual cause of unilateral proptosis identified shortly after birth. In our experience they have been more common among children born prematurely. It is likely that birth trauma is in part responsible for the production of spontaneous bleeding. Although it may be speculated that the hemorrhaging occurs in vascular hamartomas (i.e., lymphangioma, venous malformation), this has not been substantiated histologically. The degree of proptosis can vary from mild to moderate but is

not progressive, which helps to distinguish it from a malignancy. The child appears to be in no distress. Ocular function is rarely impaired. MRI identifies the blood-filled cyst (Fig. 23–4). The lesion may be difficult to distinguish from an orbital capillary hemangioma. If there is evidence of compressive optic neuropathy or slowly progressive growth, a trial of oral corticosteroids administered with the aid of a pediatrician or endocrinologist may be helpful. Left untreated the cysts will resolve spontaneously over 1 to 4 weeks. We have not needed to evacuate any of the cases that we have examined.

Encephalocele

A congenital encephalocele occurs as the result of a defect in the closure of a cranial suture that is routinely associated with a craniofacial cleft (Fig. 23–5). The cleft locations have been classified by Tessier. The clefts most commonly associated with orbital encephaloceles are the number 0, 1, 2, 3, 12, 13, and 14 clefts. Clinically the encephalocele is identified by a soft, subcutaneous nontender mass. There may be palpable pulsations coinciding with the natural pulsations of the brain. The mass does not transilluminate. If the encephalocele is located beneath the eyebrow, there may be an associated alopecia. Telecanthus is associated with midline clefts.

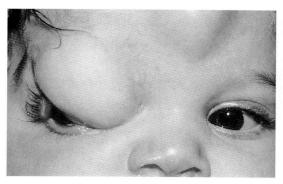

FIGURE 23–5. Encephalocele of the right superior nasal orbit.

Radiographic analysis should be performed by CT scan with particular attention to both bone and soft tissue windows that will identify the cranial bone defect and the prolapsing brain tissue.

Treatment is by craniotomy and orbital bone reconstruction with split cranial bone graft. If telecanthus exists this may be repaired at the same setting.

Microphthalmos with Cyst

At birth the microphthalmic globe is apparent. The malformation may exist in association with a cyst produced at the fourth week of embryology (Fig. 23–6). The cyst will grow slowly, which helps to distinguish it from teratomas. Imaging with ultrasound will identify the cystic nature of

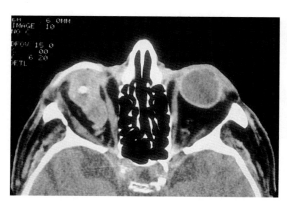

FIGURE 23–6. Microphthalmos with cyst of the left orbit; an internal calcification is noted.

the lesion. CT will exclude encephalocele by imaging of the orbital bones. MRI is helpful when examining the soft tissue contents of the cyst. Treatment is surgical excision of the cyst. The globe should be removed if rudimentary and replaced with a dermis fat graft to promote orbital bone and soft-tissue development.

Teratoma

Teratomas are defined as a tumor composed of tissues derived from all three germ cell layers. They are rare, rapidly growing lesions that may compromise normal ocular function (Fig. 23–7A). Radiographic analysis may benefit from both CT (Fig. 23–7B), which will identify the location of the lesion, and any associated bone defects and MRI, which best demonstrates the complexity of the soft-tissue structure of the lesion. If the diagnosis is not certain based on clinical and radiographic grounds, a biopsy is helpful (Fig. 23–7C). Complete resection of the lesion may be possible while preserving normal ocular function.

■ Three Months to 1 Year

Disease entities that manifest in children between 3 months and 1 year of age are listed in Table 23–2.

TABLE 23–2. Tumors Identified at 3 Months to 1 Year

Dermoid cyst
Arteriovenous malformation
Rhabdomyosarcoma
Neuroblastoma

Dermoid Cysts

Dermoid cysts are the result of ectodermal inclusions at the site of bony suture closure. Any of the orbital or periorbital sutures may be involved (Fig. 23–8A). The lesions arising from the anterior orbital sutures are generally identified within the first several months of birth. Typically the cysts arising from the deep orbital sutures present with proptosis or optic

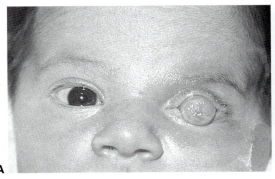

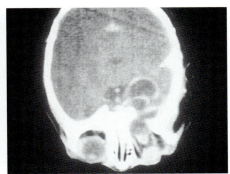

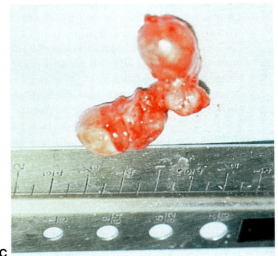

FIGURE 23–7. (A) Teratoma of the left orbit. **(B)** CT scan of an orbital teratoma demonstrating extension of the lesion into the intracranial space. **(C)** Surgical specimen of orbitocranial teratoma. (Courtesy of J.A. Katowitz, M.D.)

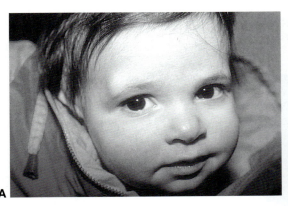

FIGURE 23–8. (A) Dermoid of right superior-temporal orbit. **(B)** CT scan of a right orbital dermoid demonstrating the cystic lesion of the right frontozygomatic suture.

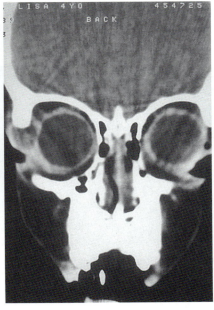

neuropathy in later decades. We have, however, seen two cases in which dermoid cysts of the sphenozygomatic suture produced proptosis in one child at 5 months and the second at 2 years of age. The most common location for the lesions are at the lateral brow (frontozygomatic suture) and the superonasal notch (frontonasal suture). We generally perform CT scans on the lesions in the superonasal quadrant to exclude the possibility of encephalocele or bone dysgenesis preoperatively (Fig. 23–8B). Excision is recommended after 6 months of age to limit anesthetic risk. Removal is advisable to eliminate the risk of rupture of the cyst, which may mimic infectious cellulitis and limit the size of the postoperative scar. To further limit the scar we have to be able to remove most anterior lesions through lid crease incisions.

Congenital Arteriovenous Malformation

Arteriovenous (AV) malformations may be of two varieties. The high flow lesions result most commonly from trauma or age-related hypertensive shunting. The congenital lesions are more often of a lower flow rate and grow slowly over decades. Unlike capillary hemangiomas, AV malformations tend to be identified several months after birth and continue to grow slowly past 1 year (Fig. 23–9D), the point at which hemangiomas will begin to involute. The AV malformations may occur as part of the Wyburn-Mason or Osler-Weber-Rendu syndromes (Fig. 23–9A–C). Examination for visceral or retinal involvement should be undertaken. In general, the lesions should be left untreated unless there

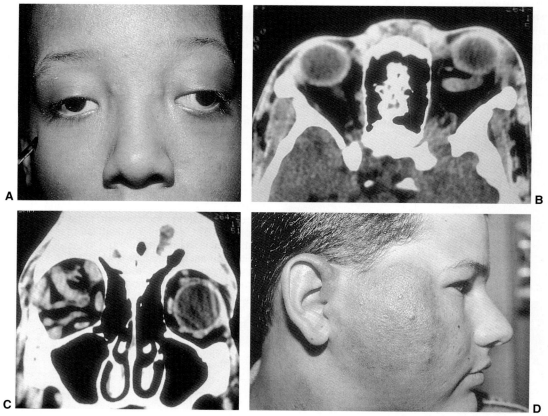

FIGURE 23–9. (A) Child with Osler-Weber-Rendu syndrome. **(B)** CT scan in axial projection of the same patient demonstrating a dilated superior ophthalmic vein of the left orbit. **(C)** Coronal CT scan demonstrating a tortuous arteriovenous malformation within the right orbit. **(D)** Subcutaneous arteriovenous malformation of the right face.

is significant visual compromise or cosmetic deformity. In such cases angiography to identify discrete arterial feeding vessels that can be occluded intravascularly may be curative. Often the lesion will arborize new vessels that will require further treatment. Surgical resection is indicated to remove devitalized tissue that produces significant residual volume after arterial occlusion or in cases of vision-threatening orbital inflammatory response to the intravascular thrombotic agent.

Rhabdomyosarcoma

Rhabdomyosarcoma is the most common orbital malignancy in the pediatric population. Over 70% of rhabdomyosarcomas are identified by the end of the first decade of life, with a high frequency within the first year. Most are identified within the first 2 decades, but occasional lesions are noted in later decades. The lesion presents clinically as a rapidly enlarging mass if superficially located in the orbit. Proptosis is common if the lesion is present behind the equator of the globe (Fig. 23–10A). Associated inflammatory signs including skin erythema and conjunctival chemosis can mimic those seen in cases of orbital cellulitis or trauma. It is rare to

identify a case in which the growth rate is slow. In such cases the diagnosis may be delayed.

The evaluation of a child with a rapidly enlarging orbital mass should include a CT scan with contrast to locate the lesion, define its anatomic extension, and identify its effect on the surrounding orbital bones (Fig. 23–10B). MRI provides added detail of the soft-tissue invasion but does not improve on the diagnostic capabilities of CT. On both CT and MR the lesion is an unencapsulated soft-tissue mass that enhances with contrast injection. The orbital structures are displaced by the mass. Bone destruction is not universal, and extension through the orbital fissures is known to occur.

The clinical radiographic features should alert the physician to the possibility of an orbital malignancy. An orbital exploration should follow almost immediately. A decision regarding the extent of surgery requires careful preoperative evaluation of the imaging studies and an intraoperative evaluation of the lesion. Tumors that appear to be poorly encapsulated on scan or intraoperatively tend to hemorrhage profusely are best managed by obtaining a representative biopsy (Fig. 23–10C). In cases where the lesion is better encapsulated and resection proceeds easily, an attempt at gross total resection is a valuable addition to the postoperative

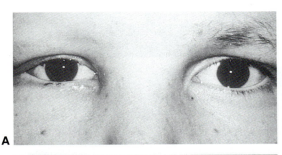

FIGURE 23–10. (A) Rhabdomyosarcoma of the left orbit featuring proptosis and upper eyelid swelling. **(B)** CT scan of patient with rhabdomyosarcoma featuring a left superior orbital soft tissue mass (arrow). **(C)** Surgical pathology specimen of rhabdomyosarcoma demonstrating muscle fibers.

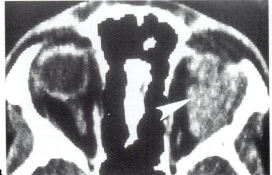

treatment planning. Specimens should be obtained for both formaldehyde and glutaraldehyde fixation and electron microscope evaluation.

There are four histopathologic subtypes of rhabdomyosarcoma: embryonal, alveolar, pleomorphic, and botryoid. The most common form is embryonal (65% of tumors). Alveolar is poorly differentiated and accounts for 30% of cases. Pleomorphic is most common in adults and is identified in only 1 to 2% of cases. It is unclear whether the histologic type of tumor bears on the survival rate. However wide tumor extension and the presence of parameningeal disease both adversely affect survival.

Prior to 1972 survival rates in cases treated with only wide local excision were only in the 20% range. Since the advent of combination therapy with radiation and chemotherapy the survival rate has increased to nearly 90%. Current protocols developed by the rhabdomyosarcoma intergroup study include multiple regimens of chemotherapy with and without adjunct radiotherapy. The final conclusions of the study will hopefully allow for reduced morbidity while preserving the high survival rate associated with the disease.

Recurrent local disease is a more difficult problem. Current recommendations include wide local excision of the involved tissue and surrounding bone and sinuses where required. This is followed by chemotherapy and, if not previously employed, radiotherapy. Long-term survival in such cases is less favorable.

The long-term effects of the treatment include orbital hypoplasia, retinopathy, optic neuropathy, and cataract. Second malignancies, frequently leukemia, are also seen.

Neuroblastoma

Neuroblastoma is the most frequently occurring metastatic tumor of childhood. Although most are identified prior to 2 years of age the rate of treatment success declines precipitously after 1 year. The classic presentation is the development of rapidly progressive proptosis with associated periorbital ecchymosis (Fig. 23–11A). Limitation of ocular rotations follows soon after with chemosis and finally compressive optic neuropathy. There may be fullness of the temporalis fossa when the lesion erodes through the sphenozygomatic suture (Fig. 23–11B). Bilateral metastatic disease has been reported in fewer than 50% of cases. Intraocular metastatic lesions are rare. A clinical examination should include abdominal palpation to inspect for the primary adrenal or paraspinal mass.

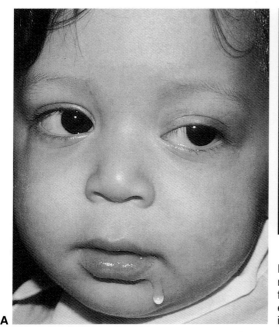
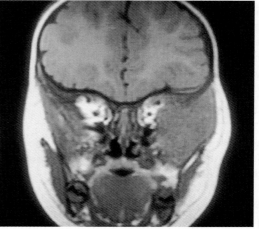

FIGURE 23–11. (A) Child with left orbital neuroblastoma. **(B)** MRI of neuroblastoma featuring soft tissue mass of the left lateral orbit extending into the temporalis fossa and down into the infratemporal fossa.

CT scan with contrast enhancement shows an enhancing lesion without encapsulation that frequently produces surrounding lytic bone destruction. The site of the metastatic lesion is most frequently the bone marrow space of the sphenoid bone. Extension into the middle cranial fossa is common. If the lesion on CT confirms the clinical suspicion for neuroblastoma, a CT of the chest and abdomen should follow. Further systemic evaluation should include blood and urine evaluation for elevated catecholamines and their metabolites.

A confirmatory diagnostic biopsy should be coordinated with a pediatric oncologist and pediatric surgeon. At the time of the orbital biopsy a bone marrow biopsy and placement of a central venous catheter can be accomplished at the same operative setting and permit rapid institution of therapy. The orbital biopsy should be performed through the safest and most direct route. Debulking the tumor is of little value and may result in damage to the surrounding normal structures.

Treatment varies among institutions but invariably involves chemotherapy (including cisplatin, cyclophosphamide, vincristine, and adriamycin). Treatment response is evaluated at 4 to 6 months and the residual tumor surgically resected. Resistant tumors have been treated with total body irradiation or high-dose chemotherapy followed by bone marrow transplantation. Success is best achieved in children less than 1 year of age (72%). After 2 years of age the survival rate falls to 12%. Children presenting with Horner's syndrome or opsoclonous appear to have a higher rate of success.

■ One to 6 Years

The most common ocular diseases that manifest in children aged 1 to 6 years are listed in Table 23–3.

Cellulitis

Infectious orbital cellulitis is the most common cause of proptosis in the pediatric population. The most common source of infection is by contiguous spread from the paranasal sinuses, although less common sources are hematogenously delivered to the orbit or by transcuta-

TABLE 23–3. Lesions Identified from 1 to 6 Years

Cellulitis
Dacryoadenitis
Lymphangioma
Neurofibroma
Schwannoma
Histiocytosis X
Optic glioma
Optic meningioma
Leukemia/lymphoma

neous puncture wounds. As such infectious orbital cellulitis generally becomes a clinically significant entity after the first year of life, when the paraorbital sinuses begin to pneumatize. The ethmoid sinuses are the first to develop followed by the maxillary sinuses within the first 2 years after birth. The frontal sinus develops between the fifth and seventh year, and the sphenoid sinuses are the last to pneumatize in the second decade.

The typical clinical picture is one of a child who has suffered an upper respiratory tract infection and develops unilateral or occasionally bilateral lid swelling (Fig. 23–12). This is followed within 1 or 2 days by proptosis and complete closure of the lids. The child is generally febrile and lethargic. Vision is often difficult to measure in these cases, but pupil reactions may be assessed to monitor for a relative afferent pupil defect. Ocular motility may be impaired if there is a subperiosteal collection. Proptosis and chemosis are often present. A leukocytosis is present, and there is a shift to immature forms. A CT scan should be obtained in cases in which the clinical examination is difficult or there is evidence of proptosis, motility impairment, or pupil defect. If lid edema and erythema are the solitary signs, medical treatment with close observation is sufficient unless the clinical picture deteriorates.

A CT scan will demonstrate opacified sinuses and, when present, a subperiosteal collection of inflammatory exudate or pus. It should be noted that in the evaluation of orbital cellulitis the findings on the CT scan will lag behind the clinical picture. This is particularly important in the resolution phase of the disease, when despite the improvements in the clinical features the CT scan may appear unchanged or worse. It is generally advisable to treat based on the clinical picture and not the CT scan find-

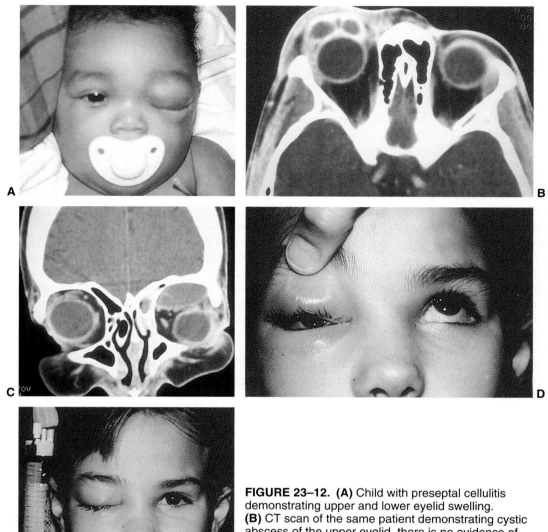

FIGURE 23–12. (A) Child with preseptal cellulitis demonstrating upper and lower eyelid swelling. **(B)** CT scan of the same patient demonstrating cystic abscess of the upper eyelid, there is no evidence of orbital inflammation or proptosis. **(C)** Child with orbital abscess featuring upper and lower eyelid edema. **(D)** Elevation of the right eye is limited by the orbital abscess. **(E)** Superior subperiosteal abscess and associated frontal sinusitis.

ings. Follow-up CT scans should be obtained if the clinical picture deteriorates despite medical therapy or there is little improvement over a long period.

Additional testing includes blood, conjunctival, and intranasal cultures. Although occasionally revealing, often the choice of antibiotic therapy is empirical.

The bacteriology of orbital cellulitis in children is generally a simple array of organisms.

The most common are staphylococcus and streptococcus. In children who have not been appropriately vaccinated against *H. influenza* this remains a more frequent organism than in adults. In a recent study by Harris et al. the population of organisms identified from subperiosteal collections was shown to increase in complexity with the age of the child. In the case of children more than 9 years of age the cultures included both gram-positive and gram-negative organisms as well as both aerobes and occasional anaerobes. In children who are immunocompromised consideration should be given to fungal organisms.

If the cellulitis solely involves the eyelid, treatment may be begun on an outpatient with oral antibiotics and nasal decongestants. If so the child should be seen daily until there are signs of improvement. If there is any clinical deterioration or when there are signs of orbital involvement, the child should be admitted for intravenous therapy. Consultation by infectious disease and otolaryngology specialists can be of assistance. The antibiotics should be chosen to treat the suspected organisms until the cultures are returned.

The children should be observed frequently in the hospital. In general children will respond well to medical treatment despite the presence of a subperiosteal collection. In our experience if the clinical picture stabilizes for a period of 24 hours this is followed by ultimate improvement. If however there is evidence of compromise of optic nerve function the patient should be rescanned and taken to the operating room to have the sinuses and any subperiosteal collection drained. Cultures should be obtained intraoperatively. Postoperatively these cases usually respond rapidly. Intravenous antibiotics should be continued for 1 to 2 weeks depending on the rapidity and completeness of the

clinical response. A further course of oral antibiotics may be indicated in some cases.

Dacryoadenitis

Dacryoadenitis is the most common form of nonspecific orbital inflammation (orbital pseudotumor) in the pediatric population. The condition features pain and swelling of the lacrimal gland and the surrounding tissues. Ptosis is a frequent finding with the typical S-shaped appearance to the eyelid (Fig. 23–13A). Less common are limited elevation of the globe, proptosis, and scleritis. Although the cause is currently unknown, the condition frequently occurs following a viral upper respiratory tract infection or during a period of seasonal allergies. The clinical picture may be confused with infectious orbital cellulitis, lymphoid infiltrate, or eosinophilic granuloma.

The evaluation should include a CT scan that will demonstrate an enlarged lacrimal gland that enhances homogeneously with intravenous contrast dye (Fig. 23–13B). There is no associated bone remodeling or destruction. There may be enhancement of the associated sclera.

Systemic evaluation including a CBC, ESR, and any measure of autoimmune disease is generally revealing.

Treatment is effective with oral corticosteroids to a dose of approximately 1 mg/kg with a rapid resolution of the pain and swelling. The

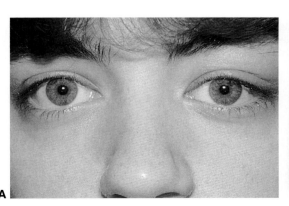

A

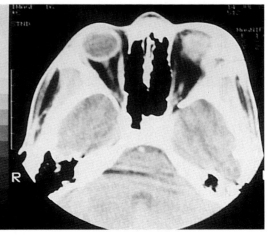

B

FIGURE 23–13. (A) Patient with dacryoadenitis of the left orbit featuring lid swelling with lateral greater than nasal ptosis. **(B)** CT scan in axial projection demonstrating enlargement of the left lacrimal gland and contrast enhancement consistent with dacryoadenitis.

corticosteroids are then tapered over a period of weeks. In some cases recurrent inflammatory signs may require a longer course of therapy. Long-term steroid therapy should be managed with a pediatrician or endocrinologist. As an alternative there are some patients that respond well to indomethacin.

Lymphangioma

At one time considered a distinct histopathologic entity, lymphangioma is now considered a vascular hamartoma that includes capillary hemangioma and venous malformation. The lesion usually becomes clinically evident after 1 year of age with an increase in the rate of identification of the tumors with increasing age. They are often first noted in association with an upper respiratory tract infection that results in the proliferation of lymphoid elements within the lesion. In other cases the sudden onset of proptosis heralds the development of a hemorrhagic cyst within the lesion (a so-called chocolate cyst). Pain, limited ocular motility, subcutaneous or subconjunctival hemorrhage, and optic neuropathy are associated clinical findings. The proptosis will cease to evolve after the initial 24 to 48 hours and will usually resolve at least partially over the subsequent several weeks. This pattern of growth helps to distinguish lymphangioma from malignant tumors, which have a rapid unrelenting growth pattern over a period of weeks, and capillary hemangioma, which tends to grow in rapid episodic spurts over the course of 1 year. Ultimately it is the tendency for the hemangioma to involute over the subsequent 4 years that may distinguish it clinically from lymphangioma.

Noninvasive evaluation is indicated by either CT or MRI. CT will reveal the location of the soft-tissue lesion, which is typically diffuse and enhances with contrast dye. It may be located intraconal, extraconal, or in some cases will extend between both the intraconal and extraconal spaces. MRI is however the most useful technique to distinguish lymphangioma from hemangioma or other solid soft-tissue tumors (Fig. 23–14). MRI will reveal the large irregular vascular spaces and when present the chocolate cysts. Ultimately, as the red blood cells separate from the serum, the layered fluid filled cyst becomes apparent on T_2-weighted images.

Treatment is generally highly conservative. In the absence of optic neuropathy, therapy is supportive. Observation, reassurance, and the occasional judicious use of a brief course of corticosteroids are warranted as the vast majority of cases will improve spontaneously over a period of weeks. Because the natural history of lymphangioma is multiple recurrent acute episodes followed by spontaneous improvement, surgical intervention is reserved for cases producing massive proptosis that threatens corneal integrity or optic neuropathy. When surgery is performed on an emergency basis, it should be limited to the evacuation of the cystic element of the lesion. If elective tumor excision is planned to reverse motility impairment or persistent proptosis, then as complete a resection as possible should be attempted. This may be aided by a CO_2 laser, which will limit intraoperative bleeding. Surgery should spare normal orbital anatomy, which is frequently intermingled with the tumor mass. Of occasional value is percutaneous or transarterial vascular thrombosis as over time some of the lesions will develop large venous lakes or high flow arterial vascular supply. In such cases the noninvasive radiologist may be of great value to the management.

Patients with lymphangioma ultimately become a career-long project with the occasional requirement for urgent treatment.

Neurofibroma

Type I versus Type II

Neurofibromas are grouped into three classes: (1) isolated, (2) diffuse, and (3) plexiform. Each will be discussed separately. Although all may be manifestations of neurofibromatosis, only the plexiform variety is uniformly associated with the syndrome. The diffuse and isolated forms are associated with neurofibromatosis in only 10% of cases. In all classes the histology features proliferation of schwannian and endoneural elements.

Neurofibromatosis

Neurofibromatosis is an autosomally inherited trait with highly variable and incomplete penetrance affecting approximately 1 in 3000 births. Diagnostic criterion include six or more

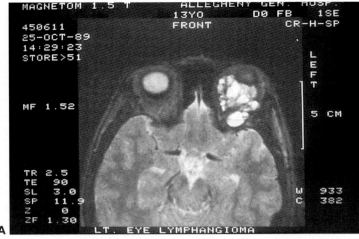

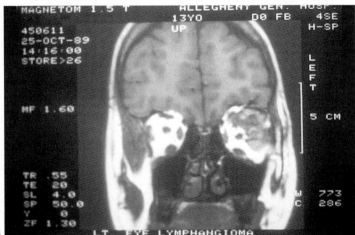

FIGURE 23–14. (A) Axial MRI of a patient with a cystic lymphangioma of the left orbit demonstrating multiple orbital cysts with fluid–fluid levels. **(B)** Coronal projection of the same MRI demonstrating interdigitation of the soft tissue lymphangioma within the orbit.

cafe-au-lait spots of greater than 15 mm in diameter, axillary freckling, cutaneous neurofibromas, and family history of neurofibromatosis. Peripheral neurofibromatosis features the appearance of cafe-au-lait spots in the first year of life followed by neurofibromas in adolescence. Visceral neurofibromas and skeletal abnormalities, most notably absence of the sphenoid wing, may be identified. Growth and mental disorders are possible. The disease may be associated with pheochromocytomas or neurilemmomas, and there is a 10% rate of malignant degeneration of neurofibromas in the setting of neurofibromatosis. Central neurofibromatosis is associated with astrocytomas, meningiomas, schwannomas, and ependymomas with few peripheral manifestations. The orbital findings of neurofibromatosis include gliomas and meningiomas of the optic nerve, orbital neurofibromas and schwannomas, and dysgenesis of the sphenoid wing (Fig. 23–15A). Lisch nodules (iris hamartomas) are present in 90% of patients with neurofibromatosis. Also seen are choroidal hamartomas, cafe-au-lait spots and neurofibromas of the eyelids, prominent corneal nerves, and glaucoma, which may produce buphthalmos.

Plexiform Neurofibromas

Plexiform neurofibromas are the most common form of the disease. They may affect any nerve, although there is a predilection for sensory nerves. Proliferation produces a "bag of worms" within the soft tissue. Management is

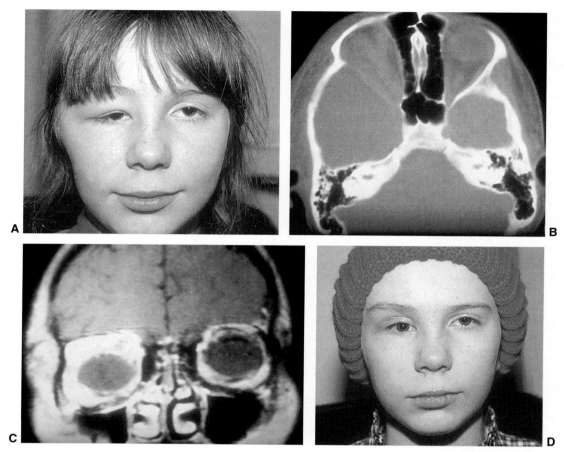

FIGURE 23–15. **(A)** A 13-year-old with neurofibromatosis featuring cutaneous extension and deep orbital neurofibroma producing an S-shaped right upper eyelid. **(B)** CT scan of the same patient with neurofibromatosis featuring typical hypoplasia of the left sphenoid wing. **(C)** MRI of the same patient demonstrating a soft tissue mass in the superior orbit displacing the globe inferiorly and expanding the bony orbit secondary to neurofibromatosis. **(D)** A postoperative picture of the same patient after resection of the subcutaneous orbital and intracranial components of the neurofibroma and reconstruction of the sphenoid bone.

complicated by the lack of encapsulation and the substantial vascularity. Malignant degeneration is rare.

CT identifies a moderately enhancing soft tissue density without clearly defined borders (Fig. 23–15B). Involvement of the extraocular muscles, intraconal sensory or motor nerves, or cavernous sinus produces nodular enlargement of these structures. Absence of the sphenoid wing is the most typical bony orbital deformity, however, long-standing soft tissue volume expansion may produce enlargement of the bony orbit when compared to the contralateral orbit. On MRI, most are hypointense on T_1 and hyperintense on T_2 and have the same gross features as seen on CT (Fig. 23–15C).

Lack of encapsulation and profound vascularity complicate management. Surgical excision is generally incomplete, bloody, and subject to significant postoperative edema that is slow to resolve. The goals of excision are to provide modest cosmetic improvement with minimal risk to normal tissues (Fig. 23–15D). This requires multiple operative procedures over the life of the patient with decreasingly satisfactory results. Use of the CO_2 laser minimizes intraoperative bleeding.

Isolated Neurofibromas

Isolated neurofibromas are rarely identified in the orbit. Generally affecting sensory nerves they enlarge slowly, producing mass occupying effects not generally appreciated until middle age. These may include proptosis, strabismus, and optic neuropathy. Although markedly adherent to the involved nerve they do not possess the substantial vascularity that exists in the plexiform variety.

CT reveals a homogeneous and well-circumscribed soft-tissue density that has uniform contrast enhancement. MRI demonstrates lesions hypo- to isointense on T_1 and hyperintense on T_2.

Treatment of these lesions is dictated by the severity of the mass effect that is produced. Resection is considered for lesions producing compressive optic neuropathy or disfigurement. The surgical approach is dictated by the location of the mass. Less vascular than the plexiform variety, solitary neurofibromas pose fewer surgical complications. Efforts should be made to identify the function of the involved nerve both prior to surgery and intraoperatively. Sensory nerve function loss is of lesser consequence than motor loss. In the latter case, attempts should be made to preserve the function of the nerve by careful dissection of the tumor from the nerve with the assistance of the operating microscope.

Diffuse Neurofibromas

Diffuse neurofibromatosis is rare, generally affecting the skin and sparing the orbit. Involvement of the orbit produces diffuse infiltration of the soft tissues. Radiologically it has much the same features as the plexiform variety. Surgical resection is subtotal and complicated by significant vascularity and lack of encapsulation. Resection should be avoided and if necessary limited in extent.

Schwannoma

Schwannomas are benign proliferations of the Schwann cell envelope of peripheral nerves. Within the orbit, they may affect any of the sensory or motor nerves. They produce slowly progressive painless proptosis. They do not affect nerve function until late in the course. Optic neuropathy is an inconsistent feature that depends on the critical size and location of the tumor producing secondary compression of the optic nerve. Small apically located tumors may produce profound visual symptoms before there is evidence of proptosis, whereas a more anteriorly located mass will feature proptosis before optic neuropathy is documented. Mass effect of the tumor may also produce choroidal folds. Rare are malignant schwannommas that appear to be degenerations of more benign histologic forms. Growth in these cases is explosive.

CT scan reveals a homogeneous well-circumscribed soft-tissue density that may be either intra- or extraconal (Fig. 23–16). It displaces surrounding structures, and long-standing lesions may produce remodeling or frank erosion of surrounding bone. Contrast dye may produce a small degree of enhancement.

MR features a discrete, homogeneous, soft-tissue density that is hypointense on T_1 and hyperintense on T_2. There is little enhancement with the use of gadolinium.

Treatment is primary excision when mass effect (i.e., optic neuropathy, proptosis) is significant or if the pattern of tumor growth accelerates, suggesting malignant degeneration. The route for orbitotomy is determined by the site of the tumor. The mass may be removed whole if small or in a fragmented fashion if larger. In such cases we find a CO_2 laser coupled to an operating neurosurgical microscope to aid the dissection and removal of the mass. Small volumes of residual tumor generally do not recur and are best left to preserve the surrounding

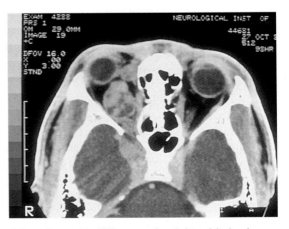

FIGURE 23–16. CT scan of a right orbital schwannoma demonstrating a knobby soft tissue mass within the orbit extending into, and enlarging, the right cavernous sinus with internal soft tissue inhomogeneity.

normal structures. If histopathologic inspection reveals a malignant schwannoma, then exenteration is recommended.

Histiocytosis X

Hand-Schuller-Christian disease, Letterer-Siwe disease, and eosinophilic granuloma (Fig. 23–17) are the triad of conditions grouped as histiocytosis X. They share the histology of abundant histiocytes and an unknown etiology.

The condition is rare and frequently misdiagnosed and treated as infectious cellulitis or an orbital malignancy before the diagnosis is revealed by orbital imaging and biopsy. The child most often presents with signs and symptoms of orbital inflammation. Pain, swelling, and redness are apparent in the superotemporal quadrant of the involved orbit. If the condition is advanced there may be swelling and pain of the temporalis fossa and pain associated with mastication. Ptosis when present is temporally based. There may be proptosis and painful limitation of ocular rotations. The orbital signs are often indolent and may remit spontaneously. Partial remissions often further confuse the

treating physician and may support the initial impression of infection. However, the child will not be febrile, and there is rarely any serum leukocytosis.

The condition is significantly different in terms of clinical behavior and prognosis depending on the age of the child. Younger patients (less than 3 years of age) tend to have more aggressive disease. Letterer-Siwe features systemic histiocytic disease, Hand-Schuller-Christian multifocal bone lesions, and eosinophilic granuloma focal orbital lytic lesions. Eosinophilic granuloma is the most common of the group. It is more common in boys and generally is identified by 10 years of age (although we have seen some cases in teenage children). The etiology of the lesion is unknown, but it is suspected to be a disregulation of the immune system.

CT imaging is most helpful in reaching a diagnosis. A rather dramatic picture is often revealed featuring a superotemporal soft-tissue mass that enhances with contrast injection. Surrounding lytic bone destruction is the rule. There may be extension of the lesion into the extradural–intracranial space.

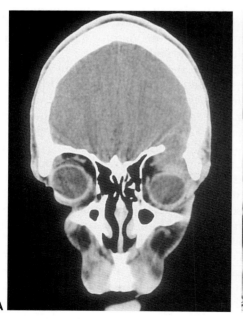
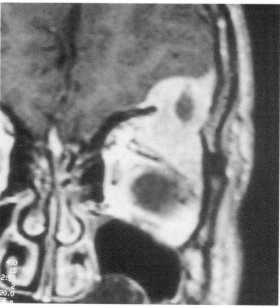

FIGURE 23–17. (A) CT scan in coronal projection of a patient with eosinophilic granuloma. The soft tissue mass in the superior temporal orbit has displaced the globe inferiorally, eroded through the roof of the orbit, and extended into the intracranial space. The lesion remains extradural. **(B)** MRI of a patient with eosinophilic granuloma demonstrating intracranial extension and intralesional cystic degeneration.

Treatment planning requires a biopsy of the most readily available tissue. Children should undergo a systemic evaluation. If there is systemic disease, chemotherapy is delivered by a pediatric oncologist. If the disease is localized to the orbit, surgery can be approached through the orbit despite the size of the lesion. The goal is biopsy for diagnosis and curettage of the readily accessible lesion and surrounding bone. There is no need routinely to reconstruct the bone defect. If the periosteum is replaced and the lesion is effectively treated the bone will reform over a period of months.

Medical treatment of the solitary orbital lesion is generally successful with a tapering dose of oral corticosteroids. Rarely are chemotherapeutic agents or low-dose orbital radiotherapy required.

Optic Nerve Glioma

The biologic behavior of the group of lesions grouped histologically as gliomas varies to such an extent that making predictions regarding the growth potential of a given tumor or conclusions of a retrospective analysis is imprecise. All attempts at identifying clinical, radiographic, or histologic markers that consistantly predict behavior or outcome have failed. Most gliomas are solitary lesions. The tumor may be located solely within the orbit, bridge the orbitocranial space, or reside within the intracranial space alone. Modern imaging permits noninvasive diagnosis and localization, which are keystones to management.

Retrospective studies offer conflicting data. Alvord and Lofton compiled the data of 623 previously reported cases of optic nerve or chiasmal glioma and applied a mathematical model to derive more statistically significant results. They found that, whereas the behavior of the tumors varied overall, there was a general trend toward declining growth rate over time. This result argues for the classification of these tumors as low-grade pilocytic astrocytomas. The majority of tumors are diagnosed within the first 2 decades of life. Increasing age at the time of diagnosis correlates with a poorer long-term prognosis. Those younger than 20 years of age at the time of diagnosis had a 20-year survival rate of 65%, whereas the group diagnosed at older than 50 years had an 80% 10-year mortality rate. Mortality rates were higher among patients with chiasmal involvement at the time of diagnosis and higher still when involving the hypothalamus or ventricles.

In Alvord and Lofton's study, 25% of tumors had invaded the chiasm at the time of surgical excision. Although this figure may represent cases that involved the chiasm early in the course it also includes cases from the pre-CT era when data from plain film radiographs and tomograms came late in the course of the disease. Earlier diagnosis with MRI and the ability to closely monitor the growth of the tumor may yield different statistics.

Recurrences developed in 5% of cases in which a "complete" intraorbital resection was performed. We would strongly advocate a combined intracranial and intraorbital approach for excision of the involved optic nerve from the globe to the chiasm to minimize such reccurences.

In 15 to 50% of cases associated with neurofibromatosis (NF) multifocal disease is found. Bilateral optic nerve glioma is nearly uniformly associated with NF. Investigators differ regarding prognosis in the multifocal cases. Although most have no long-term increase in mortality, there is an increase in the rate of distant sarcomas or glioblastoma mutiformae, unrelated to the treatment rendered.

The clinical signs and symptoms depend on the size and location of the tumor. Intraorbital gliomas produce axial proptosis and visual loss (Fig. 23–18A). The vision loss varies and is often severe and out of proportion to the proptosis. In young children, the vision loss may be manifest as amblyopia or strabismus. Profound proptosis may limit ocular rotations and produce corneal decompensation and spontaneous prolapse of the globe. Papilledema is generally present, although long-standing disease may produce optic disc pallor.

Tumors predominantly within the intracanalicular segment of the optic nerve, the chiasm, or optic radiations may be difficult to detect in the pediatric population. In the absence of proptosis, vision loss is the sole clinical barometer.

Similarly, tumors involving the optic radiations will not produce proptosis; typical visual field defects will, however, be present.

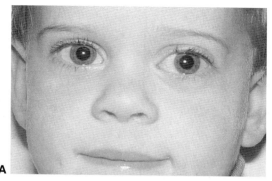

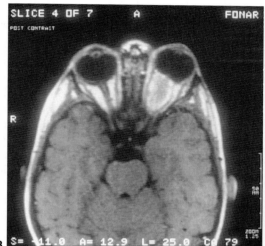

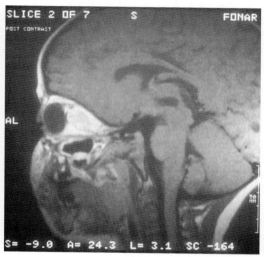

FIGURE 23–18. **(A)** Patient with left optic nerve glioma featuring mild proptosis. **(B)** MRI in axial projection of the patient demonstrating enlargement of the left optic nerve with mild enhancement. **(C)** Saggital section MRI of an optic nerve glioma demonstrating enlargement of the optic nerve from the posterior globe to the optic canal. (Courtesy of J.S. Kennerdell, M.D.)

The increased risk of optic nerve gliomas in patients with NF mandates baseline neurooph-thalmic examination and radiologic investiga-tion when indicated by the clinical findings.

CT has been the standard diagnostic imaging modality for optic gliomas. Images should be rendered in the axial and coronal planes both with and without contrast. Optic nerve gliomas produce fusiform enlargement of the optic nerve. The optic nerve is not identified within the tumor, and calcification is rarely present. The nerve and sheath are often kinked at nearly 90 degrees in the anterior one third of the orbit. Invasion of the optic canal, chiasm, or optic radiations is best imaged by MRI (Figs. 23–18B and C). Enlargement of the optic canal may be seen with parasaggital views in the plane of the canal. Optic gliomas are hypo- or isoin-tense on T_1 and hyperintense on T_2.

Treatment is guided by the location of the tumor and visual potential. Bilateral optic nerve or chiasmal involvement precludes surgical treatment. We generally monitor these cases closely. Those that appear static are not treated. Measurements of optic nerve function, propto-sis, corneal decompensation, and optic disc edema are made quarterly. Deterioration of the clinical picture or radiographic evidence of disease progression necessitates treatment. Obstructive hydrocephalus requires shunting; chiasmal involvement may produce pituitary insufficiency, which may require treatment. Multicenter trials are being conducted to determine the efficacy of radiotherapy and chemotherapy in such cases. A description of the early results of the trials is included in the oncology chapter.

Surgery is reserved for unilateral cases that radiographically invade the optic canal but spare the chiasm or when proptosis produces medically uncontrollable corneal decompensa-tion or gross disfigurement. We prefer a tran-scranial approach and resection of the optic nerve from the globe to the chiasm to assure complete extirpation of the tumor. Should tumor be evident at the proximal end of the resected specimen at the time of histopathologic inspection we do not attempt to resect the residual tumor within the chiasm as surgical damage to the contralateral visual pathway may result. Additionally, there is no assurance that further resection into the chiasm will obtain a tumor-free margin. Although guarded, the prognosis is unclear in individual cases. Each is monitored closely, and if clinical or radiographic progression is noted careful consideration is given to treatment with radiotherapy or chemotherapy. The use of radiotherapy to treat chiasmal lesions is, however, relatively contraindicated in children less than 5 years of age.

Meningioma

Orbital meningiomas involve either the optic nerve or the sphenoid bone. Lesions of the sphenoid bone are identified almost exclusively in adults.

Meningiomas of the optic nerve are also more frequently identified in women in the third or fourth decade; however, in most studies they are the second most common optic nerve tumors in the pediatric population. Early in the course of the disease, visual loss may be mild. Strabismus or unexplained or refractory amblyopia may be the earliest clinical signs. More profound visual loss evolves over decades. Although proptosis is occasionally seen it, too, is generally a late finding. The slow evolution of signs and symptoms argues for a conservative approach to management.

CT identifies two morphologic tumor types. The en-plaque variety is generally first identified after the third decade. It appears as a focal exophytic tumor that may be present at any point along the course of the intraorbital segment of the optic nerve. The tumor enhances with intravenous contrast dye. The morphologic MRI findings are much the same as CT. The tumor is intense on both T_1 and T_2 sequences and is hyperintense with gadolinium contrast.

The second, more common variety produces a fusiform enlargement of the optic nerve. On CT the tumor is denser than the normal nerve and is often identified by the classic "railroad

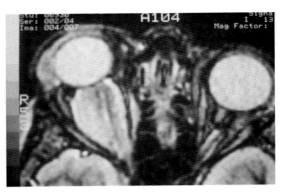

FIGURE 23–19. MRI of an optic nerve meningioma featuring a fusiform enlargement of the optic nerve sheath with preservation of the optic nerve.

track" sign produced by calcification within the tumor. This sign is not, however, uniformly identified. As imaged by MR, the tumor is isointense on T_1 and hyperintense on T_2 and enhances with contrast (Fig. 23–19). Generally, the normal centrally located optic nerve is identified within a circumferentially expanded tumor mass. This finding helps distinguish a meningioma from a glioma. MRI provides the earliest evidence of optic canal invasion by tumor.

Treatment is dictated by the degree of visual acuity loss, development of proptosis, and evidence of intracranial extension. Although there have been isolated reports of surgical removal of en-plaque optic nerve tumors with preservation or improvement in vision, complete loss of vision is most common. Decompression of the nerve sheath has been advocated. We avoid this approach as it has been associated with massive orbital extension requiring exenteration. We avoid surgery except to prevent intracranial extension. Invasion of the optic canal is identified by MRI and associated with rapid vision loss. Resection is approached through a cranioorbitotomy to permit complete removal of the tumor and prevent intracranial spread. If intracranial extension occurs treatment is more complicated and less successful. We favor the same surgical approach if resection is performed to treat profound proptosis.

As an alternative some have applied radiotherapy in adult patients to halt the progression of visual loss. We generally avoid radiotherapy in pediatric cases because of the high rate of secondary malignancies in the irradiated field.

Leukemia/Lymphoma

Involvement of the orbit by lymphoproliferative disease in the pediatric population is rare. Most are B-cell lymphomas. The most common lymphoma to invade the orbit is Burkitt's; most frequently identified in Africa it is associated with infection by the Epstein-Barr virus. Tumorous infiltration may occur from the paraorbital sinuses. In the United States the variant of Burkitt's lymphoma is not associated with Epstein-Barr virus infection, is identified later in life, and rarely involves the orbit. The lesion may invade the intracranial space to produce cranial neuropathies and CSF pleocytosis. Rapidly evolving proptosis can ultimately produce optic neuropathy. Imaging with CT or MRI will demonstrate a widely infiltrative soft-tissue mass that enhances with intravenous contrast injection. A biopsy for diagnosis will demonstrate the typical "starry-sky" histiocytes. Treatment with systemic chemotherapy (cyclophosphamide, vincristine, methotrexate, and corticosteroids) is combined with brain irradiation in cases in which bone marrow disease is identified. Tumor remission is achieved in 50% of cases.

Childhood leukemias more typically metastasize to the intraocular tissues (retina and choroid) as opposed to the orbit. In such cases the 5-year survival is 50% of the rate among children without ocular involvement. Acute myeloid leukemia is the most likely form of leukemia to involve the orbit. Often the disease is first identified in the orbit when it produces proptosis (Figs. 23–20A and B) and may not be identified in the peripheral blood or bone for

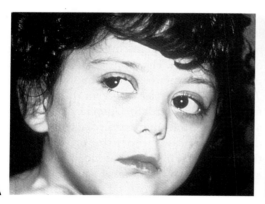

A

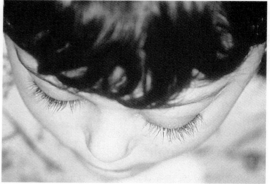

B

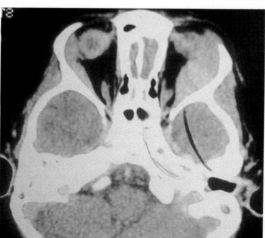

C

FIGURE 23–20. (A) Patient with metastatic left orbital leukemia. **(B)** A view from above demonstrating left proptosis. **(C)** CT scan demonstrating large left lateral orbital soft tissue mass consistent with the leukemic process. (Courtesy of J.A. Katowitz, M.D.)

months. In such cases early identification and treatment are associated with improved prognosis. Clinically the child will present with rapidly evolving proptosis. The CT scan (Fig. 23–20C) or MRI will define the infiltrative soft-tissue mass that does not produce bone destruction. The lesion enhances with contrast dye. A biopsy is diagnostic if the diagnosis is considered, and appropriate stains for esterase activity are performed with a Leder stain, which aids in the distinction of this lesion from rhabdomyosarcoma and neuroblastoma.

If the lesion is confined to the orbit, orbital radiotherapy is indicated. The patients are subsequently monitored for the development of systemic lesions that require chemotherapy.

■ Ages 7 to 15 Years

The most commonly presenting lesions in the 7- to 15-year age group are listed in Table 23–4.

TABLE 23–4. Lesions Identified from 7 to 15 Years

Orbital pseudotumor
Osteoma
Fibrous dysplasia
Graves' orbitopathy
Lacrimal gland tumors

Orbital Pseudotumor

Orbital pseudotumor is a term applied to a group of nonspecific orbital inflammatory processes without defined etiologies. Among them is dacryoadenitis described previously. Although the lacrimal gland appears to be more frequently targeted in younger children, the remainder of the orbital tissues become targets as patient age increases. Specific names are given to particular forms of pseudotumor, including scleritis, myositis optic neuritis, and Tolusa-Hunt (when affecting the orbital apex/cavernous sinus). When a more diffuse process affecting the orbital tissues is present the term *orbital pseudotumor* or *nonspecific orbital inflammation* is applied (Figs. 23–21A and B). Although each entity may ultimately prove to result from a distinct etiology we currently have no way to distinguish one from the next on his-

tologic grounds. The histopathologic pattern is typically a mixture of acute and occasionally chronic inflammatory cells. Polyclonality is the rule, and there is no evidence of infectious elements that are cultured from the specimen despite long-standing suspicion that viral infection may play a role.

Clinically the patient presents with signs of diffuse orbital inflammation except in cases where a particular subset of the orbital tissues is affected. Pain is a hallmark of the disease. Lid swelling and erythema are typical. Limitation of ocular rotations and chemosis is identified if the process is fulminant. Proptosis may be present as well as upper eyelid ptosis. Ptosis in the presence of orbital inflammation can be helpful in attempting to distinguish orbital pseudotumor from Graves' orbitopathy. The latter is uniformly associated with eyelid retraction. Optic neuropathy when present may be the result of primary optic nerve inflammation or may occur secondary to compression from diffuse orbital edema. Focal inflammations of the posterior sclera, extraocular muscles, or optic nerve do not uniformly result in clinically apparent signs of inflammation. However, they always produce pain and dysfunction of the involved structure. *Tolusa-Hunt syndrome* is a term used to characterize painful ophthalmoplegia resulting from a benign inflammatory process. It was first described in cases where the process involved the cavernous sinus but has more recently been applied to inflammations of the orbital apex.

The diagnosis of orbital pseudotumor is the same in each entity. A careful attempt to exclude specifically treatable diseases must be undertaken. These include infection, neoplasia, and autoimmune disease. Generally the evaluation proceeds beyond the clinical examination to noninvasive imaging. In cases of suspected pseudotumor an MRI is generally of greatest value. It provides the greatest soft-tissue resolution within the orbit and especially of the optic nerve and cavernous sinus. It should be performed both with and without contrast enhancement to best delineate the inflammatory process. In addition to excluding intraorbital malignancy the paraorbital sinuses should be inspected for the presence of disease. Typically in the case of diffuse orbital inflammation a poorly delimited

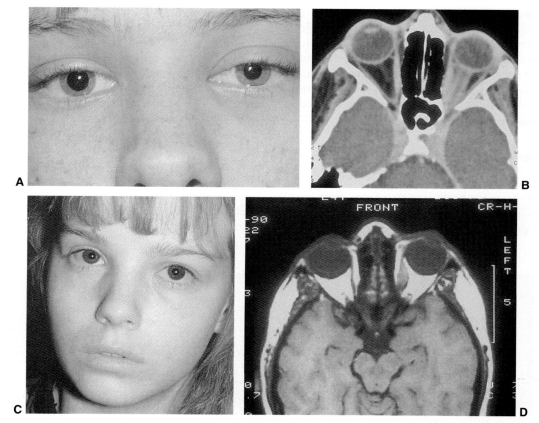

FIGURE 23–21. (A) Patient with left orbital pseudotumor. **(B)** CT scan of the patient demonstrating left optic nerve enhancement. **(C)** Patient with left orbital myositis. **(D)** MRI demonstrating fusiform enlargement of the left medial rectus muscle.

enhancing soft-tissue mass will be identified. Focal disease of the extraocular muscles produces swelling of both the belly of the muscle and in general the tendonous insertion into the globe. This is in contradistinction to the swelling of extraocular muscle affected by Graves' orbitopathy, which spares the tendons. Optic neuritis produces a dramatic enhancement of the optic nerve sheath that appears to spill over to the surrounding orbital fat in shaggy fashion (Figs. 23–21A and B). This is similar in appearance to the inflammation produced in the posterior sclera. The sclera enhances, the choroid is usually thickened, and the surrounding orbital fat enhances with contrast. In cases of Tolusa-Hunt the MR is critical in excluding malignancy or aneurysm (a rare cause in the pediatric population) as a cause of the clinical signs and symptoms.

The serologic evaluation should include a CBC, ESR, Lyme antibody titer, ANA, rheumatoid factor, ANCA, ACE, and Ca. If there is evidence of intracranial disease a lumbar puncture may be indicated. If the paraorbital sinuses and serological testing is normal a trial of oral corticosteroids is indicated. The dose is generally begun at the level of 1 mg/kg of prednisone. This is coordinated with the pediatrician or endocrinologist. The clinical response should be rapid, on the order of days to a week. The dose should then be tapered over the course of 4 to 6 weeks. If the process reoccurs the serologic testing and MRI may need to be repeated, and consideration of an open orbital biopsy and culture should be undertaken to rule out malignancy. If the biopsy is performed and excludes a specific cause of the inflammation, a more prolonged course of corticosteroids may be undertaken. As an alternative to corticosteroids the use of nonsteroidal antiinflammatory drugs (in particular indomethicin) was found in several series to be effective in the treatment of orbital pseudo- tumor. Ultimately the disease may last for 1 month to several years with occasional bouts of recurrence before it becomes quiescent.

Ossifying Lesions

Osteoma (Fibrous Osteoma)

Osteomas are bony lesions of unknown etiology. They are unusual lesions in the pediatric age group representing less than 1% of tumors

in our experience. In general, the lesions become clinically apparent in the second decade of life or later. The clinical signs and symptoms vary depending upon the site of bone from which they arise (Fig. 23–22A). Proptosis is usually nonaxial and slowly progressive. In a few cases the proptosis may progress rapidly resulting from an associated acute sinusitis or adjacent hemorrhage. In addition to acute sinusitis resulting in orbital cellulitis and meningitis we have seen one case in which acute dacryocystitis resulted from obstruction of the nasolacrimal duct. Optic neuropathy can occur if cellulitis occurs acutely or if the lesion grows slowly to a critical size.

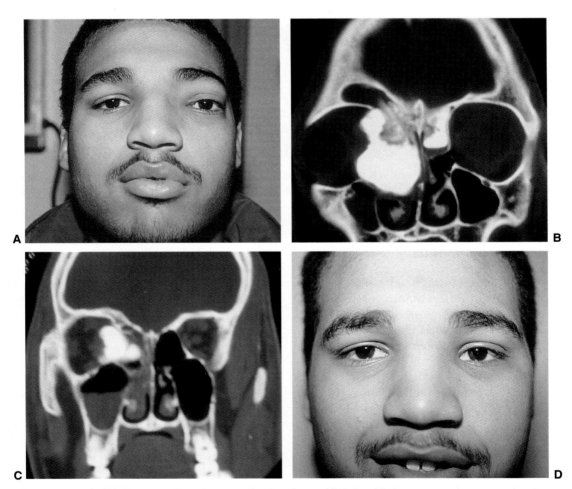

FIGURE 23–22. (A) Preoperative photograph of patient with left orbital osteoma demonstrating hypertelorism. **(B)** CT scan of anterior orbit demonstrating an osteoma of the left ethmoid and right frontal sinus. **(C)** Posterior orbital coronal CT scan demonstrating osteoma of the left ethmoid sinus. **(D)** Postoperative photograph of the same patient demonstrating restoration of normal intraorbital dimensions.

CT scanning provides the best noninvasive imaging technique (Figs. 23–22B and C). The use of bone window density in the axial and coronal planes reveals the interface of normal bone and tumor. Osteomas will appear uniformly hyperintense, but bone windows reveal internal inhomogeneity repesenting fibrous material.

Histologically osteoid predominates, however, there may be a variable amount of fibrous tissue accounting for the areas of lucency identified on bone windows of the CT scan. Although pathologists will variably describe the lesions as osteoma or fibrous osteoma, we feel this reflects a spectrum of disease without clinical significance.

Excision is performed by the approach that provides most direct access. We have been able to approach lesions that extend from frontal to maxillary sinus through a bifrontal craniotomy. However, smaller lesions may be approached more directly. The lesions routinely cleave from the surrounding normal bone, which is easy to identify intraoperatively. If difficulty is encountered the lesion may be drilled centrally and the peripheral edges removed with rongeurs. Reconstruction of the bony orbital wall that reseced with the osteoma is only required if its absence will result in functional or cosmetic deformity. Examples are the orbital rim, the anterior third of the orbital roof, and the medial wall of the orbit.

If the osteoma is completely excised we have not seen a recurrence (Fig. 23–22D). Subtotal resections can be expected to regrow; however, the generally slow growth pattern may make it clinically insignificant.

Ossifying Fibroma

The spectrum of bony osseous lesions includes ossifying fibroma. Clinically the lesion grows slowly and produces signs and symptoms by mass effect in similar fashion to osteomas. They are often not identified until the second decade of life and grow slowly over decades. CT scanning features a predominantly osseous lesion with a greater relative soft-tissue component. On occasion the radiographic picture can be confused with fibrous dysplasia. However, the distinction between normal and abnormal bone tends to be better defined in the case of ossifying fibroma. Histologically a well-vascularized fibrous stroma distinguishes it from osteoma.

Treatment is surgical excision. Indications for excision include disfiguring proptosis, exposure keratitis, and compressive optic neuropathy. Surgical excision is accomplished by the same means as described for osteoma. Similarly, the lesion is easy to distiguish from the surrounding normal bone intraoperatively. Complete surgical resection is rarely complicated by recurrence.

Fibrous Dysplasia

Fibrous dysplasia is likely to represent a developmental process that is generally first identified in the first decade of life. Fibrous dysplasia may represent one manifestation of a clinical complex of Albright's syndrome, which includes endocrine abnormalities, long bone deformities, cutaneous pigmentation, and facial fibrous dysplasia (Fig. 23–23A). The growth of the orbital lesions can be sporadic and may be linked to growth hormone because the rapid growth phase tends to conclude by the end of the second decade. With the exception of cases associated with Albright's syndrome most involve only one facial bone. However, unlike osteomas these lesions are difficult to distinguish from the surrounding normal bone either intraoperatively or by preoperative neuroimaging. This feature complicates the management of the disease. Imaging is best performed with CT (Figs. 23–23B and C). However, in cases in which the diagnosis is obscure and the differentiation from meningioma unclear an MRI with contrast enhancement is helpful. The characteristic dural enhancement seen in meningiomas of the sphenoid bone distinguishes the lesion from fibrous dysplasia, which does not involve the dura.

Management is expectant. Careful attention is paid to the development of proptosis, facial deformity, and optic neuropathy. The latter generally results from rapidly expanding mucocele of the sphenoid and occasionally the posterior ethmoid air cells. The rapid deterioration of vision loss is an emergency, requires noninvasive imaging, and may necessitate urgent evacuation of the mucocele and decompression of the optic nerve. It is not our belief that prophylactic decompression of the optic canal is of

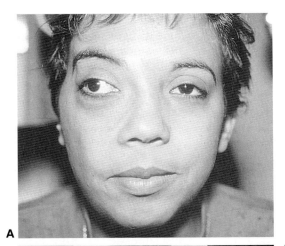

A

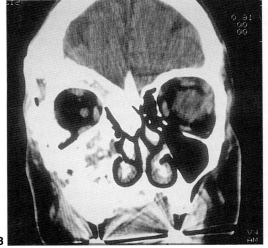

B

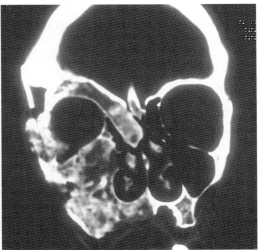

C

FIGURE 23–23. (A) Photograph of patient with fibrous dysplasia demonstrating right proptosis and exotropia due to a blind right eye. **(B)** CT scan of the same patient demonstrating hyperostosis of the right paraorbital bones. **(C)** CT scan with bone windows demonstrating the ground glass appearance of the bony hyperostosis.

value in avoiding permanent vision loss. In some cases the efforts required to remove the hyperostotic bone may result in traumatic optic neuropathy and complete and irreversible vision loss. In other cases the resection of tumor should be reserved for cases in which the facial deformity is profound.

Graves' Orbitopathy

Graves' orbitopathy is an autoimmune manifestation of a systemic process (Graves' hyperthyroidism) that is the most common cause of both unilateral and bilateral proptosis in adults. In children it is a rare cause of proptosis (Fig. 23–24A). The youngest case we have treated is in a 6-year-old. Identification of the condition is made more difficult in the pediatric population because the clinical manifestations frequently differ from those in adults. In children the systemic hyperthyroidism is often difficult to diagnose because of the tendency for children to have naturally high metabolic rates and activity levels. The proptosis and associated soft-tissue inflammation are often mistaken for signs of infectious orbital cellulitis. Frequently lacking is the extraocular motility impairment. Upper lid retraction is a variable finding. CT imaging is vital to exclude infectious and neoplastic causes of proptosis (Fig. 23–24B). Expansion of the orbital fat compartment is typical of

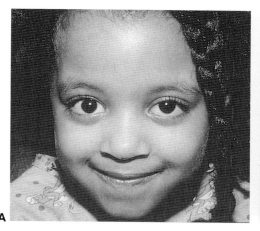
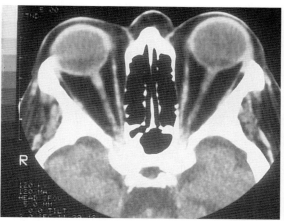

A   **B**

FIGURE 23–24. (A) Child with acute Graves' orbitopathy featuring right upper eyelid retraction and mild proptosis. **(B)** CT scan on the same patient demonstrating mild proptosis but, as is typical, no extraocular muscle enlargement.

the pediatric patient with Graves' orbitopathy. Enlargement of the extraocular muscles is not routinely identified. Serologic testing will typically reveal elevation of T3 and T4 levels and suppression of the TSH.

Treatment is aimed at supportive care until the systemic thyroid disease is stabilized. This more frequently ameliorates the orbital signs than in adults. Fortunately, exposure keratitis is rare in children. When present, topical lubrication is indicated. Diplopia can be treated with prism lenses until the disease is stabilized. Optic neuropathy is treated with corticosteroids and decompressive surgery in the acute phase of disease to prevent permanent vision loss.

The acute phase of the disease can last from 6 months to 2 years. In the stable phase of the disease surgery can help to reverse the proptosis, lid retraction, and diplopia.

Lacrimal Gland Tumors

Epithelial tumors of the lacrimal gland are exceedingly rare in childhood. Occasional reports of both benign mixed tumors and malignant adenoid cystic tumors exist in the pediatric population. The benign tumors produce painless enlargement of the lacrimal gland and may be associated with proptosis and displacement of the globe inferiorly and nasally. CT scanning

reveals a homogeneous soft-tissue enlargement of the lacrimal gland (Fig. 23–25). If present for a sufficient length of time it will be associated with thinning of the surrounding orbital bone. Treatment is complete surgical excision. In view of the rarity of the lesion in the pediatric population, the preoperative diagnosis may be difficult. In such instances intraoperative inspection of the lacrimal gland may be helpful. A hard lacrimal gland should raise the surgeon's suspicion. The capsule of the lesion should not be violated if possible. If necessary a biopsy may be performed, but a frozen section should be obtained, the tumor walled off while awaiting the pathologist's report, and the remainder of the lesion ultimately removed during the same operation.

Adenoid cystic carcinoma is an equally rare tumor among children. It presents clinically with pain, proptosis, and a firmly enlarged lacrimal gland. CT scan reveals an enlarged lacrimal gland that may be associated with either relatively normal orbital bones if early in the course of the disease or, if identified later, significant bone destruction with direct invasion into the intracranial space. Treatment involves biopsy to confirm the diagnosis. The extent of surgical resection that is required for effective treatment is debated. The limits include local resection followed by radiotherapy to transcranial

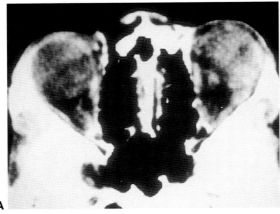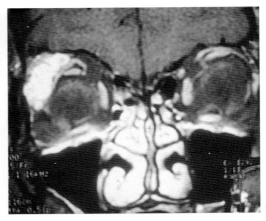

FIGURE 23–25. (A) CT scan of patient with left benign mixed tumor featuring knobby enlargement of the lacrimal gland and remodeling of the lacrimal fossa. **(B)** MRI of patient with a right lacrimal gland tumor featuring enhancement and displacement of the globe and extraocular muscles inferiorly and nasally.

orbitectomy. Failures after even the most aggressive forms of treatment have limited the enthusiasm for radical resections. Ultimately 80% of patients will die by 15 years. Tumor metastasis occurs by perineural and hematogenous spread.

REFERENCES

1. Henderson JW, ed. *Orbital Tumors.* New York: Decker; 1980.
2. Rootman J, ed. *Diseases of the Orbit.* Philadelphia: JB Lippincott; 1988.
3. Rootman J, Stewart B, Goldberg RA, eds. *Orbital Surgery.* Philadelphia: Lippincott-Raven; 1995.
4. Beard C. Dermolipoma surgery, or, "An ounce of prevention is worth a pound of cure." *Ophthalmol Plast Recons Surg.* 1990; 6:153.
5. Lo AKM, et al. The role of tissue expanders in an anophthalmic animal model. *Plast Recons Surg.* 1990; 86:399.
6. Bartlett SP, et al. The surgical management of orbitofacial dermoids in the pediatric patient. *Plast Reconstr Surg.* 1993; 91:1208.
7. Fry CL, Leone CR. Safe management of dermolipomas. *Arch Ophthalmol.* 1994; 112:1114.
8. Liu GT, et al. Prominent proptosis in childhood thyroid eye disease. *Ophthalmology.* 1996; 103:779.
9. Mottow LS, Jakobiec FA. Idiopathic inflammatory orbital pseudotumor in childhood. I. Clinical characteristics. *Arch Ophthalmol.* 1978; 96:1410.
10. Weiss A, et al. Bacterial periorbital and orbital cellulitis in childhood. *Arch Ophthalmol.* 1978; 96:1410.
11. Harris GJ. Subperiosteal abscess of the orbit: age as a factor in the bacteriology and response to treatment. *Ophthalmology.* 1994; 101:585.
12. Harris GJ. Subperiosteal abscess of the orbit: computed tomography and the clinical course. *Ophthal Plast Reconstr Surg.* 1996; 12:1.
13. Leone CR, Lloyd WC. Treatment protocol for orbital inflammatory disease. *Ophthalmology.* 1985; 92:1325.
14. Collison JMT, et al. Involvement of orbital tissues by sarcoid. *Am J Ophthalmol.* 1986; 102:302.
15. Jordan ER, et al. Eosinophilic granuloma. *Arch Ophthalmol.* 1993; 111:134.
16. Power WJ, et al. The value of combined serum angiotensin-converting enzyme and gallium scan in diagnosing ocular sarcoidosis. *Ophthalmology.* 1995; 102:2007.
17. Jakobiec FA, et al. Conjunctival adnexal cysts and dermoids. *Arch Ophthalmol.* 1978; 96:1404.
18. Ilani K, et al. Conservative surgery in orbital teratoma. *Orbit.* 1986; 5:61.
19. Shapiro A, et al. A clinicopathologic study of hematic cysts of the orbit. *Am J Ophthalmol.* 1986; 102:237.
20. Loeffler M, Hornblass A. Hematic cyst of the orbit. *Arch Ophthalmol.* 1990; 108:886.
21. Font RL, Ferry AP. The phakomatoses. *Int Ophthalmol.* 1972; 12:1.
22. Williams HB. Facial bone changes with vascular tumors in children. *Plast Recons Surg.* 1979; 63:309.
23. Williams HB. Facial bone changes with vascular tumors in children. *Plast Recons Surg.* 1979; 63:309; Thomson HG, et al. Hemangiomas of the eyelid: visual complications and prophylactic concepts. *Plast Recons Surg.* 1979; 63:641.
24. Kushner BJ. Local steroid therapy in adnexal hemangioma. *Ann Ophthalmol.* 1979; 11:1005.
25. Haik BG, et al. Capillary hemangioma of the lids and orbit: an analysis of the clinical features and therapeutic results in 101 cases. *Ophthalmology.* 1979; 86:760.
26. Kushner BJ. Intralesional corticosteroid injection for infantile adnexal hemangioma. *Am J Ophthalmol.* 1982; 93:496.

27. Rootman J, et al. Orbital-adnexal lymphangiomas. *Ophthalmology*. 1986; 93:1558.

28. Zucker JJ, Levine MR, Chu A. Primary intraosseous hemangioma of the orbit. *Ophthal Plast Recons Surg*. 1989; 5:247.

29. Harris GJ, et al. An analysis of thirty cases of orbital lymphangioma: pathophysiologic considerations and management recommendations. *Ophthalmology*. 1990; 97:1583.

30. Glatt HJ, et al. Adrenal suppression and growth retardation after injection of periocular capillary hemangioma with corticosteroids. *Ophthal Surg*. 1991; 22:95.

31. Kazim M, et al. Orbital lymphangioma: correlation of magnetic resonance images and intraoperative findings. *Ophthalmology*. 1992; 99:1588.

32. Walker RS, Custer PL, Nerad JA. Surgical excision of periorbital capillary hemangiomas. *Ophthalmology*. 1994; 101:1333.

33. Scheepers JH, Auaba AA. Does the pulsed tunable dye laser have a role in the management of infantile hemangiomas? Observations based on 3 years' experience. *Plast Reconstr Surg*. 1995; 95:305.

34. Cruz OA, et al. Treatment of periocular capillary hemangioma with topical clobetasol propionate. *Ophthalmology*. 1995; 102:2012.

35. Hoyt WF, Baghdassarian SA. Optic glioma of childhood: natural history and rationale for conservative management. *Br J Ophthalmol*. 1969; 53:793.

36. Wright JE. Primary optic nerve meningiomas: clinical presentation and management. *Trans Am Acad Ophthal Oto*. 1977; 83:617.

37. DeSousa AL, et al. Optic chiasmatic glioma in children. *Am J Ophthalmol*. 1979; 87:376.

38. Charles NC, et al. Pilocytic astrocytoma of the optic nerve with hemorrhage and extreme cystic degeneration. *Am J Ophthalmol*. 1981; 92:691.

39. Rootman J, Goldberg C, Robertson W. Primary orbital schwannomas. *Br J Ophthalmol*. 1982; 66:194.

40. Lewis RA, et al. von Rechlinghausen neurofibromatosis. II. Incidence of optic gliomata. *Ophthalmology*. 1984; 91:929.

41. Imes RK, Hoyt WF. Childhood chiasma gliomas: update on the facts of patients in the 1969 San Francisco study. *Br J Ophthalmol*. 1986; 70:179.

42. Haik BG, et al. Magnetic resonance imaging in the evaluation of optic nerve gliomas. *Ophthalmology*. 1987; 94:709.

43. Bullock JD, et al. Primary orbital neuroblastoma. *Arch Ophthalmol*. 1989; 107:1031.

44. Wright JE, McNab AA, McDonald WI. Optic nerve glioma and the management of optic nerve tumours in the young. *Br J Ophthalmol*. 1989; 73:967.

45. Maurer HM, et al. The intergroup rhabdomyosarcoma study: update—November, 1978. *J Natl Cancer Inst*. 1981; 56:61.

46. Wharam M, et al. Localized orbital rhabdomyosarcoma: an interim report of the intergroup rhabdomyosarcoma study committee. *Ophthalmology*. 1987; 94:251.

47. Shields CL, et al. Clinicopathologic review of 142 cases of lacrimal gland lesions. *Ophthalmology*. 1989; 96:431.

48. Grove AS. Osteomas of the orbit. *Opth Surg*. 1978;9:23.

49. Ehrlich WW. Orbital fibrous dysplasia: current diagnosis and management. In: Henkind P, ed. *ACTA: XXIV. International Congress of Ophthalmology*. Philadelphia: JB Lippincott; 1983:1030–1035.

50. Moore AT, Brincic JR, Munro IR: Fibrous dysplasia of the orbit in childhood. *Ophthalmol*. 1985;92:12.

51. Weisman JS, Hepler RS, Vinters HV. Reversible visual loss caused by fibrous dysplasia. *Am J Ophthalmol*. 1990; 110:244.

52. Bullock JD, Goldberg SH, Rakes SM. Orbital tumors in children. *Ophthalmol Plast Recons Surg*. 1989; 5:13.

53. Shields JA, et al. Space-occupying orbital masses in children: a review of 250 consecutive biopsies. *Ophthalmology*. 1986; 93:379.

54. Kodsi SR, et al. A review of 340 orbital tumors in children during a 60-year period. *Am J Ophthalmol*. 1994; 117:177.

Pediatric Ophthalmology
Edited by P. F. Gallin
Thieme Medical Publishers, Inc.
New York © 2000

24

Plastic Surgery

MARTIN L. LEIB

This chapter details congenital ptosis and naso-lacrimal duct obstructions, which together constitute the majority of nontumorous pediatric ophthalmology/plastic surgery cases. More detailed and global information can be obtained in the many superb and detailed ophthalmic plastic surgery texts referenced herein.

■ Congenital Ptosis

In addition to a host of associated clinical issues including amblyopia, anisometropia, strabismus, and blepharophimosis, the cosmetic appearance of the child with ptosis is objectionable to parents and may affect social interaction with other children. Severe bilateral ptosis that produces the head-back and chin-up posture may interfere with the child's ability to walk and delay general motor development. Included in this discussion of congenital ptosis are those cases secondary to developmental dystrophy without any innervational abnormality.

After a comprehensive physical examination is performed to exclude other congenital anomalies, meticulous history taking and ophthalmic examination are imperative to arrive at the proper diagnosis and the best management plan. All phases of examination and management must be carefully balanced with the needs of the child and parents, including the child's general development.

Evaluation

One initiates the evaluation of a child with congenital ptosis with a careful history. Although generally rare, a family history of congenital ptosis may be elicited. Blepharophimosis syndrome (including telecanthus, epicanthus inversus, and often lateral ectropion of the lower eyelids) constitutes 3 to 6% of cases of bilateral congenital ptosis and is transmitted as a dominant hereditary trait. Because of the intimate embryologic association of the levator and superior rectus muscles, some cases of congenital ptosis may be seen with ipsilateral weakness of the superior rectus muscle.[1,2]

The parents' observations are always important in determining the child's level of impairment and variability. The ophthalmologist must conduct thorough discussions with parents to rule out the possibility of birth trauma, myasthenia gravis, or synkinetic causes.

Physical Examination

After a complete general physical examination is performed by a pediatrician, the ophthalmologist should first perform a general inspection including head and chin position, brow, and frontalis muscle elevation. The examiner should take care to note the chin-up head position, furrows on the forehead, and markedly arched eyebrows. These features underscore the functional impairment the ptosis has upon the child. Variation of the degree of ptosis with jaw or extraocular muscle movement suggests synkinetic ptosis. From 4 to 6% of all congenital ptosis cases are associated with the jaw-winking phenomenon of Marcus-Gunn. This syndrome is characterized by ptosis that is either reduced or overcompensated with chewing movements. Infants sucking on a bottle or pacifier will often elicit these synkinetic movements. Old photographs may also assist the ophthalmologist in assessing the history and possible variability.

Visual acuity and cycloplegic refraction must be performed to evaluate for the presence of amblyopia either secondary to lid occlusion or anisometropia from unilaterally oblique astigmatism. A careful neuroophthalmic exam will identify superior rectus or congenital oculomotor palsy or Horner's syndrome.

A meticulous data sheet must be devised for each patient with congenital ptosis. While the patient fixates at a distant target, the following signs should be noted. Palpebral fissure height, marginal reflex distance, upper lid crease position, levator function, and tarsal width should be measured; the presence of Bell's phenomenon, jaw winking, or Cogan's lid twitch sign (as seen in myasthenia gravis) should be noted. In the appropriate setting, pharmacologic testing (including phenylephrine hydrochloride 2.5%, cocaine, and hydroxyamphetamine) should be performed.

The degree of levator function should be carefully measured. The frontalis muscle's contribution to eyelid elevation is eliminated by exerting mild pressure with the examiner's open hand upon the forehead and brow. A millimeter ruler is held in front of the patient's eye, and the patient is then instructed to look downward. In this position, the millimeter ruler is lined up with the lid margin, and then the patient is instructed to look in extreme upgaze. The amount of excursion between these two positions is noted as the levator function.

At times a pharmacologic agent is instilled in the fornices and the levator function is remeasured. This determines if the sympathetic lid receptors correlating with Muller's muscle are functioning.

Drawings, photographs, and basic tear production tests are also of paramount importance before arriving at a diagnosis and developing a treatment plan.

Treatment

Once diagnosis of congenital ptosis is made, a management plan must be devised based primarily on the magnitude of the ptosis and visual disability and secondarily on cosmetic consequences (Table 24–1).

Indications

Mild Unilateral or Bilateral Ptosis

Mild ptosis that does not encroach upon the visual axis is a cosmetic issue and can be approached surgically after a child reaches 4 to 5 years of age, when measurement can be more readily obtained and social interaction at school becomes an issue. The parents, in conjunction with the physician, determine the optimal time.

This type of ptosis is associated with good levator function (10 to 11 mm or more) and is easily treatable with a Fasanella-Servat tarsectomy or relieved by a small (10 to 13 mm) levator resection performed either via the skin or conjunctival route.[1]

TABLE 24–1. Ptosis Procedures

	Fasanella-Servat	Levator Resection	Brow Suspension
Ease of performance	Relatively easy	Difficult	Moderately difficult
Surgical option			
Treatment for mild ptosis	+	+; limited role	−
Treatment for moderate ptosis	−	+; procedure of choice	−
Treatment for severe ptosis	−	+; limited role	+
Complications	Limited	Potential	Potential

+ = can be utilized; − = cannot be utilized

Moderate Ptosis

Moderate ptosis is both functionally and cosmetically important because it often causes the child to adopt a head-back, chin-up position to compensate. If the child has fair levator function (5 to 7 mm), a large levator resection of 18 to 22 mm should be considered. If the levator function is good (8 mm or more), a moderate amount of levator resection (14 to 17 mm) is performed.[1]

Severe Ptosis

This type of ptosis is most functionally disabling and usually requires intervention between 1 and $1\frac{1}{2}$ years of age. This form is usually associated with poor levator function (4 mm or less). It is probably best to first attempt a maximal levator resection (23 to 24 mm or more) by the skin approach. If this procedure fails, the most definitive procedure is a fascia lata brow suspension.[1]

Surgical Options
Fasanella-Servat Tarsectomy

This rather simple operation has been modified by many and is an invaluable procedure in the management of mild ptosis associated with good levator function (10 to 11 mm or more). Although some of the levator aponeurosis is included, this procedure is largely a tarsectomy with shortening of Muller's muscle.

The details of this operation can be briefly described (Fig. 24–1). The upper lid involved is everted over a Desmarres retractor, and the upper 3 mm of tarsus and palpebral conjunctiva are clamped within two small curved hemostats. A double-armed 6-0 plain catgut suture is run in a mattress fashion at right angles, first entering the skin side temporally and then through the conjunctiva, passing beneath the clamp and toward the nasal limits. With the lid fixated, the hemostats are removed, and Wescott scissors excise the tissue within the crush marks.

In a meticulous subconjunctival fashion, the nasal end of the suture is then passed in a running manner, uniting the palpebral conjunctiva to the upper tarsal edge, carrying the final pass through the full thickness of the lid and out through the skin adjacent to the initial entrance site temporally. The ends are tied, antibiotic

ointment is instilled, and a simple patch dressing is applied for 48 hours' duration.[1, 8]

Levator Resection (Skin Approach)

This is the procedure of choice for moderate to severe ptosis. The details of this operation can be briefly described (Fig. 24–2). The upper lid is incised with a #11 Bard Parker blade along a previously noted lid fold that matches the height of the fold in the opposite upper eyelid. One then undermines beneath the preseptal orbicularis for a distance of approximately 7 mm. At the two extreme ends of the skin incision the blade penetrates the full thickness of the upper lid and emerges through the palpebral conjunctiva.

A ptosis clamp is inserted between these two incisions in a position just above the tarsus. The tissues within the clamp are then divided from their tarsal attachment with a sharp Wescott scissor.

The conjunctiva is separated from the other tissues within the clamp by injecting normal saline into the subconjunctival space and then incising the conjunctiva at the clamp, draping it downward toward its original position. A running 6-0 plain catgut suture is used to reapproximate it to the exposed tarsal edge.

The orbital septum is identified and is separated off the levator aponeurosis. The medial and lateral horns of the levator are severed in line with the levator's orientation.

Three double-armed 5-0 chromic catgut sutures are placed equidistant in the anterior tarsal face 3 to 4 mm beneath the superior tarsal border. These three same sutures are passed through the levator muscle at the predetermined height and then tied. The excess levator is excised. Any redundant eyelid skin can be excised above the lid fold incision. To re-create the lid fold, the three tied sutures are then passed through the upper and lower skin borders. Several additional interrupted skin sutures are placed to complete the closure. A Frost suture is inserted and taped to the brow for several days to enhance the levator resection.[1]

Brow Suspension

Severe unilateral congenital ptosis associated even with poor (4 mm or less) levator function can best be addressed with a "super maximum"

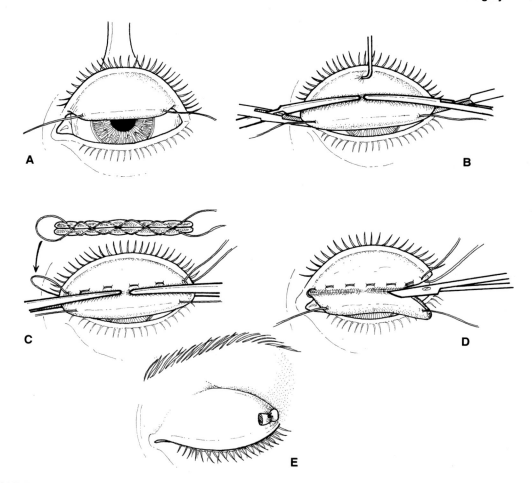

FIGURE 24–1. Fasanella-Servat tarsectomy. **(A)** The upper lid is everted with the assistance of a Desmarres retractor. Two small, curved hemostats are placed 2 to 3 mm beneath the superior tarsal border. A 6-0 plain catgut suture is placed in a 90 degree angled mattress fashion running the initial suture temporally through the skin and toward the nasal aspect of the eyelid beneath the hemostats. **(B)** The running mattress suture is shown from the palpebral conjunctival side. **(C)** The assistant secures the eyelid in the everted position, and the first hemostat is removed. Wescott scissors are utilized to excise the crushed area of tarsoconjunctiva, tarsus, Muller's muscle, levator aponeurosis, and palpebral conjunctiva. The second hemostat is then removed, and a similar excision is performed. **(D,E)** In a meticulous subconjunctival fashion, the nasal end of the suture is then passed in a running manner, uniting the palpebral conjunctiva to the upper tarsal edge, carrying the final pass through the full-thickness of the lid and out through the skin adjacent to the initial entrance site temporally.

levator resection by the aforementioned skin approach. However, should this fail, unilateral brow suspension should be considered.

The details of this operation can be briefly described (Fig. 24–3). Using a #11 Bard Parker blade, two stab incisions are made into the upper lid to the depth of tarsus 2 mm above the lash line. Two similar stab incisions are made just above the eyebrow to the depth of the periosteum overlying the frontal bone slightly medial and lateral to a vertical line from the

medial and lateral lid incision. A third incision is made midway between the brow incisions, 1 cm superior to them.

With a Wright fascia needle, a single long strip of fascia lata (either banked or harvested autogenous) is carried through all of the aforementioned incisions with the ends emerging from the top of the pentagon. (Some surgeons have used supramid. At times this becomes resorbed, thus collapsing the lid elevation. In addition, the patient can have severe inflammatory reactions

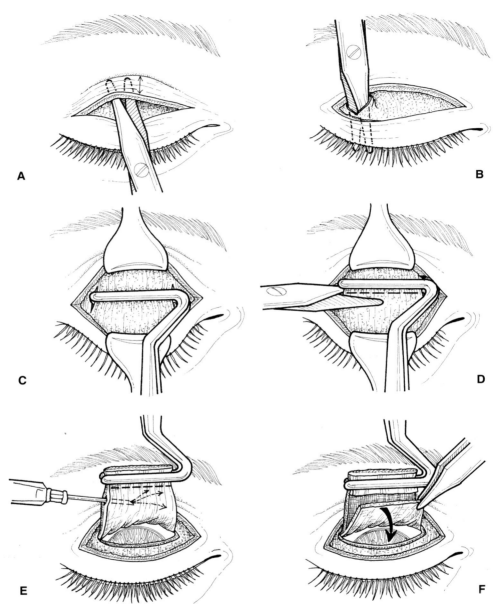

FIGURE 24–2. Levator resection (skin approach). **(A)** The upper lid is incised with a #11 Bard Parker blade along a previously noted lid fold that matches the height of the fold in the opposite upper eyelid. One then undermines beneath the preseptal orbicularis for a distance of approximately 7 mm. **(B)** At the two extreme ends of the skin incision the blade penetrates through the full thickness of the upper lid and emerges through the palpebral conjunctiva. **(C)** A ptosis clamp is inserted between these two incisions in a position just above the tarsus. **(D)** The tissues within the clamp are then divided from their tarsal attachment with a sharp Wescott scissor. **(E,F)** The conjunctiva is separated from the other tissues within the clamp by injecting normal saline into the subconjunctival space and then incising the conjunctiva at the clamp, draping it downward toward its original position.

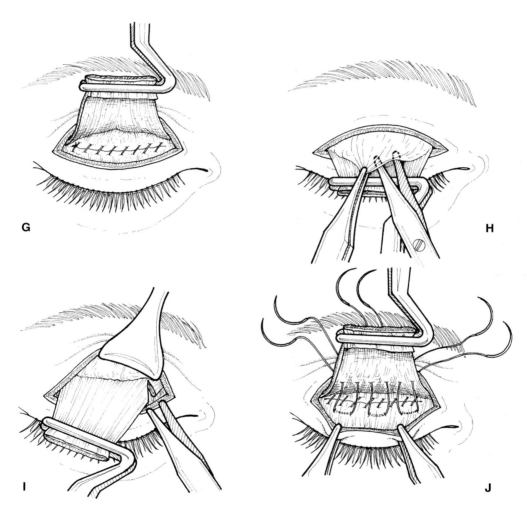

FIGURE 24–2. *(continued)* **(G)** A running 6-0 plain catgut suture is used to reapproximate it to the exposed tarsal edge. **(H)** The orbital septum is identified and is separated off the levator aponeurosis. **(I)** The medial and lateral horns of the levator are severed in line with the levator's orientation. **(J–K)** Three double-armed 5-0 chromic catgut sutures are placed equidistant into the anterior tarsal face 3 to 4 mm beneath the superior tarsal border. These three same sutures are passed through the levator muscle at the predetermined height and then tied. The excess levator is excised. *(Figure continued on page 330.)*

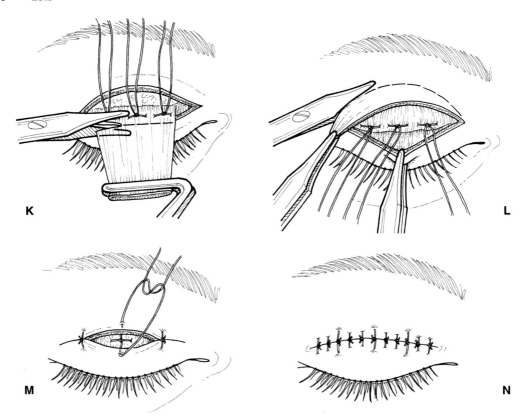

FIGURE 24–2. *(continued)* **(L)** Any redundant eyelid skin can be excised above the lid fold incision. **(M)** To re-create the lid fold, the three tied sutures are then passed through the upper and lower skin borders. **(N)** Several additional interrupted skin sutures are placed to complete the closure.

to the suture itself. Fascia lata is *the* preferred material.) Traction is placed on these two ends to adjust the lid margin contour to the height desired. A ligature of 5-0 chromic gut is tied firmly around the two fascia strips at the skin level and is fixed by passing the suture needle deep in the upper brow incision to the level of the frontalis muscle. The excess fascia is then excised. Only the brow skin incisions are closed with fine nylon or catgut sutures.

Here too Frost sutures are inserted and taped to the forehead for several days to enhance the eyelid elevation.[1]

■ Congenital Nasolacrimal Duct Obstruction

Congenital obstruction of the lacrimal drainage system is a relatively common condition that

may become clinically evident in 2 to 4% of all full-term newborn infants between 1 and 2 weeks of age. The diagnosis is based on a history of tearing, or wet eye, when the child is not crying, with or without mucopurulent discharge. This obstruction is usually secondary to a membranous blockage of the valve of Hasner at the distal portion of the nasolacrimal duct, although there may be multiple small obstructions. Most of the obstructions open spontaneously within 4 to 6 weeks after birth. The majority (80%) of nasolacrimal duct obstructions clear spontaneously by 10 to 12 months of age. However, occasionally obstruction persists, and intervention is required.[2,3]

Evaluation

The etiologies of epiphora in the pediatric population are numerous. It is imperative that

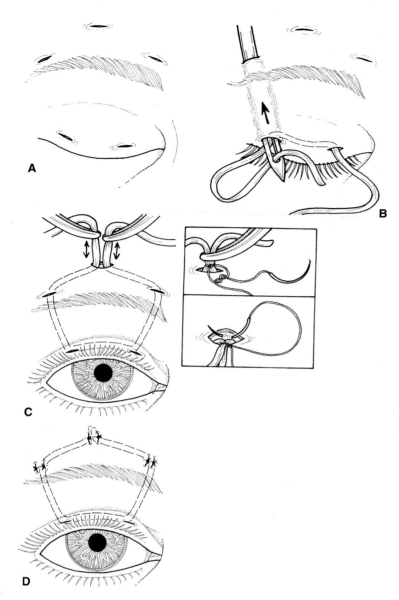

FIGURE 24–3. Brow suspension. **(A)** Using a #11 Bard Parker blade, two stab incisions are made into the upper lid to the depth of tarsus 2 mm above the lash line. Two similar stab incisions are made just above the eyebrow to the depth of the periosteum overlying the frontal bone slightly medial and lateral to a vertical line from the medial and lateral lid incision. A third incision is made midway between the brow incisions, 1 cm superior to them. **(B)** With a Wright fascia needle, a single long strip of fascia lata (either banked or harvested autogenous) is carried through all of the aforementioned incisions with the ends emerging from the top of the pentagon. **(C)** Traction is placed on these two ends to adjust the lid margin contour to the height desired. A ligature of 5-0 chromic gut is tied firmly around the two fascia strips at the skin level and is fixed by passing the suture needle deep in the upper brow incision to the level of the frontalis muscle. The excess fascia is then excised. **(D)** Only the brow skin incisions are closed with fine nylon or catgut sutures.

meticulous examination be undertaken to exclude the other causes, including punctal occlusion or agenesis, foreign body, conjunctivitis, distichiasis, trichiasis, epiblepharon, entropion, ectropion, keratitis, iritis, glaucoma, and seventh nerve palsy.[4]

Parents and grandparents are usually good sources for eliciting a history of tearing and/or mucopurulent discharge and matting beginning at birth or shortly thereafter. Direct inspection in the office setting often reveals frank epiphora, discharge, or increase in the lacrimal lake. Any other nasal or facial abnormalities should be noted, including cleft lip, nasal malformation, facial asymmetry, etc.

Physical Examination

The punctae should be assessed, and the size and patency of the openings should be determined. Accessory punctae should be noted, as should the presence and location of fistulas.

Lacrimal excretory evaluation should include a fluorescein dye disappearance test, which, after instilling a drop into the conjunctival sac, can give indirect evidence about nasolacrimal patency. In addition, 5 minutes postinjection, one can perform a Jones 1 test by inspecting the nares using a light source with cobalt blue filter.

Though nasolacrimal irrigation would provide definitive assessment of patency, this procedure is impractical with infants in the office. The single most important maneuver is digital pressure over the nasolacrimal sac. If mucopurulent reflux is present, obstruction at the distal conduit of the duct is the working diagnosis.

Treatment

The initial treatment of congenital nasolacrimal obstruction is a conservative one and should include properly performed Crigler massage over the sac several times daily to encourage increased hydrostatic pressure within the duct, topical antibiotics during periods of mucopurulent discharge, and occasional nasal decongestants. Periodic cultures should be performed to rule out recalcitrant organisms. Most (80%) obstructions clear spontaneously by 10 to 12 months of age.[5]

If there is no evidence of acute dacryocystitis and the symptoms are not extreme, the ophthalmologist can wait until the child is 12 to 13 months of age before performing nasolacrimal probing and irrigation under general anesthesia. Probing also should be used as the primary procedure in older children with congenital nasolacrimal duct obstruction who have not received previous treatment. The failure rate in older children (over $1\frac{3}{4}$ years of age) is much higher, thus often requiring a second procedure (Fig. 24–4).[3,5,6]

Occasionally, during the 13-month period of observation and massage, acute dacryocystitis (infection of the nasolacrimal sac) may occur with adjacent cellulitis. Treatment in such an instance requires systemic antibiotics and, if an abscess develops, surgical drainage may be required. Under such circumstances, following complete resolution of the infectious process, an earlier probing and irrigation is performed to prevent recurrence of dacryocystitis. Prior to 6 months of age if necessary, one could consider an in-office probing without irrigation.[4]

Surgery

If the first probing fails and the child continues to be symptomatic, one should wait a minimum of 3 months before considering an additional probing. Although some surgeons may argue to simply repeat the probing, I think it prudent on the second attempt to include medial infracturing of the inferior turbinate with a Freer periosteal elevator and silicone intubation left in place for 3 months' duration.[7]

If one cannot successfully probe initially or if on the second procedure one cannot pass the tubes, the surgeon should be prepared to perform a dacryocystorhinostomy (DCR). DCR is the surgical procedure reserved for management of nasolacrimal sac-duct obstruction that cannot be successfully treated permanently by probings without and then with silastic tubes. The surgical goal is to create a new epithelial lined conduit to carry tears from the nasolacrimal sac into the nose through an area adjacent to the medial turbinate.

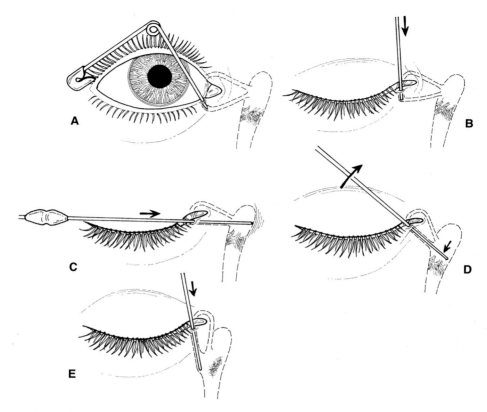

FIGURE 24–4. Technique for probing the nasolacrimal system. **(A)** After adequate anesthesia, the inferior and superior puncta are dilated with a sterile, blunted safety pin or other fine punctum dilator. **(B)** A Bowman probe No. 0 or 00 is bent to a slight "J" configuration. The tip is lubricated with ointment and is then inserted vertically into the dilated punctum. **(C)** After passing 1.5 to 2 mm vertically, the probe is directed medially 12 to 14 mm until bone is encountered. **(D)** The Bowman probe is then raised vertically while the tip remains in contact with the medial wall of the sac. **(E)** When the entrance to the lacrimal duct is encountered, the probe is directed straight downward for as much as 15 degrees posteriorly for 12 to 15 mm. At this point some obstruction may be encountered. The probing is complete when it encounters the floor of the nasal cavity. Patency is then confirmed by irrigation of fluorescein-stained balanced salt solution, which can be identified with suction in the posterior pharynx.

REFERENCES

1. Beard C. *Ptosis.* St. Louis, MO: Mosby; 1976:42–111.
2. Helveston EM, Ellis FD. *Pediatric Ophthalmology Practice.* St. Louis, MO: Mosby; 1984:129–153, 179–213.
3. Kushner BJ. Congenital nasolacrimal system obstruction. *Arch Ophthalmol.* 1982;100:597–600.
4. Hurwitz JJ. *The Lacrimal System.* Philadelphia: Lippincott-Raven; 1996: 61–62, 237–241.
5. Jones LT, Wobig JL. *Surgery of the Eyelids and Lacrimal System.* Birmingham, AL: Aesculapius; 1976:163–169.
6. Dortzbach RK, France TD, Jushner BJ, et al. Silicone intubation for obstruction of the nasolacrimal duct in children. *Am J Ophthalmol.* 1982; 94:585–590.
7. Robb RM. Probing and irrigation for congenital nasolacrimal duct obstruction. *Arch Ophthalmol.* 1986; 104:378–379.
8. Ramsey RB and Leib ML. Clothesline operation for ptosis. In: Wesley RE ed, *Techniques in Ophthalmic Plastic Surgery.* New York: Wiley Medical Publication; 1986:311–314.

Pediatric Ophthalmology
Edited by P. F. Gallin
Thieme Medical Publishers, Inc.
New York © 2000

25
■■■

Use of Ophthalmic Laser in Children

MARC G. ODRICH*, STEPHEN L. TROKEL*, STEPHEN A. ODRICH, AND WILLIAM M. SCHIFF

Corneal Laser Surgery

Excimer lasers used for corneal surgery are a relatively newly developed class of lasers with output in the ultraviolet range. The term *excimer* is derived from a contraction of "excited dimer." An excited dimer is a reference to the electrically excited complex of a noble gas such as argon and a halide such as fluorine that occurs in the laser cavity. The wavelength of light is determined by the constituents of the dimer. The clinically most used excimer utilizes argon and fluorine to make up this dimer and produces 193-nm light. When the high-energy photons emitted strike the exposed corneal tissue, a unique interaction occurs, termed ablative photodecomposition. When this process occurs, molecular fragments are ejected from the surface at over 3000 m/s. There is little heat generated in this reaction and consequently almost none of the tissue distortion that is more typical of other laser tissue interactions.

Laser Equipment

In the United States, three laser manufacturers have approval to market and sell their devices.

*Both Marc G. Odrich and Stephen L. Trokel are paid consultants to VISX and have a financial interest in that company.

TABLE 25–1. Lasers Approved for Use in the United States

Specification	Summit	VISX	ATCI*
Wavelength (nm)	193	193	193
Repetition rate	10	5–6	100
Energy (mJ/cm^2)	180	160	180

* Autonomous Technologies Corporation.

Table 25–1 lists the differences among the three approved lasers. Note that two of these lasers are wide-area ablaters and one is a spot scanner. The VISX system is illustrated in Figure 25–1. There are other types of lasers and delivery systems such as scanning slit and flying spot lasers. These other lasers are in various phases of the FDA approval process.

All calibration and centering procedures for each individual laser must be followed precisely to be sure that a beam of known energy and sufficiently high quality is delivered to the cornea. Typically, this calibration process requires ablating a material, such as a piece of plastic, and measuring the quantity of material ablated and the quality of the remaining cut. Each manufacturer has proprietary methods for calibration. Excimer lasers are more demanding in terms of maintenance than other lasers that ophthalmologists typically use (Fig. 25–2). As a result the technician who runs the machine has a very important role in its operation and calibration and is an integral member of the surgical team.

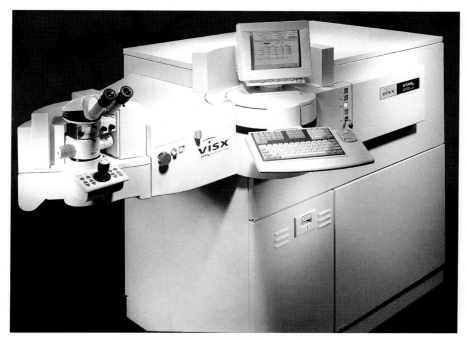

FIGURE 25–1. VISX STAR excimer laser system.

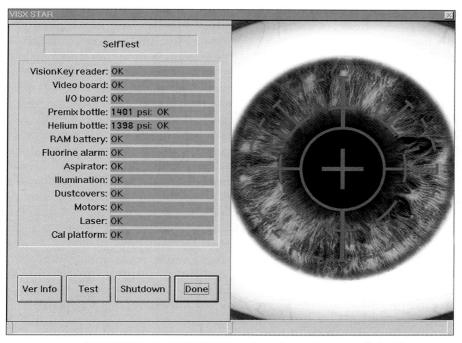

FIGURE 25–2. VISX STAR excimer laser system self-check.

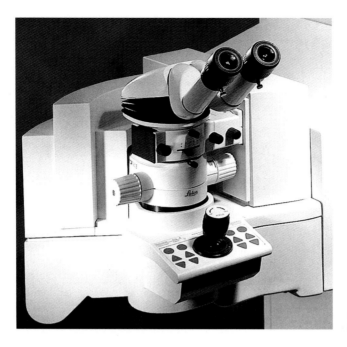

FIGURE 25–3. Surgeon controls of the VISX STAR excimer laser system.

It is, however, the surgeon's responsibility to ensure that all calibration and operating parameters are correct for the individual patient. Operating information including the desired treatment is entered into a computer, which contains the laser's execution. Regardless of who enters the data into the computer (surgeon or technician), the operating surgeon is entirely and solely responsible for the patient's treatment. This includes the verification of the data entered into the system for a particular treatment. The surgical parameters should be confirmed by the operating surgeon both visually and verbally prior to the initiation of any treatment (Fig. 25–3).

Specific Uses

These 193-nm excimer lasers are approved for the correction of scars and corneal irregularities (phototherapeutic keratectomy, PTK), the correction of mild to moderate myopia (photorefractive keratectomy [PRK]), the correction of mild to moderate myopia with concomitant astigmatism of between 0.75 and 4.0 diopters (PRKa), and the correction of high degrees of myopia (VISX only) and hyperopia (VISX only). However, none of these refractive modalities is approved for use in children in the United States. The minimum age for PRK to 6 diopters of myopia is 18 years, and for higher myopia and astigmatism (PRKa) it is 21 years. There is a recommended minimum age of 18 years for PTK, although there were patients treated in the clinical trials of these lasers who were less than 18 years and had obtained appropriate consent. There is, however, a growing body of international experience with these lasers in the pediatric population. This experience is entirely anecdotal with no prospective trials currently under way, although there is a university-based study soon to be started[1,2] (E. Bluestein, M.D., personal communication). A second difficulty in describing the experience of children treated with the excimer laser is that it requires an extremely cooperative patient. The use of flammable anesthetics in and around this laser is specifically contraindicated. There are rare cases, however, where mask anesthesia or ketamine was used to temporarily immobilize the child outside of the laser suite, and then the essentially unconscious child is treated while in this "twilight" state.

There is very little published or reported about the use of the excimer laser to correct refractive errors in the pediatric population. Many surgeons are concerned about the developmental significance of Bowman's layer, and its removal could precipitate a corneal ectasia. Laser in situ keratomileusis (LASIK) could also cause a similar ectasia through removal of stromal tissue and the near complete severing of Bowman's layer, not to mention the added difficulty of placing the required instrumentation into a small, pediatric fissure. The peer-reviewed literature describes only two indications for PRK.

1. Anisometropia, which threatens to be amblyopiagenic, both hypermetropic and myopic.
2. Progressive and extreme myopia and refractive changes after pediatric cataract surgery.

Although not the only indications, these indications appear in the peer-reviewed literature. Administration of ketamine anesthesia is described in one of these reports for patients who are unable to cooperate with the treatment.

Results obtained thus far are very encouraging, with all patients reporting a reduction in refractive error. There is an improvement in best-corrected visual acuity in almost all patients. Significant haze is also reported, particularly in patients who are noncompliant with steroid regimens. The use of topical steroid medications in the pediatric population to prevent the formation of haze and subsequent visual acuity loss may be important. However, one should remember that this is only anecdotal information with very limited follow-up; that better study is warranted.

There were also pediatric patients treated in the United States under the PTK guidelines. These are patients who had posttraumatic scarring and leukoma, band keratopathy, or penetrating corneal trauma with a stepped wound.

Patients with Posttraumatic Scarring and Leukoma

Corneal trauma resulting in leukoma formation, which may be amblyopiagenic, can be effectively treated with the excimer laser. The principle behind any scar-reducing procedure is to remove as little tissue as possible to allow good vision. It is also important to avoid areas of corneal depression as the excimer laser removes and does not replace any tissue. The cornea does not need to be crystal clear to allow for the development of good visual acuity. It is important to reduce dense, confluent opacity to nonconfluence. This will allow visual improvement while minimizing unwanted induced hyperopic or other refractive change (induced myopia or astigmatism). An important relationship exists between the diameter and depth of tissue ablated and the anticipated refractive change, even in a theoretically nonrefractive keratectomy such as PTK. Generally, the larger the diameter of tissue to be removed, the more tissue needs to be removed to effect a 1-diopter hyperopic shift. In normal (nonscarred) corneas, this translates to 12 μm of tissue at a 6.0-mm diameter causing a 1-diopter shift, whereas at a 3.0-mm diameter this is only 3 μm per diopter. This relationship is for a refractive cut (PRK) and does not apply to the PTK-type cuts, although a similar yet nonlinear relationship appears to exist. Careful planning of tissue removal and avoiding hyperopic shifts from excessive tissue removal will allow the best clinical results.

One must be vigilant to ensure that leukoma formation in a pediatric patient is not caused by herpetic keratitis. A careful history and record review (where available) may alert the clinician to possible herpetic keratitis as a cause of leukoma formation. This is important because oral acyclovir prophylaxis has been shown to be effective controlling herpetic reactivations due to ultraviolet light in the adult population (the excimer lasers are intense sources of ultraviolet radiation). Additionally, topical antivirals are used over a 10- to 14-day taper period while the fresh epithelium closes the newly formed defect. One should not use the excimer laser to clear acute, active infections or inflammation (e.g., Thygeson's and epidemic keratoconjunctivitis that are active). The laser expels tissue and does not necessarily destroy viral DNA; in fact, it may actually aerosolize these particles. It also causes a significant amount of inflammation in the healing of the keratectomy.

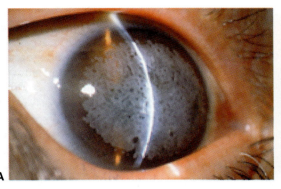 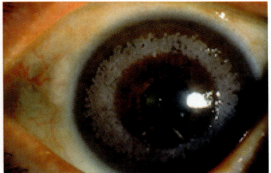

FIGURE 25–4. Calcific band keratopathy. **(A)** Preoperative. **(B)** Postoperative.

Band Keratopathy

If appropriately selected, patients with calcific band formation can be treated with the excimer laser (Fig. 25–4). Large, calcific changes are best handled with a chelation treatment or other manual debulking. However, feathery epithelial and subepithelial band formation can be removed quite easily with a very shallow transepithelial ablation. The principle of "less is better" also applies here. Patients must be carefully monitored at the slit lamp, if possible, during treatment. The cornea is not made completely clear, but rather the opacity is made nonconfluent so that the child will have better vision without unnecessary refractive shifts. It is important to recognize that the surgeon is, most likely, not curing the disease process but rather staving off amblyopia or making the child more comfortable to allow better vision. This process can be repeated several times on an eye as long as there is little or no stromal thinning.

Penetrating Corneal Trauma with a Stepped Wound

Following primary repair of laceration of the cornea (with or without tissue avulsion) in children, there can be an unevenness to the wound that does not occur in slower-healing, but comparable adult trauma. Once all the sutures are removed and the wound is deemed sufficiently stable (via refraction, keratometry, and/or videokeratography), one can ameliorate the corneal irregularity in one of any of a number of ways. The following are just two examples of these techniques:

1. A small spot size (1.5 to 2.0 mm) can be used in the PTK circle mode to smooth the scar and even the elevated spots, and a surface-modulating agent such as Tears Naturale II™ (0.3% methylcellulose) can be used to prevent ablation of depressed areas.

2. A slit sized to encompass the scar can be used to smooth and induce cylinder where appropriate (this variable slit mode is available on the VISX instrument as the PTK slit mode).

Both techniques are advanced and require a thorough understanding of optics and corneal responses and wound healing in pediatric patients. These techniques should only be undertaken by one well versed in the use of the excimer laser because the potential exists to worsen the problem through the induction of cylinder. A postoperative course of steroid and antibiotic is recommended to decrease chances of infection and corneal haze.

■ Glaucoma

Pediatric glaucoma broadly encompasses two types of disease: congenital glaucoma, which manifests and, it is hoped, is diagnosed within the first months of life, and infantile glaucoma, which becomes evident somewhat later in life, usually between ages 6 months and 1 year. Together these may be called developmental glaucomas. These glaucomas may be part of widespread syndromes, metabolic derangements, or localized abnormalities such as the phakomatoses (Sturge-Weber syndrome and neurofibromatosis). It is important to recognize the presence of a systemic condition both to institute possible treatment (e.g., dietary restriction in homocystinuria) and to understand the pathophysiology of the intraocular pressure abnormality (e.g., raised episcleral venous pressure in Sturge-Weber syndrome). Recognizing that there are various possible pathophysiological causes of intraocular pressure elevation in the pediatric population, one should also be aware that the vast majority of developmental glaucomas are open-angle glaucomas with some form of decreased outflow due to microscopic angle abnormality. The "congenital angle," that is, the angle of patient with a developmental glaucoma, is variously described as being covered by a transparent membrane (Barkan's membrane), having a high iris insertion, and having prominent iris processes, to name three of the more common descriptions. However it is described, the open angle and, more specifically, the trabecular meshwork (TM) are widely felt to be primary sites of disease in developmental glaucoma.

This knowledge allows us to understand why a particular laser application may or may not be appropriate. For example, laser iridotomies are rarely, if ever, performed primarily in developmental glaucoma because it is almost always an open angle form of glaucoma. Although it is true that some children develop iris bombe following intraocular surgery, even then laser iridotomy is rarely performed due to the inability of most infants and children to sit cooperatively at a laser with a goniolens coupled to their cornea. At most facilities, it is far easier to perform a surgical iridotomy in the operating room setting where general or mask anesthesia is administered than a laser iridotomy. Thus, laser iridotomy is not a procedure that is performed regularly in treating developmental glaucoma.

Laser trabeculoplasty (LTP), a mainstay in the treatment of adult open-angle glaucoma, is another procedure that is rarely used in the pediatric population. Knowing that developmental glaucoma is caused by an abnormal and sometimes poorly visible TM allows us to understand why LTP is not used in this setting. It is certainly impossible to treat the TM when there is a broad sheet of iris swept over the very structure targeted for LTP. The damage done to the iris and the secondary inflammation that is induced, which is usually quite exuberant in infants and children, make this procedure inappropriate in this group. Furthermore, in settings where the cornea is clear and the iris is not anteriorly inserted, it is questionable whether laser applications to the abnormal TM would have a beneficial effect. It is more likely that a paradoxical rise in intraocular pressure would result. The logistics of actually delivering a focused laser on the microscopic structure of a pediatric patient's TM in the operating room setting (very different from the slit-lamp delivery systems normally used in adults) are also problematic.

The primary treatment in developmental glaucoma is surgery, which actually does not involve the use of a laser. Trabeculotomy and goniotomy are procedures aimed at cleaving the TM and the putative blocking "membrane" that may cover it. When performed early in the course of developmental glaucoma, this surgical treatment can be curative. Trabeculectomy also may be performed when initial trabeculotomy and goniotomy are unsuccessful.

Laser Endocyclophotocoagulation

In cases in which several attempts at surgical correction failed, there is a laser procedure that meets with some success in the pediatric population. This procedure is called endoscopic cyclophotocoagulation (ECP). Described by Uram in 1992,[3,4] this procedure has several advantages over transscleral cyclophotocoagulation, a procedure that is inappropriate in all but the most dire of developmental glaucoma cases. ECP allows the surgeon to see target tissue directly and avoid the "shotgun" approach characteristic of transscleral procedures, which are shown to be only variably successful in achieving ablation of targeted ciliary processes. Collateral tissue damage can be particularly damaging in the pediatric population, given children's tendency to respond with large amounts of inflammation. Additionally, the surgeon has the ability, endoscopically, to obtain an excellent magnified view of the optic nerve and retina, which may be otherwise unviewable due to media opacity commonly associated with developmental as well as secondary pediatric glaucomas.

For ECP, a 20-gauge (0.88 mm) opening is created in the sclera over the pars plana after the overlying conjunctiva is dissected. The laser endoscopic probe is introduced, and the posterior chamber is examined. If examination reveals features that warrant lowering of the intraocular pressure, the probe is directed toward the pars plicata of the ciliary body 180 degrees away. Usually, 90 to 180 degrees of the ciliary processes is treated. The energy is varied to achieve the end points of shrinkage and whitening of each treated process (200 to 300 mW). Two areas of treatment per ciliary process are usually necessary. The laser energy transmitted through the probe is generated by a diode laser.

Successful intraocular pressure management with one such treatment is the rule. A low incidence of hypotony and phthisis is reported. It should be noted, however, that, although this is a destructive procedure, it is appropriate as a first-line treatment. It is unclear why early (immediately postoperatively) and late (up to 1 year postoperatively) visual loss occurs in a very low but definite number of patients. There are also reports of sympathetic ophthalmia following contact and noncontact cyclodestructive procedures. Initial studies describe incidences of up to 5% for sympathetic ophthalmia,[5,6] but these are not reproduced. Nonetheless, the possibility (probably very low likelihood) of these potentially devastating complications should be weighed in the overall clinical decision process.

The patients most likely to benefit from ECP are those with cloudy cornea and intraocular pressure evaluation. These children pose the difficult problem of allowing little or no viewing of the optic nerve and retina in the setting of intraocular pressure elevation. There may be primary corneal opacity (Peter's anomaly, endothelial dystrophy, sclerocornea, corneal scars, etc.) or secondary corneal edema. Clinical decision making becomes difficult without knowledge of the status of the optic nerve in these patients. ECP represents a solution, both diagnostic and therapeutic, to this difficult situation.

■ Retinal Laser Photocoagulation

Laser delivery to the retina can be an important prophylactic and therapeutic modality. Similar to laser treatment for glaucomatous processes, it is important to identify the etiology of the retinal aberration and then to decide upon appropriate treatment, always bearing in mind the age of the patient and the ability of that patient to cooperate with the treatment course. A variety of chorioretinal diseases affecting the pediatric population is shown to benefit from laser treatment. An understanding of the various delivery systems, indications for therapy, and treatment techniques specific to retinal laser photocoagulation will enable the clinician to comfortably manage a host of disorders effectively.

Laser Surgery Principles and Techniques

Thermal Interaction

When incident laser light is absorbed by intraocular tissues, heat is generated, and the temperature of the specific tissue is elevated. With sufficient tissue temperature elevation, proteins and other large molecules are denatured causing thermal damage, and a photocoagulation lesion is produced. This process is the basis for conventional retinal laser photocoagulation.

Parameters

Several treatment parameters are available to the surgeon, and an understanding of these is essential for safe and optimal treatment.

1. Exposure time—A short and intense exposure of laser light to ocular tissue produces high temperatures in the center of the lesion. The risk of tissue rupture and hemorrhage is therefore increased. A longer and less-intense exposure of light creates a less defined lesion.
2. Power—The choice of laser power determines the intensity of the laser spot and the extent of thermal damage.
3. Spot size—When one wishes to increase the spot size, a proportional increase in laser power must be made to manufacture a laser spot of similar intensity. If large areas of the retina require photocoagulation, a large spot is required (i.e., panretinal photocoagulation for proliferative diabetic retinopathy). Conversely, when precise and accurate application of light is required and tissue destruction is to be

avoided, a smaller spot may be utilized (i.e., focal laser photocoagulation for clinically significant diabetic macular edema).

4. Wavelength—When choosing which color wavelength to use, the clinician must consider two principles, scatter and absorption. The components of the eye that can scatter light are basically the cornea, the lens, and a turbid vitreous. A longer wavelength will minimize the effects of scattering in posterior segment laser photocoagulation and will optimize tissue reaction, making the desired spot more predictable. Absorption of light occurs when incident light interacts with pigmented tissue. Ocular pigments include macular xanthophyll, melanin (found in the retinal pigment epithelium, choroid), and hemoglobin (red blood cells). Blue light should be avoided when lasering in the macula due to its absorption by xanthophyll. Red light, due to the relatively longer wavelength, is scattered less and is optimal for hazy media (i.e., cataract). Yellow light is absorbed by blood, is scattered only minimally, and is ideal for blood-containing lesions.

5. Lens type—Contact lenses are currently used with standard, slit lamp delivery systems. Flat macular lenses are generally used for laser photocoagulation in the macula. For peripheral laser photocoagulation, a mirrored contact lens (Goldmann lens) or an inverted image lens system (Rodenstock, Mainster, Quadraspheric) can be used. It is important to note that the inverted image lens system inverts the image the observer sees and magnifies the chosen spot on the retina.

Delivery Systems

A discussion of the various delivery systems (parafocal and defocusing) is beyond the scope of this chapter. Laser delivery via indirect ophthalmoscopy (argon or diode laser capability) is essential for laser photocoagulation in the neonate or young child. The adolescent and young adult are usually sufficiently cooperative, and laser photocoagulation delivered at the slit lamp is possible. Laser endophotocoagulation (argon and diode laser capability) can be per-

formed at the time of pars plana vitrectomy if necessary. In addition, the location of a particular lesion requiring laser photocoagulation may influence the mode of delivery. Retinal tears, dialysis, and angiomas in the anterior retina may require laser delivery via an indirect ophthalmoscope, whereas small lesions in the macula are safely treated with a slit lamp delivery system.

Anesthesia

The level of anesthesia and sedation required for standard posterior segment laser photocoagulation varies according to the age of the patient and the specific laser procedure being performed. In general, the level of cooperation determines the need for sedation or anesthesia. In the cooperative patient, topical or, infrequently, retrobulbar anesthesia is required. Focal laser photocoagulation for diabetic macular edema is painless, whereas a patient undergoing panretinal photocoagulation for proliferative diabetic retinopathy may experience considerable pain and can benefit from retrobulbar anesthesia. Neonates requiring indirect laser photocoagulation do not generally require intravenous sedation, although this may vary depending on specific institutional guidelines and patient medical status. Topical or retrobulbar anesthesia is often utilized.

Diseases Amenable to Laser Photocoagulation

Macular Edema

Important diseases in the pediatric population complicated by macular edema are diabetes, retinal vasculitis, retinal vein occlusion, pars planitis, and hypertension, to name a few. Laser photocoagulation may be of benefit when macular edema is caused by diabetes or vasoocclusive diseases.

Retinal Ischemia (Neovascularization)

Diabetes, hypertension, sickle cell disease, hyperviscosity syndromes, intraocular inflammation, and other ophthalmic diseases can be causative. Neovascularization is the retinal response to ischemia. Laser photocoagulation is shown to cause regression of retinal and anterior (iris and angle) neovascularization and is also used as a prophylaxis against its occurrence.

Choroidal Neovascularization

Macular choroidal neovascularization in the pediatric population can be secondary to trauma (Bruch's membrane rupture), pathologic myopia, presumed ocular histoplasmosis syndrome (POHS), inflammatory diseases [punctate inner choroidopathy (PIC), multifocal choroiditis with panuveitis], and choroidal osteoma, to name a few. When a well-defined choroidal neovascular membrane is juxta- or extrafoveal, laser photocoagulation may be of benefit.

Vascular Malformations

Retinal exudative vasculopathies (Coats' disease, retinal capillary hemangiomas) are characterized by the occurrence of multiple vascular anomalies that can lead to massive tissue exudation. Laser photocoagulation is of benefit in these disease entities.

Malignancy

In the proper clinical setting, retinoblastoma and malignant choroidal melanoma respond favorably to laser photocoagulation. Lesions must be small and in the appropriate anatomic location.

Rhegmatogenous

A hole or tear in the retina may lead to the development of a retinal detachment. Tears may be due to vitreoretinal traction, trauma, and retinal necrosis. Some patients are at higher risk for the development of retinal detachment; this includes patients with high myopia, hereditary vitreoretinal degeneration (Stickler syndrome, lattice degeneration), and a prior history of giant retinal tears. Cytomegaloviral retinitis is a specific infectious entity that causes necrosis of the retina and subsequent holes and tears. Prophylactic laser photocoagulation can often prevent or limit the extent of a retinal detachment when performed in the appropriate clinical setting.

Miscellaneous

Entities such as optic pit-related macular detachments may respond favorably to laser photocoagulation.

Management of Common Diseases

Diabetic Macular Edema

Laser therapy, as described in the Early Treatment Diabetic Retinopathy Study (ETDRS), tends to reduce the rate of visual loss in eyes with clinically significant diabetic macular edema (CSME).[7-9] However, relatively few eyes show significant improvement in vision. CSME is defined as the presence of one or more of the following criteria:

1. Thickening of the retina located less than 500 μm from the center of the macula.
2. Hard exudates, with thickening of the adjacent retina, located less than 500 μm from the center of the macula.
3. A zone of retinal thickening one disc area or larger in size, any portion of which is located less than one disc diameter from the center of the macula.

Based on the findings in the ETDRS, several recommendations are advocated. When macular edema is not clinically significant, observation is preferred. If CSME is present with foveal involvement, laser photocoagulation should be performed. Eyes with CSME should be considered for treatment even in the setting of good central vision.

Focal laser photocoagulation is generally performed when the macular edema is localized and well defined, arising predominantly from foci of microaneurysms. The microaneurysms are treated with a moderately intense, 75- to 100-μm spot, for 0.1 seconds several times. We prefer the yellow wavelength due to its predictability (discussed previously). A "grid"-type laser procedure is performed when the macular swelling is more diffuse. Adjacent regions of capillary nonperfusion were also treated in the ETDRS. Mild to moderate intensity laser spots (50- to 200-μm size) are placed in a grid pattern, one burn width apart, to the area of swelling. Smaller spots are placed closer to the center of the macula, and larger spots are placed in the periphery. We usually wait approximately 3 months to re-treat to allow the prior treatment to have its effect.

Side effects of treatment include small central isolated or grid-like scotomas. Choroidal neovascularization, retinochoroidal anastamosis, hemorrhage, and avascular submacular fibrosis are some of the complications reported with laser photocoagulation in the macula.

Proliferative Diabetic Retinopathy

Panretinal photocoagulation can significantly reduce the rate of severe visual loss as demonstrated by the Diabetic Retinopathy Study (DRS).[10–14] Severe visual loss is defined as visual acuity less than 5/200. Eyes with high-risk characteristics are at a greater risk for severe visual loss unless treated with laser. High-risk characteristics include

1. Disc neovascularization (NVD) less than one fourth to one third disc area, with vitreous hemorrhage
2. NVD greater than one fourth to one third disc area, with or without vitreous hemorrhage
3. Neovascularization elsewhere (NVE) equal or greater than one half disc area, with vitreous hemorrhage

It is unclear whether performing panretinal photoablation in eyes with severe nonproliferative diabetic retinopathy (NPDR) or PDR is preferable to careful observation with prompt treatment once high-risk characteristics develop.

Generally, prompt treatment should be performed in eyes with PDR with well-established NVD, vitreous or preretinal hemorrhage, or iris or angle neovascularization. Consideration for early treatment depends on the patient's ability to seek medical attention, the status of the fellow eye, and the retinopathy status in the eye being considered for treatment. The end point of treatment is the regression of neovascularization and the prevention of new vessel formation. The clinical response to treatment determines the amount of laser photocoagulation needed.

Panretinal photoablation is performed at the slit lamp when possible. Five hundred-micron burns of moderate intensity are generally placed between one half to one burn width apart beginning outside the major vascular arcades. Treatment should be performed over multiple sessions and usually begins nasally and/or inferiorly. Complications and side effects include reduction in night vision, color vision, peripheral vision, and accommodation. The patient may complain of glare and photopsia. Visual acuity and macular edema may worsen. Fibrovascular contraction and extension can result in macular and peripheral traction retinal detachment, rhegmatogenous detachment, and vitreous hemorrhage.

Venous Occlusive Diseases
Branch Retinal Vein Occlusion

Branch retinal vein occlusion (BRVO) in the pediatric population is often a complication of a preexisting intraocular problem. Patients with retinal vasculitis, ocular complications of systemic lupus erythematosus (SLE), Eales' disease, ocular sarcoidosis, and ocular toxoplasmosis are at risk for venous occlusive disease. Complications include macular edema, macular ischemia, retinal neovascularization, and vitreous hemorrhage.

The collaborative Branch Vein Occlusion Study (BVOS) demonstrated the efficacy of laser photocoagulation in the setting of chronic macular edema and retinal neovascularization.[15,16] In eyes with macular edema present for 3 to 18 months following occlusion, intact perfusion to the fovea, and visual acuity 20/40 or worse, argon laser grid treatment to the areas of leakage resulted in a significant improvement in the visual outcome.

The BVOS demonstrated that scatter laser photocoagulation in the setting of significant retinal capillary nonperfusion and ischemia (greater than 5 disc diameters) can reduce the risk of retinal neovascularization, and when neovascularization exists scatter laser photocoagulation can reduce the risk of subsequent vitreous hemorrhage. The BVOS recommended that eyes at risk for neovascularization be observed, with scatter laser treatment initiated only with the development of neovascularization.

A grid laser treatment for macular edema is placed at the areas of leakage, which are demonstrated by fluorescein angiography. Treatment is placed outside the foveal avascular zone (FAZ) and within the major vascular arcade. One hundred-micron, 0.1-second, moderately intense spots are recommended. Scatter treatment for neovascularization covers the entire area of nonperfusion, beginning 2 disc diameters from the center of the FAZ. Two hundred to 500 moderately intense burns are placed 1 burn width apart. The complications of these procedures are discussed previously.

Central Retinal Vein Occlusion

Central retinal vein occlusion (CRVO) occurs infrequently in the pediatric population and like BRVO can complicate an underlying intraocular problem (i.e., ocular sarcoid, SLE). Risks of CRVO include extensive retinal ischemia resulting in iris (INV) and anterior chamber angle neovascularization (ANV), neovascular glaucoma, macular edema, macular ischemia, and retinal neovascularization.

The collaborative Central Retinal Vein Occlusion Study (CRVOS) does not support prophylactic panretinal photocoagulation for ischemic CRVO, although there is a direct relationship between the amount of retinal capillary nonperfusion and the risk of developing INV or ANV.[17] Should eyes develop INV or ANV, prompt panretinal photoablation is recommended. Macular grid photocoagulation for persistent macular edema due to CRVO is not effective in improving visual acuity, although angiographic evidence of macular edema is dramatically reduced.[18] The mean age in the study group is 65 years.

Retinal Vasculitis and Other Vascular Occlusive Diseases

Eyes with significant vasoocclusion with secondary ischemia and retinal neovascularization (retinal vasculitis and Eales' disease, SLE) may respond favorably to laser photocoagulation. Panretinal photoablation or scatter treatment to areas of nonperfusion is frequently performed.[19] The treatment technique is previously described.

Sickle Cell Retinopathy

Sickle cell retinal abnormalities, when proliferative, respond to laser photocoagulation.[20-22]

Treatment probably decreases the rate of complications from proliferative disease, including vitreous hemorrhage, traction, and rhegmatogenous detachments. Treatment options include direct photoablation of the feeder arteriole or scatter laser photocoagulation around the sea fan. Direct ablation of the feeder vessel is associated with a significant incidence of complications, including vitreous hemorrhage, retinal detachment, subretinal fibrosis, chorioretinal anastomosis, choriovitreal anastomosis, and choroidal neovascularization. Large burns of low intensity and long duration are utilized.

Scatter treatment is effective and has a lower complication rate. Light to moderately intense 500-μm spots are placed one burn width apart around the sea fan. Ischemic regions in close proximity to the frond (involved quadrant) are usually treated.

Retinopathy of Prematurity

Due to incomplete retinal vascularization, local ischemia and secondary neovascularization develop. The Cryotherapy-Retinopathy of Prematurity Study (CRYO-ROP Study) found significantly more unfavorable outcomes when cryotherapy is performed on eyes with posterior (zone I or II) stage 3 ROP, with five or more continuous or eight cumulative clock hours of involvement in the presence of plus disease.[23,24] Transscleral cryopexy spots are directed at the area of anterior, avascular retina. Favorable macular anatomic outcomes with treatment are significant. Unfavorable outcomes included retinal detachment, retinal folds extending into macula, and abnormal retrolental tissue.

Laser photocoagulation using the binocular laser indirect system (diode or argon) is utilized in place of cryopexy to ablate the anterior, avascular retina in eyes that meet criteria for treatment based on the CRYO-ROP Study with favorable results.[25] Adequate visualization for treatment is a prerequisite. In one series, the diode laser delivery system is used.[26] Sedation is required for larger, healthier neonates. Topical anesthesia is used if scleral indentation is necessary. Gray burns are placed anterior to the shunt, one-half burn width apart. If additional therapy is necessary, spots are placed between previous photocoagulation sites. Mean burn duration was 252 ms, and mean power was 360 mW.

Complications of treatment include intraretinal and vitreous hemorrhage, inadvertent foveal burns, and other complications found with scatter laser photocoagulation.

Coats' Disease

Coats' disease and other exudative vasculopathies can be treated quite effectively with angiography guided ablation to abnormal vessels and lesions.[27] Exudative lesions are treated directly with large, moderately intense spots (200 to 500 μm). Vessels are ablated as previously discussed. For anterior lesions, indirect laser photocoagulation can be performed. Cryopexy is usually necessary when the retina is elevated.

Choroidal Neovascularization

Choroidal neovascularization (CNV) in the pediatric population is usually secondary to trauma with secondary rupture to Bruch's membrane, choroiditis (POHS, PIC, multifocal choroiditis with panuveitis), pathologic myopia, and choroidal osteoma. Systemic steroids may be of benefit in selected entities. Laser photocoagulation of a well-defined, extrafoveal or juxtafoveal membrane can be beneficial in preventing or delaying visual loss.[28] Some diseases are more amenable to treatment.

The borders of the membrane beginning at the inferior edge, as determined angiographically, are treated with moderately intense, 200-μm burns for a duration of at least 0.2 seconds. The center of the lesion is then treated with moderately intense, 200- to 500-μm overlapping burns (0.5 to 1.0 second) to produce marked retinal whitening. Retrobulbar anesthesia may be necessary when fixation is problematic. When peripapillary CNV is treated, several clock hours of the temporal papillomacular bundle should be spared, and treatment should probably not extend within several hundred microns of the disc.

Complications include preretinal, retinal, subretinal, and choroidal hemorrhage, vascular occlusion, retinal detachment, inadvertent foveal burns, and thermal necrosis of the optic nerve.

Radiation Retinopathy

Radiation retinopathy is an occlusive microangiopathy that is complicated by macular edema, macular ischemia, and retinal neovascularization. Generally, the treatment guidelines of the ETDRS and DRS are applied to eyes with these complications.[29]

Retinal Capillary Hemangioma and von Hippel-Lindau Disease

Retinal angiomas due to retinal capillary hemangioma or von Hippel-Lindau disease are treated successfully with laser photocoagulation.[30] Due to the potential for exudation and secondary tissue destruction, photoablation of these lesions should be performed early. Angiomas are treated directly with large size (500 μm), low-intensity spots for 0.2 to 0.5 seconds. Smaller, more-intense spots increase the risk of hemorrhage and exudation. Multiple treatment sessions may be required for larger lesions. Cryoablation is usually reserved for anterior lesions.

Rhegmatogenous Conditions

Retinal holes and tears, localized retinal detachments, and necrotic retina at risk for detaching (acute retinal necrosis) can be demarcated with laser photocoagulation. Delivery is performed at the slit lamp or via indirect ophthalmoscopy when anterior treatment is indicated. Generally, two rows of moderately intense, 200- to 500-μm burns one half burn width apart are placed surrounding the region in question. Anterior treatment extending to the ora serrata is necessary for most retinal tears and localized detachments.

Retinal and Choroidal Tumors

Retinoblastoma, malignant choroidal melanoma, and localized choroidal hemangioma were treated successfully with laser photocoagulation. The indications for therapy and techniques are beyond the scope of this chapter.

■ Conclusion

A variety of disorders can be managed effectively with laser photocoagulation. An understanding and recognition of the specific disease processes and a familiarity with the various techniques discussed will enhance treatment outcomes and limit complications.

■ Acknowledgment

Drs. Odrich and Trokel wish to thank Normal Medow, M.D., for help in preparing this chapter.

REFERENCES

1. Singh D. Photorefractive keratectomy in pediatric patients. *J Cataract Refract Surg*. 1995; 21:630–633.
2. Nano H, Muzzin S, Irigaray F. Excimer laser photorefractive keratectomy in pediatric patients. *J Cataract Refract Surg*. 1997; 23:736–739.
3. Uram M. Ophthalmic laser microendoscopic ciliary process ablation in the management of neovascular glaucoma. *Ophthalmology*. 1992; 99:1823–1828.
4. Uram M. Ophthalmic laser microendoscope endophotocoagulation. *Ophthalmology*. 1992; 99:1829–1832.
5. Brancato R, Giovanni L, Trabucchi G, Pietroni C. Contact transscleral cyclophotocoagulation with Nd:YAG laser in uncontrolled glaucoma. *Ophthal Surg*. 1989; 20:547–551.
6. Edward DP, Brown SV, Higgenbottom E, Jennings T, Tessler HH, Tso MO. Sympathetic ophthalmia following Nd:Yag cyclotherapy. *Ophthal Surg*. 1989; 20(8): 544–546.
7. Early Treatment Diabetic Retinopathy Study Research Group. Photocoagulation for diabetic macular edema: Early Treatment Diabetic Retinopathy Study report number 1. *Arch Ophthalmol*. 1985; 103:1796–1806.
8. Early Treatment Diabetic Retinopathy Study Research Group. Treatment techniques and clinical guidelines for photocoagulation of diabetic macular edema: Early Treatment Diabetic Retinopathy Study report number 2. *Ophthalmology*. 1987; 94:761–774.
9. Early Treatment Diabetic Retinopathy Study Research Group. Photocoagulation for diabetic macular edema. *Int Ophthalmol Clin*. 1987; 27:265–272.
10. Diabetic Retinopathy Study Research Group. Preliminary report on effects of photocoagulation therapy. *Am J Ophthalmol*. 1976; 81:383–396.
11. Diabetic Retinopathy Study Research Group. Photocoagulation treatment for proliferative diabetic retinopathy: the second report of Diabetic Retinopathy Study findings. *Ophthalmology*. 1978; 85:82–106.
12. Diabetic Retinopathy Study Research Group. Four risk factors for severe visual loss in diabetic retinopathy: the third report from the Diabetic Retinopathy Study. *Arch Ophthalmol*. 1979; 97:654–655.
13. Diabetic Retinopathy Study Research Group. Photocoagulation treatment of proliferative diabetic retinopathy: clinical application of Diabetic Retinopathy Study (DRS) findings, DRS report number 8. *Invest Ophthalmol Vis Sci*. 1981; 88:583–600.
14. Diabetic Retinopathy Study Research Group. Indications for photocoagulation treatment of diabetic retinopathy: DRS report number 14. *Int Ophthalmol Clin*. 1987; 27:239–253.
15. Branch Vein Occlusion Study Group. Argon laser photocoagulation for macular edema in branch vein occlusion. *Am J Ophthalmol*. 1984; 98:271–282.
16. Branch Vein Occlusion Study Group. Argon laser scatter photocoagulation for prevention of neovascularization and vitreous hemorrhage in branch vein occlusion. *Arch Ophthalmol*. 1986; 104:34–41.
17. Central Vein Occlusion Study, Group N Report. A randomized clinical trial of early panretinal photocoagulation for ischemic central vein occlusion. *Ophthalmology*. 1995; 102:1434–1444.
18. Central Vein Occlusion Study, Group M Report. Evaluation of grid pattern photocoagulation for macular edema in central vein occlusion. *Ophthalmology*. 1995; 102:1425–1433.
19. Spitznas M, Meyer-Schwickerath G, Stephan B. Treatment of Eales' disease with photocoagulation. *Grafes Arch Clin Exp Ophthalmol*. 1975; 194:193–198.
20. Jampol LM, Condon P, Farber M, Rabb M, Ford S, and Serjeant G. A randomized clinical trial of feeder vessel photocoagulation of proliferative sickle cell retinopathy. I. Preliminary results. *Ophthalmology*. 1983; 90: 540–545.
21. Condon P, Jampol LM, Farber M, Rabb M, and Serjeant G. A randomized clinical trial of feeder vessel photocoagulation of proliferative sickle cell retinopathy. II. Update and analysis of risk factors. *Ophthalmology*. 1984; 91:1496–1498.
22. Rednam KRV, Jampol LM, Goldberg MF. Scatter retinal photocoagulation for proliferative sickle cell retinopathy. *Am J Ophthalmol*. 1982; 93:594–599.
23. Cryotherapy for Retinopathy of Prematurity Cooperative Group. Multicenter trial of cryotherapy for retinopathy of prematurity: preliminary results. *Arch Ophthalmol*. 1988; 106:471–479.
24. Cryotherapy for Retinopathy of Prematurity Cooperative Group. Multicenter trial of cryotherapy for retinopathy of prematurity: three month outcome. *Arch Ophthalmol*. 1990; 108:195–204.
25. Laser-ROP Study Group. Laser therapy for retinopathy of prematurity. *Arch Ophthalmol*. 1994; 112:154–156.
26. Goggin M, O'Keefe M. Diode laser for retinopathy of prematurity—early outcome. *Br J Ophthalmol*. 1993; 77:559–562.
27. Pauleikhoff D, Kruger K, Heinriech T, Wessing A. Epidemiologic features and therapeutic results in Coats' disease. *Invest Ophthalmol*. 1988;29:335.
28. Macular Photocoagulation Study Group. Argon laser photocoagulation for ocular histoplasmosis syndrome: results of a randomized clinical trial. *Arch Ophthalmol*. 1983; 101:1347–1357.
29. Kinyoun JL, Chittum ME, Wells CG. Photocoagulation treatment of radiation retinopathy. *Am J Ophthalmol*. 1988; 105:470–478.
30. Lane CM, Turner G, Gregor ZJ, Bird AC. Laser treatment of retinal angiomatosis. *Eye*. 1989; 3:33–38.

Index

Note: pages in boldface indicate figures and tables.